T0257881

Encyclopedia of DNA Repair and Human Health

Volume I

Encyclopedia of DNA Repair and Human Health

Volume I

Encyclopedia of DNA Repair and Human Health
Volume I

Edited by **Nas Wilson**

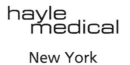

New York

Published by Hayle Medical,
30 West, 37th Street, Suite 612,
New York, NY 10018, USA
www.haylemedical.com

Encyclopedia of DNA Repair and Human Health
Volume I
Edited by Nas Wilson

International Standard Book Number: 978-1-63241-000-9 (Hardback)

Printed in the United States of America.

Contents

Preface

Every book is initially just a concept; it takes months of research and hard work to give it the final shape in which the readers receive it. In its early stages, this book also went through rigorous reviewing. The notable contributions made by experts from across the globe were first molded into patterned chapters and then arranged in a sensibly sequential manner to bring out the best results.

This book provides comprehensive information regarding DNA repair and human health. Over the past decades, significant developments have been made in comprehending the cellular DNA repair pathways. Simultaneously, a wealth of elucidative knowledge of human diseases has been compiled. Now, the fundamental research of the mechanisms of DNA repair is integrating with clinical research, placing the action of the DNA repair pathways in light of the whole organism. Such integrative approach allows understanding of the disease mechanisms and is useful in enhancing diagnostics and prevention. This book throws light on the primary role of DNA repair in human health and well-being. The chapters consist of detailed elucidations of DNA repair mechanisms. It will appeal to a huge audience, ranging from molecular biologists working on DNA repair to the medical researchers.

It has been my immense pleasure to be a part of this project and to contribute my years of learning in such a meaningful form. I would like to take this opportunity to thank all the people who have been associated with the completion of this book at any step.

Editor

DNA Repair Mechanisms

DNA Repair, Human Diseases and Aging

Vaidehi Krishnan, Baohua Liu and Zhongjun Zhou
Department of Biochemistry, The University of Hong Kong
Hong Kong

1. Introduction

One of the most fundamental functions of a cell is the transmission of genetic information to the next generation, with high fidelity. On the face of it, this seems a challenging task given that cells in the human body are constantly exposed to thousands of DNA lesions every day both from endogenous and exogenous sources. Yet, for long periods of time, the DNA sequences are one of the most invariable and stable components of a cell, a task achieved by an arsenal of DNA damage detection and repair machinery that detects and fixes DNA lesions with high fidelity at each and every round of cell division. In this chapter, we describe how normal cells cope with DNA damage and the manner in which a defective DNA damage response can lead to human disease and aging.

2. The types and sources of DNA damage

All livings cells of the human body have to constantly contend with DNA damage. Due to its chemical structure itself, the DNA is sensitive to spontaneous hydrolysis which leads to damage in the form of abasic sites and base deamination. Single strand breaks (SSBs) and oxidative damage such as 8-oxoguanine lesions in DNA are generated by endogenous by-products of metabolism like reactive oxygen species (ROS) and their highly reactive intermediates. For example, it is estimated that about 100-500 8-oxoguanine lesions form per day in a human cell (Lindahl, 1993). The formamidopyrimidine lesions, 2,6-diamino-4-hydroxy-5-formamidopyrimidine (FapyG) and 4,6-diamino-5-formamidopyrimidine are also formed at similar rates as 8-oxoG after oxidative stress. Spontaneous DNA alterations may also arise due to dNTP misincorporation during DNA replication. Put together, it is estimated that each human cell can face up to 10^5 spontaneous DNA lesions per day (Maynard et al., 2009).

Apart from endogenous sources, DNA can also be damaged by exogenous agents from the environment. These include physical genotoxic stresses such as the ultraviolet light (mainly UV-B: 280-315 nm) from sunlight which can induce a variety of mutagenic and cytotoxic DNA lesions such as cyclobutane-pyrimidine dimers (CPDs) and 6-4 photoproducts (6-4PPs) (Rastogi et al., 2010). DNA damage in the form of double strand breaks (DSBs) can be incurred as a result of medical treatments like radiotherapy, ionising radiation (IR) exposure from cosmic radiation or as a result of the natural decay of radioactive compounds. For example, uranium decay produces radioactive radon gas, which accumulates in some houses to cause an increased incidence of lung cancer (Jackson and Bartek, 2009). Nuclear disasters like the Chernobyl nuclear disaster, nuclear detonations during World War II or more recently, the radiation leakage from the Fukushima power plant in Japan are examples of other sources of severe exposure to exogenous radiation. Chemical sources of DNA damage include chemotherapeutic drugs used in cancer therapy or for other medical conditions. Alkylating agents such as methyl methanesulfonate (MMS) induce alkylation of bases, whereas drugs such as mitomycin C, cisplatin and nitrogen mustard cause DNA interstrand cross links (ICLs), and DNA intrastrand cross links. Chemotherapeutic drugs like camptothecin and etoposide are topoisomerse I and II inhibitors respectively, and give rise to SSBs or DSBs by trapping topoisomerase–DNA complexes. Other exogenous DNA-damaging sources, that are carcinogenic as well, are foods contaminated with fungal toxins such as the aflatoxin and overcooked meat products containing heterocyclic amines. Another common source of environmental mutagen is tobacco smoke, which generates DNA lesions in the form of aromatic adducts on DNA and SSBs (Jackson and Bartek, 2009).

3. DNA repair pathways

To maintain genomic integrity, a cellular machinery composed of multi-protein complexes that are capable of detecting and signalling the presence of DNA lesions and delaying cell cycle progression to promote DNA repair is activated, called as the DNA damage response (DDR) (Harper and Elledge, 2007). To accomplish DNA repair, cells utilise biochemically distinct pathways specific of the DNA lesion, which are integrated with appropriate signalling systems to delay cell division until the completion of repair (Figure.1). Small chemical alterations caused by the oxidation of bases is detected and repaired by the base excision repair system (BER), through the direct excision of the damaged base. DNA replication errors or polymerase slippage errors that commonly result in single base mismatches and insertion-deletion loops are corrected by the mismatch repair system (MMR). Lesions such as pyrimidine dimers and intrastrand cross links are corrected by the nucleotide excision repair (NER) pathway. SSBs are removed by the SSB repair pathway whereas DSBs are repaired by the DSB repair systems, which itself could be either by homologous recombination (HR) or non-homologous end joining (NHEJ) pathway (Ciccia and Elledge, 2010).

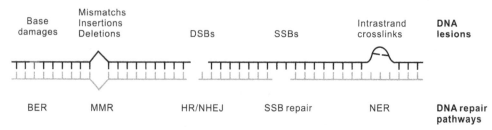

Fig. 1. Summary of DNA repair pathways

3.1 Base excision repair and single strand break repair

Base excision repair (BER) is the major pathway responsible for handling the mutagenic and cytotoxic effects of DNA damage that can arise due to spontaneous hydrolytic, oxidative, and non-enzymatic alkylation reactions. (Wilson and Bohr, 2007). This pathway focuses on

DNA lesions that do not tend to cause structural distortions of the DNA double helix. The BER target lesions can be classified as oxidised/reduced bases such as 8-oxo-G/FapyG, methylated bases, deaminated bases or bases mismatches. There are two types of BER: short patch and long patch. During short patch BER, only the damaged nucleotide is replaced, whereas in long patch BER, 2-6 new nucleotides are incorporated.

The very first step in BER involves the use of DNA glycosylases that cleave the N-glycosyl bond between the damaged base and sugar to generate an abasic site, called as the AP (apurinic/apyrimidinic) site. Similar AP sites may also arise due to the spontaneous depurination or depyrimidination of bases. The DNA glycosylases that perform this function are classified as monofunctional or bifunctional, depending on their mode of action. Monofunctional glycosylases such as UNG only possess the glycosylase activity and therefore a second enzyme called the APE1 lyase is required to cut base-free deoxyribose to generate the 5'-deoxyribose phosphate termini (dRP). The next step involves the action of DNA polymerase β (polβ) which removes the dRP group left behind by APE1 incision in the short-patch pathway. However, if the 5' terminal is refractory to polβ activity, strand displacement synthesis is required in order to incorporate multiple nucleotides by long-patch pathway. In this case, several enzymes such as proliferating cell nuclear antigen (PCNA), FEN1 and polβ and/or polδ/ε act together to remove the blocking terminus. The final step of BER consists of ligation of the remaining nick, by either Lig1 alone or Lig3–XRCC1 complex (Maynard et al., 2009).

SSB repair pathway is a major pathway responsible for the repair of SSBs that arise directly as a result of ROS-induced disintegration of oxidized deoxyribose or genotoxic stresses such as IR. SSBs may also arise spontaneously due to the erroneous activity of DNA topoisomerase 1 (TOP1). TOP1 creates a cleavage complex intermediate which contains a DNA nick to allow DNA relaxation during DNA replication and transcription. Usually, the nick generation is transient and is rapidly sealed by TOP1. However, if the nick inadvertently collides with RNA polymerase, SSBs may be generated in the process. In addition to the above scenarios where SSBs are generated directly within cells, SSBs may also arise indirectly as BER intermediates due to the lyase activity of bifunctional glycosylases such as OGG1 and NEIL1.

Single strand break repair (SSB) involves the activation of PARP (poly ADP ribose polymerase) family members PARP1 and PARP2, which act as sensors of SSBs, through the two PARP1 zinc finger motifs (Caldecott, 2008). Upon activation of PARP1 and PARP2, poly (ADP-ribose) chains are synthesized within seconds, and assembled on target proteins such as histone H1 and H2B and PARP1 itself (Schreiber et al., 2006). Histone PARylation contributes to chromatin reorganization and helps in the recruitment of DNA repair and chromatin remodelling proteins to DNA damage sites. Three types of PAR-binding motifs have been identified: the PBZ (PAR-binding zinc finger), the macrodomain and an 8 amino acid basic residue-rich cluster. Many DDR factors such as p53, XRCC1, Lig3, MRE11 and ATM have the 8 amino acid basic residue-rich cluster, whereas macrodomains containing proteins include PARP9, PARP14, PARP15, the histone variant macroH2A1.1, and the chromatin remodeling factor ALC1. PBZ motifs have been identified in the nucleases APLF and SNM1 and in the cell cycle protein CHFR.

Once SSBs are detected, they undergo end processing, where the 3' and/or 5' termini of SSBs are restored to conventional 3'hydroxyl and 5' phosphate moieties for gap filling and DNA ligation to occur. XRCC1 has a particularly important role during DNA end processing step, since XRCC1 directly interacts with enzymes such as   pol β, PNK (polynucleotide kinase) and the nucleases APTX and indirectly with DNA ligase III α and TDP1 (tyrosyl-DNA phosphodiesterase) to facilitate end processing. Damage termini present at indirect BER-induced SSB are repaired by APE1, Pol β, PNKP and APTX. Direct sugar damage-induced SSBs are repaired by APE1, PNKP and APTX. SSBs generated by TOP1 are repaired by TDP1. Finally, end processing is followed by gap filling and ligation, and the enzymes utilized during these two steps overlap with BER (as described above).

It is interesting that ~30% of all human tumors examined express a variant form of DNA polymerase β (Starcevic et al., 2004) Moreover, at least two proteins, TDP1 and APTX, involved in SSB repair are mutated in an inherited form of human neurodegenerative disease (discussed in Section 5.1).

3.2 Mismatch repair

The replication of DNA sequences in the S phase of cell cycle is subjected to a low but significant level of error that includes the inadvertent incorporation of chemically altered nucleotides in place of the normal counterparts. The cell has two main strategies to detect and remove the miscopied nucleotides. In a 'proofreading' type of monitoring executed by the DNA polymerase δ (pol- δ), the stretch of DNA that has been newly synthesized is scanned, and if misincorporation of nucleotides is detected, the enzyme uses it 3'-5' exonuclease activity to remove the aberrant nucleotide and resynthesize the DNA stretch. However, if the miscopied DNA sequence is overlooked by DNA pol-δ, the MMR pathway is activated that detects and corrects misincorporated nucleotides. The action of this pathway becomes especially critical in regions of DNA that carry repetitive sequences such as mono or dinucleotide repeats. The resulting base substitution mismatches and insertion-deletion mismatches (IDLs) may escape correction by the proofreading mechanism described above, making the repair of such defects the prime function of the MMR machinery (Kunkel and Erie, 2005).

The 'Mut' proteins are the principle active components of the mismatch repair pathway (Kolodner and Marsischky, 1999). The main function of the Mut proteins lies in the ability to detect bulges and loops in the newly formed DNA and in being able to distinguish between recently synthesized DNA from the complementary parent strand. In mammalian cells, two components of the MMR apparatus, MutS and MutL collaborate to correct mismatched DNA. MutS homologs form two major heterodimers, Msh2/Msh6 (MutSα) and Msh2/Msh3 (MutSβ) which scan for the mismatched base on the newly formed daughter strand and bind directly to the mutated DNA. The main difference between the two MutS complexes is that MutSα pathway is mainly involved in the repair of base substitution and small loop mismatches, while the MutSβ pathway is also involved in large loop repair. After the recruitment of MutS, MutL dimer is loaded to the mutated site through its binding to the MutS-DNA complex. MutL has three forms designated as MutLα, MutLβ, and MutLγ. The MutLα complex is made of two subunits MLH1 and PMS2, the MutLβ heterodimer is made of MLH1 and PMS1, while MutLγ is made of MLH1 and MLH3. MutLα is an endonuclease that facilitates strand-discrimination and nicks the discontinuous strand of the mismatched duplex in a PCNA, RFC and ATP-dependent manner. Lastly, the excision reaction is performed by the 5'-3' single-stranded exonuclease EXO1, whose exonuclease activity is increased by its direct interaction with MutSα. The resulting fragment is excised and a fresh attempt at resynthesizing DNA using DNA pol-δ is made using the parent strand as the template (Fukui, 2010; Larrea et al., 2010).

The MMR pathway is particularly important in mammals, where the mutator phenotype conferred by loss of MMR activity contributes to the initiation and promotion of multistage-carcinogenesis (Venkatesan et al., 2006)

3.3 Nucleotide excision repair

The activation of NER pathway seems to require two distinct structural changes in DNA: a significant distortion to the native conformation of DNA and the presence of a chemically altered base. NER is accomplished by a large multisubunit complex composed of almost two dozen subunits. NER comprises of two distinct subpathways that mainly differ in the molecular mechanism used to identify the damaged base. Global genome repair (GGR) repairs DNA damage throughout the genome, whereas transcription-coupled repair (TCR) repairs lesions in regions that are undergoing transcription (Nouspikel, 2009).

Historically, the NER pathway was discovered through the study of a human syndrome involving a severe burning of the skin after only a minimal exposure to sun light. These individuals show dry, parchment like skin (Xeroderma) and freckles (pigmentosa). Individuals suffering from Xeroderma Pigmentosa (XP) have a 1000-fold greater risk of developing skin cancers and inherited defects in any of the so-called XP genes cause this syndrome. Subsequently, elegant somatic cell genetic experiments were performed and seven genetic complementation groups of the human XP, designated XPA to XPG were identified in mammalian cells. According to current understanding, two independent complexes, one composed of the DDB1/DDB2 heterodimer, and the other containing the XPC/HR23B/Centrin 2 proteins are required for the early steps of base damage recognition during NER (Guo et al., 2010; Nouspikel, 2009).

UV-damaged DNA-binding protein (UV-DDB) is a heterodimeric complex composed of DDB1 and DDB2 which upon binding to UV-damaged sites activates a UV-DDB-associated ubiquitin ligase complex that recruits XPC protein to the lesion and promotes ubiquitination of DDB2 and XPC proteins (Sugasawa et al., 2005). Upon polyubiquitination, DDB2 loses its ability to bind to UV-irradiated DNA, whereas XPC upon ubiquitination shows increased DNA binding. In turn, XPC recruits the multiprotein transcription-repair complex called as the TFIIH (transcription factor IIH). Subsequent recruitment of RPA and XPA drive detachment of cyclin-dependent kinase activating (CAK) subcomplex of TFIIH which is essential for GGR. The two helicases within the TFIIH complex (XPB and XPD) unwind the DNA by about 20 bp around the damage to form a stable complex called pre-incision complex 1 (PIC1). Localized unwinding around the damaged base then leads to the exit of XPC-HR23 and the entry of XPG to form PIC2. Finally, XPF-ERCC1 is recruited to form PIC3. At each of these steps ATP is hydrolyzed, and the free energy of ATP hydrolysis is used to unwind the helix as well as to amplify the damage recognition specificity of the enzyme system. Within PIC3, XPG and the ERCC1/XPF complex are both structure-specific endonucleases that carry out dual excision and cut the damaged strand of DNA 3' and 5' to the lesion, respectively. This generates a single-stranded oligonucleotide 24–32 nucleotides in length. The incisions are asymmetrical, such that the 3' incision occurs 2 to 8 nucleotides from the damaged base and the 5' incision occurs 15 to 24 nucleotides from the damaged base. The resulting gap is filled in by the combined actions of DNA polymerase δ or ε, proliferating cell nuclear antigen (PCNA), RPA, and DNA ligase I (or a complex of XRCC1and DNA ligase III) (Hanawalt and Spivak, 2008).

Bulky lesions consisting of UV-induced pyrimidine dimers in transcribed regions can lead to RNA polymerase II stalling, evoking the activation of TCR. In TCR, the stalled RNA polymerase is removed and DNA damage is repaired, through a process initiated by the Cockayne syndrome proteins, CSA and CSB. The CSA protein belongs to the 'WD repeat' family of proteins and exhibits structural and regulatory roles while CSB protein which is an ATP-dependent chromatin remodelling factor in the SWI/SNF family. CSB, in turn recruits additional factors such as the histone acetytransferase p300, the CSA-DDB1 E3 ubiquitin/COP9 signalosome complex (O'Connell and Harper, 2007). Similar to GGR, the subsequent steps involve the binding of TFIIH and XPA/RPA to the lesion and the nucleases XPG and XPF/ERCC1 carry out the incision 3'and 5' to the damaged lesion. The generated oligonucleotide is removed and the gap is filled in by the combined action of DNA polymerases δ or ε, PCNA, RPA, and DNA ligase I or XRCC1/ DNA ligase III.

3.4 DNA replication stress and ATR

Replication stress is a unifying term used to denote large unprotected regions of ssDNA generated during the course of DNA replication or formed at the resected region of DSBs (Lopez-Contreras and Fernandez-Capetillo, 2010). Both situations converge with the generation of a RPA-coated ssDNA intermediate which is the triggering signal for the DNA replication checkpoint. The ssDNA-RPA complex plays two critical roles: it recruits ATR by directly binding to the ATR partner, ATRIP. Secondly, it recruits and activates the Rad17 clamp loader which then loads the PCNA-like heterotrimeric ring 9-1-1 (Rad9-Hus1-Rad1) complex to DNA. The 911 complex binds to the ATR activator TopBP1, thus bringing it in close proximity to ATR-ATRIP, leading to ATR activation. Once activated, ATR initiates the DNA replication checkpoint through the phosphorylation of its downstream substrates. In addition to replication checkpoint signalling, ATR is also required for stabilization of stalled replication forks. In the absence of ATR, forks undergo a 'collapse' and are unable to resume replication upon the withdrawal of replication stress (Friedel et al., 2009). The absence of ATR also results in a specific type of genomic instability, named as DNA Fragile site expression. DNA fragile sites (DFS) are large (>100 Kb) genomic regions that exhibit breaks under conditions of replication stress. DFS sites are 'hot spots' for sister chromatid exchanges and are involved in gene amplification events via a breakage-fusion-bridge cycle. Breakage at DFS is associated with several cancers (Dillon et al., 2010).

3.5 Interstrand cross link repair (ICL repair)

ICLs are generated by cross linking agents like mitomycin C and these lesions covalently connect the two strands of DNA to form a barrier to replication fork progression. Important components of the ICL repair pathway are 13 genes mutated in the genetic syndrome, Fanconi anemia (FA). FA is an autosomal recessive cancer predisposition disorder characterized by progressive bone marrow failure, congenital developmental defects, chromosomal abnormalities and hypersensitivity to ICL agents (Kitao and Takata, 2011). The gene products of FA constitute a common pathway called the FA pathway, whose main role is in the repair of ICL lesions to maintain genomic integrity (Moldovan and D'Andrea, 2009). Eight of the FA proteins (FANCA, B, C, E, F, G, L and M) form the so-called FA core complex, an E3 ubiquitin ligase that monoubiquitinates downstream FANCD2-FANCI dimer. The core complex also incorporates FAAP100 and FAAP24 and the heterodimer MHF1/MHF2 as crucial components. Upon monoubiquitination, the ID complex accumulates at the sites of crosslinks and co-localizes with three additional FA proteins, Brca2 (FANCD), PALB2 (FANCN), and BACH1 (FANCJ). Monoubiquitinated ID complex is required for the incision and translesion synthesis steps of ICL repair by promoting the recruitment of DDR factors required for ICL repair (Moldovan and D'Andrea, 2009). Recently, another level of regulation was revealed in the FA pathway, in that ID complex is phosphorylated first by ATR and this step was shown to be critical for further monoubiquitination by the core complex. Subsequently, factors required for HR are also recruited to repair the DSBs generated during the repair process. Thus, ICL repair requires the coordinated recruitment and concerted action of several DNA repair pathways.

3.6 Double strand break repair

DNA double strand breaks are the most deleterious type of DNA damage and cells have evolved at least four types of repair pathways to detect and correct DSBs. These pathways include homologous recombination (HR), non-homologous end joining (NHEJ), alternative NHEJ pathway. The main factor influencing pathway choice is the extent of DNA processing. While NHEJ does not require DNA end resection, HR and alternative NHEJ pathways are dependent on end resection (Ciccia and Elledge, 2010).

NHEJ is an error-prone process, where broken ends are recognised and sealed together and mainly occurs in G0, G1 and early S phase of the cell cycle and requires the DNA-PK (DNA protein kinase) complex and the Lig4 complex (Lieber, 2010). The DNA-PK complex consists of the Ku70 and Ku80 heterodimer which recognises and binds to the DSB and recruits DNA-PKcs, the catalytic subunit of DNA-PK. Following DSB binding, DNA-PKcs autophosphorylation on the six-residue ABCDE cluster (T2609) causes destabilization of the DNA-PKcs interaction with DNA thus providing access to end processing enzymes such as ARTEMIS (Goodarzi et al., 2006). On the other hand, to prevent excessive end processing, DNA-PKcs is also autophosphorylated at the five-residue cluster called as the PQR cluster at S2056, which helps protect DNA ends. Thus, two reciprocally acting phosphorylation clusters regulate end processing by DNA-PKcs (Cui et al., 2005).

Following the recognition of DSBs, ends must be transformed into 5'phosphorylated ligatable ends to complete repair. One key enzyme required for end processing is ARTEMIS, which might be recruited to DSBs through its ability to interact with DNA-PKcs. End processing is also carried out by APLF nucleases and the PNK kinase/phosphatase prior to ligation (Mahaney et al., 2009). Next, the end processing of complex lesions might lead to the generation of gaps which are filled in by DNA polymerase μ, polymerase λ and terminal deoxyribonucleotidyltransferase. The final step involves the ligation of DNA ends, a step carried out by X4-L4 (a complex containing XRCC4, DNA ligase IV and XLF) (Hartlerode and Scully, 2009).

Interestingly, when the classical NHEJ pathway is inhibited, an alternative end-joining pathway operates in cells. This substitution is called as alternative end joining (alt-EJ), backup NHEJ (B-NHEJ) or microhomology mediated end joining (MMEJ) (Lieber and Wilson, 2010). This pathway functions even in the absence of classical NHEJ factors such as Ku, XRCC4 or DNA ligase IV. For example, the alt-NHEJ pathway is robustly activated in mice lacking X4-L4. Alt-NHEJ is mediated by the annealing of ssDNA microhomology regions followed by LIG3-dependent DNA end ligation (Ciccia and Elledge, 2010; Hartlerode and Scully, 2009). Microhomologies are short stretches of complementary "microhomology" sequences (1–10 base pairs) that often appear at repair junctions. This suggests that even limited base pairing between two ends of a double-strand break is exploited during alt-NHEJ repair (Lieber and Wilson, 2010). Alt-NHEJ pathway is error-prone and frequently results in small deletions/insertions around the region of double strand breaks or could even result in deleterious translocations (Zhang and Jasin, 2011).

Unlike NHEJ, HR is an error-free process that involves the use of the undamaged homologous sister chromatid as the template to facilitate DNA repair of the damaged strand and is carried out in cells that are in the late S and G2 phases of cell cycle (Moynahan and Jasin, 2010). Homologous recombination (HR) provides an important mechanism to repair double strand breaks during mitosis and meiosis. Defective HR can potentially transform cells by disrupting their genomic integrity. HR involves the detection of DSB by the MRN (MRE11-Rad50-NBS1) complex which promotes activation of ATM (Ataxia-telangiectasia mutated). In addition to stabilizing DNA ends, MRE11 has endonuclease and exonuclease activities which are important to mediate 5'-3' resection along with CtIP to generate single strand DNA (ssDNA). ssDNA is coated by the ssDNA-binding protein, RPA which is a heterotrimeric complex (RPA1, RPA2, RPA3) that stabilizes ssDNA regions generated during both DNA replication, repair and recombination. At the double strand break, the RPA-coated ssDNA recruits ATR-ATRIP to chromatin, an event critical for the activation of the ATR-chk1 pathway. Similar to the trimeric RPA complex, the newly identified human ssDNA binding protein, hSSB1 is thought play a role in checkpoint activation and repair (Richard et al., 2008). The next critical step in HR is the assimilation of Rad51 to ssDNA in a Brca2 and PALB2 (Partner and localizer of Brca2) dependent manner to form the Rad51-coated nucleoprotein filament. Rad51-mediated homology search and strand invasion follows where the Rad51 recombinase utilizes the sister chromatid as the homologous template and together with Rad51 paralogs (Xrcc2, Xrcc3, Rad51L1, Rad51L2 and Rad51L3), Rad52 and Rad54 promotes strand invasion and recombination. Strand invasion and migration involve the formation of a structure termed as the Holliday junction. Following DNA polymerase δ-mediated DNA synthesis, resolution of Holliday junction occurs via Rad54/Mus81/Emc1 and Rad51C/Xrcc3 (San Filippo et al., 2008).

It is now becoming increasingly clear that the choice between the various DNA repair pathways is dictated by negative regulation of on one pathway by another. For example, DSB resection promoted by CtIP is inhibited by 53BP1 (Bunting et al., 2010). 53BP1 itself promotes NHEJ by increasing the stability of DSBs during ligation. Another example of this regulation was highlighted by a recent study where defective DSB resection in Brca1 mutant cells results in NHEJ-dependent chromosomal rearrangements which could be overcome by 53BP1 loss, suggesting that Brca1 might somehow overcome 53BP1 function at DSBs to promote HR (Bunting et al., 2010). Also, abnormal activity of alt-NHEJ in the absence of NHEJ induces chromosomal translocation in mammalian cells (Simsek and Jasin, 2010). Thus, the right choice of DSB repair pathways can be a critical determinant of genomic stability and alterations in the appropriate repair pathway choice can lead to DSB repair defects with deleterious consequences.

3.7 Double strand break signalling

Amongst the various classes of DNA repair, perhaps the best studied pathway with respect to DNA lesion sensing and signalling is the DSB repair signalling response. The response to DSBs has been characterised by the rapid localization of repair factors to DSB sites into subnuclear foci called ionizing radiation-induced foci (IRIF) (Bekker-Jensen and Mailand, 2010). At a more mechanistic level, the DDR proteins can be divided into three major classes of proteins that act together to translate the DNA damage signal into an appropriate response. These consist of (a) sensor proteins that recognize abnormal DNA lesions and initiate the signalling cascade (b) transducers that amplify the damage signal and (c) effectors proteins that participate in a number of downstream pathways such as cell cycle, apoptosis and senescence (Figure 2: DNA damage signalling and response) (Jackson and Bartek, 2009).

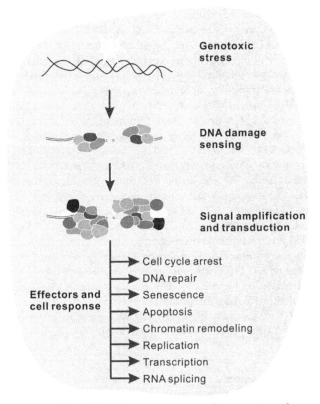

Fig. 2. Basic organization of the DNA damage response: Sensors, transducers and effectors

3.7.1 Sensing the damage

The efficient sensing of DSBs is achieved by Mre11-Rad50-Nbs1 (MRN) protein complex (Stracker and Petrini, 2011). The MRE11 (Meiotic Recombination 11) protein is an evolutionarily conserved protein that is involved in HR, NHEJ, meiosis and in the maintenance of telomeres. RAD50 is a homolog of *S.cerevisiae* Rad50 and is a member of the structural maintenance of chromosome (SMC) protein family. The third protein in the MRN complex is NBS1 (Nijmegen breakage syndrome 1) protein also known as Nibrin and p95. Structural and biochemical studies have elucidated the architecture of the MRN complex and have proposed the biochemical events that lead to the activation of the DDR. The key protein in the MRN complex is the Mre11 homodimer. This protein has the ability to bind free DSBs and also has an intrinsic 3'-5' exonuclease activity that can help in the resection of broken ends. The Mre11 dimer can interact with two molecules of Rad50 and with the scaffolding protein Nbs1. The extended coiled-coil domains of Rad50 permit it to extend out from DNA breaks and bridge with another Rad50 protein through the Zn^{2+}-binding CXXC motif, like a 'hook'. Thus, Rad50 might act as a molecular tether to bridge the DSBs.

The MRN complex interacts with the N-terminal of ATM and recruits it to DSBs (Lee and Paull, 2004). ATM belongs to the phosphatidylinositol-3-like kinase-related kinases (PIKK) family and plays an important role in the propagation of the initial DSB lesion by phosphorylating a number of downstream substrates. The PIKK family of proteins have a conserved kinase domain and three other domains: FAT (FRAP-ATM-TRRAP) domain, FATC domain (FRAP-ATM-TRRAP-C-terminal) and the PIKK regulatory domain that regulate the kinase activity of the protein. Apart from ATM, the other two PIKK proteins essential for DNA damage signalling are ATR (ATM and Rad3 related) and DNA-PKcs. ATM and DNA-PKcs are primarily involved in the signalling of DSBs and ATR is mainly required in response to stalled DNA replication forks. The interaction between the C-terminus of NBS1 and ATM leads to the recruitment of ATM to DSBs leading to its activation. In undamaged cells, ATM forms inactive dimers or multimers. However, upon the induction of DSBs, ATM is autophosphorylated at serine 1981, leading to its dissociation into activated monomers (Bakkenist and Kastan, 2003). Apart from ser1981, ATM is also autophosphorylated at serine 367 and serine 1983 and mutations at these sites reduce ATM activity. However, observations that transgenic mice carrying alanine substituted autophosphorylation serine sites 1987, 367 and 1899 of ATM (corresponding to human ATM serine 1981, 367 and 1893) display normal ATM-dependent responses, brought into question the function of ATM autophosphorylation *in vivo* (Daniel et al., 2008). This issue has been reconciled with the observation that autophosporylation of ATM at 1981 is not needed for the initial recruitment of ATM to DSBs, but for the stable association of activated ATM with the damaged chromatin (So et al., 2009). The regulation of ATM autophosphorylation is under the control of three serine/threonine phosphatases, PP2A, PP5 and Wip1, so that ATM is not activated in an untimely manner in the absence of DSBs. Interestingly, defects in the activity of these phosphatases also lead to disease phenotypes in knock-out mice (Peng and Maller, 2010).

3.7.2 Amplification of the signal

Activated ATM rapidly phosphorylates and activates several DNA repair factors to directly promote their recruitment to sites of DNA damage. Perhaps, the most important event is the ATM-dependent phosphorylation of the histone variant, H2AX at the C-terminal of the protein, corresponding to Ser139 (γ-H2AX) (Rogakou et al., 1998). Remarkably, in mammalian cells, this phosphorylation spreads over a 2 Mb domain of chromatin surrounding the DSB. γ-H2AX flanked DSB creates a specialized chromatin compartment capable of recruiting and retaining DNA repair factors. Indeed, mice deficient for H2AX develop genomic instability and cancers (Celeste et al., 2002). A large number of proteins have been identified as substrates for activated ATM and this list includes the proteins SMC1, NBS1, CHK2, p53, BRCA1 and MDC1 (Harper and Elledge, 2007). Key amongst these substrates are the Chk2 kinase and p53 which act to reduce cyclin-dependent kinase (CDK) activity. The direct consequence of reduced Cdk activity is that cells arrest in the various stages of cell cycle to allow time of the completion of DNA repair. Amongst the various ATM substrates, MDC1, in particular, is an important mediator of DSB signalling because it recognizes and binds γ-H2AX via its tandem BRCA1 C-terminal (BRCT) domains. The MDC1 C-terminal domain has been crystallized with γ-H2AX and the importance of this interaction was shown by experiments where mutations either in the phospho-acceptor site or in the conserved residues of BRCT domain impaired repair foci recruitment after DSB induction. Moreover, accumulation of several other repair factors such as NBS1, 53BP1 and the phosphorylation of ATM were reduced when MDC1-γ-H2AX interaction was abrogated. The serine-aspartic acid-threonine (SDT) repeats near the N-terminus of MDC1 are phosphorylated by Casein kinase 2, and this enables the interaction of MDC1 with NBS1. This interaction is not controlled by DNA damage, and MDC1 and MRN already exist as a complex in undamaged cells. Upon the generation of γ-H2AX, MDC1 together with MRN is recruited via the BRCT domain of MDC1. The concentrated binding of ATM to MDC1 and MRN further promotes the phosphorylation of H2AX, resulting in the amplification of the DDR. Thus, MDC1 is an important mediator of the DDR that regulates both the recruitment and retention of several downstream proteins (Huen and Chen, 2010).

Elegant work from the Misteli laboratory has established that the stable tethering of MDC1, MRN or ATM to DNA is sufficient to induce the DDR, even in the absence of DSBs. Upon targeted binding of MRN to a repetitive array, MDC1 and 53BP1 were recruited in an H2AX-dependent manner (Soutoglou and Misteli, 2008). These and other studies have given rise to the current model that MRN binding causes ATM recruitment and activation which initiates γ-H2AX formation. When MDC1 interacts with γ-H2AX, it provides a platform for the recruitment of MRN and ATM resulting in further propagation and spreading of γ-H2AX. Interestingly, when the kinetics of recruitment of DDR factors to DSBs was studied by live-cell imaging, NBS1 and MDC1 were the first factors to get recruited, seconds after DSB induction. The appearance of 53BP1 and BRCA1 was significantly slower that the MDC1 and NBS1 and more significantly, 53BP1 and Brca1 recruitment were abolished in MDC-null cells. This gave rise to a hierarchical model that the recruitment of 53BP1 and Brca1 was dependent on the stable recruitment of MDC1 through its interaction with γ-H2AX (Bekker-Jensen et al., 2006).

3.7.3 Recruitment of 53BP1 and Brca1

How exactly are Brca1 and 53BP1 recruited to DSB sites? A flurry of papers in recent years solved this conundrum through the identification of a ubiquitination cascade at DSB lesions. The product of the tumor suppressor gene *BRCA1* plays a central role in the maintenance of genomic integrity. Brca1 has been shown to regulate several cellular processes including transcriptional regulation, centrosome duplication, HR, NHEJ and checkpoint control. *BRCA1* encodes a large protein of 1863 amino acids and contains tandem BRCT domains in its C-terminal region (Huen et al., 2010). In its N-terminus, it harbours a RING finger domain that specifically interacts with the structurally related protein Bard1 (BRCA1-associated ring domain protein 1) to heterodimerize and form a functional E3 ubiquitin ligase which forms a complex with E2 UBCH5C to promote the formation of K6-linked ubiquitin chains, an unusual chain linkage. The Brca1-Bard1 heterodimer form three non-overlapping complexes with distinct functions. The complexes are formed between Brca1 and phosphorylated proteins through the BRCT domain. The complexes include Brca1-BRIP, Brca1-CtIP and Brca1-Abraxas-Rap80-BRCC36 complexes. The Brca1-Abraxas-Rap80 complex mainly accumulates at DSBs and promotes the G2/M checkpoint. BRCC36 is a deubiquitinating enzyme and it is speculated that it might regulate Brca1-Bard1 ubquitination activity. The key mediator of Brca1 recruitment to DSB sites is Rap80. It was found that Rap80 depletion abolished Brca1 focus formation, whereas Brca1 depletion did not affect Rap80 focus formation. This strongly suggested that Rap80 controlled Brca1 focus formation. Upon mapping the site required for focus formation, it was found that the UIM motifs of Rap80 are required. The ubiquitin-binding function of the UIM motif is important to facilitate BRCA1-Rap80 recruitment to DNA lesions and the introduction of mutations that reduce ubiquitin binding also impair Brca1 and Rap80 focus formation. These studies led to the idea that a ubiquitin-dependent signalling system is important for Brca1 recruitment to sites of DSBs (Al-Hakim et al., 2010).

An important breakthrough in this area of research was made upon the identification of RNF8, the first of the three E3 ubiquitin ligases that catalyze regulatory ubiquitination at DNA lesions (Mailand et al., 2007). Importantly, the ubiquitin ligase activity of RNF8 was found to be absolutely essential for the recruitment of both Brca1 and 53BP1 to DSBs. RNF8 contains an FHA domain at its N-terminus and a RING finger motif at its C-terminus. The FHA domain of RNF8 recognises the ATM phosphorylated site of MDC1, leading to its recruitment to IRIF. The FHA domain of RNF8 also interacts with the HECT domain of the second E3 ligase HERC2, thus recruiting HERC2 to DSB sites. RNF8 together with HERC2 facilitates the assembly of the E2 ubiquitin conjugating enzyme Ubc13 to initiate K63-linked ubiquitin chains on H2A and its variants. The third E3 RING domain ubiquitin E3 ligase RNF168 recognizes and binds to K63-linked ubiquitin chains on H2A and H2AX through its two MIUs ((Motif Interacting with Ubiquitin). This amplifies the local concentration of K63-linked ubiquitin resulting in the recruitment and retention of 53BP1 and BRCA1 at the sites of lesions. Interestingly RNF168 was first identified as the gene mutated in RIDDLE syndrome (Stewart et al., 2009). RIDDLE (Radiosensitivity, immunodeficiency, dysmorphic features and learning difficulties) is a novel human immunodeficiency disorder associated with defects in DSB repair and Brca1/53BP1 recruitment defects.

Recently, another layer of complexity has emerged in the scenario of post translational modifications occurring following DSB induction. DSB-induced ubiquitylation and the recruitment of BRCA1 and other repair proteins to the sites of damage are also regulated by SUMOylation, placing SUMOylation as a critical post-translational modification necessary for optimal ubiquitylation at DSBs (Tang and Greenberg, 2010). Apart of ubiquitination and sumoylation, methylation of histones is also important for 53BP1 recruitment. According to a recent study, the loading of 53BP1 to DNA lesions is enabled by a local increase in H4K20 dimethylation surrounding the DSBs and this step is catalysed by the histone methyltransferase MMSET (Pei et al., 2011).

3.8 Coordinating DDR with cell cycle transitions

One important cellular consequence of DNA damage is the activation of cell cycle checkpoints which are surveillance mechanisms that arrest the cell cycle until repair is satisfactorily accomplished. The cell cycle is regulated through oscillations in cyclin dependent kinase activity (CDK) whose activity is upregulated by cyclins and inhibited by cyclin-dependent kinase inhibitors (CKI) and inhibitory phosphorylation of CDKs (Guardavaccaro and Pagano, 2006). At the molecular level, the DNA damage checkpoint arrests cell cycle transitions by directly reducing CDK activity through various mechanisms mainly initiated by ATM and ATR. Two ATM-dependent G/S checkpoints have been described. ATM activation by DSBs in G1 leads to Chk2 phosphorylation and consequent phosphorylation of the phosphatase CDC25A. This results in the formation of a phosphodegron which marks CDC25A for ubiquitin-mediated degradation and prevents the Thr14/Tyr15 dephosphorylation-mediated activation of CDK2. A second mechanism underlying the G1/S checkpoint involves the phosphorylation and stabilization of p53, either directly by ATM or indirectly by Chk2, which in turn acts as the transcription factor for the CKI, p21. This results in delayed G1/S transition after DNA damage. Together, CDC25A degradation and p21 upregulation form the basis for G1/S checkpoint maintenance (Bartek and Lukas, 2007).

During the S phase checkpoint, ATR is activated in response to stalled replication forks leading to the phosphorylation of Chk1 and the subsequent phosphorylation mediated degradation of Cdc25A by the SCF (Skp1-Cullin-F-box) β-TRCP ubiquitin ligase (Guardavaccaro and Pagano, 2006). This causes the inhibition of CDK2-Cyclin E/A activity preventing the initiation of new replication origins to slow down DNA replication. The failure to regulate Cdc25 leads to hyperactive Cdk activity and defective intra-S phase checkpoint. Yet another regulatory circuit to prevent DNA replication during repair involves the targeted degradation of Cdt1 which loads the replicative helicases MCM2-7 to form the pre-replication complex (Arias and Walter, 2007).

The G2/M checkpoint is initiated by the phosphorylation of checkpoint kinases, Chk1 and Chk2, which phosphorylate and inactivate CDC25C phosphatase by promoting its inhibitory sequestration by 14-3-3 proteins. This prevents the dephosphorylation-mediated activation of CDK1-Cyclin B complex required for mitotic progression (Lukas et al., 2004). Another target of the G2/M checkpoint are the Wee1 kinases. During a normal G2/M transition, Polo kinase 1(Plk1) phosphorylates Wee1 to create a phosphodegron that targets Wee1 for ubiquitin-mediated proteolysis. In the wake of G2/M checkpoint activation, Plk1 is negatively regulated by ATM/ATR and Wee1 accumulates in the cell to maintain CDKs in their inhibited form. Together, these mechanisms act in concert to halt cell cycle progression until the completion of DNA repair (Harper and Elledge, 2007).

3.9 Identification of novel ATM/ATR substrates using proteomic approaches

Recently, it has become apparent that DNA damage-activated kinases do not simply contact key individual proteins in a process, but phosphorylate multiple proteins of individual pathways. Importantly, understanding such linkages could have tremendous implications for human disease. In a large scale proteomic study, about 900 phosphorylation sites containing a consensus ATM and ATR phosphorylation motif were identified in 700 substrates that were inducibly phosphorylated after irradiation (Matsuoka et al., 2007). Based on the rationale that ATM and ATR phosphorylate substrates at the consensus SQ/TQ motifs, a phospho-antibody specific directed against this consensus site was used to immunoprecipitate peptides and mass spectrometric analyses was performed. The identified proteins were clustered into modules based on their known function. Multiple modules involved in DNA replication were identified such as the Orc module consisting of Orc3 and Or6, MCM module, including Mcm2, Mcm3, Mcm6, Mcm7 and Mcm10, RFC clamp-loader module consisting of Rfc1 and Rfc3 and the DNA polymerase module composed of the catalytic subunit of DNA polymerase epsilon, its interacting protein PolE4 and two translesion polymerases PolL and PolQ. Other modules included the mismatch repair module consisting of the proteins, Msh2, Msh3 and Msh6 and Exo1, excision repair module included XPA, XPC, RPA1, CSB, components of the transcription factor IIH, a fanconi anaemia module and a HR module. Interestingly, three components of the COP9 signalosome involved in the regulation of SCF (Skp1-Cullin-F-box) E3 ligase function and a novel cell cycle module comprising Cyclin E and its negative regulators FBW7, p27kip1 and CIZ1 were also identified as ATM/ATR substrates. Other proteins included components of the spindle checkpoint pathway comprising of Bub1, Mad1, Sgo1 and Mad2BP, Cdc26, separase, and cohesion subunits SMC1 and SMC3. Perhaps, the most interesting group of substrates were proteins in the insulin–IGF-1 (insulin-like growth factor)–PI3K (phosphatidylinositol 3-kinase)–AKT pathway, including the adaptor molecule IRS2 (insulin receptor substrate 2), the kinase AKT3, two regulators of AKT, HSP90 (heat shock protein 90), and PP2A (protein phosphatase 2A), and several downstream effectors of AKT such as FOXO1, and proteins involved in translation control such as TSC1 (tuberous sclerosis 1), 4E-BP1 (eIF4E binding protein 1), and p70S6K (ribosomal protein S6 kinase). This indicates that the DDR is likely to control the insulin-IGF pathway in multiple ways and further studies in this direction will shed light on the role of ATM/ATR pathway in human metabolic syndromes such as diabetes and other age-associated metabolic disorders.

4. Physiological roles of DDR

It has now become apparent that the DDR pathway is not just activated in response to genotoxic stress, but that it is essential for several physiological processes. Examples where genome alterations are induced in a programmed manner are V(D)J recombination (Bassing and Alt, 2004), class switch recombination (CSR) (Stavnezer et al., 2008) and somatic hypermutation (SHM) (Di Noia and Neuberger, 2007). These processes occur in developing T and B lymphocytes to generate T-cell receptor and immunoglobulin diversity, to allow the recognition of pathogens (Jackson and Bartek, 2009). In the meiotic cells, the DDR plays an important role when homologous chromosomes align and exchange genetic information by recombination. Meiotic HR is generated by the topoisomerase II-like enzyme Spo11, which generates DSBs. In subsequent steps that require MRN complex, HR recombination occurs which requires all mitotic HR proteins along with a Rad51-like protein, DMC (Richardson et al., 2004). In the developing nervous system, high levels of oxidative and metabolic stress are effectively repaired by the DDR. During infections with pathogens such as the avian influenza virus, the DDR proteins modulate the virulence properties of the virus through recombination (Jackson and Bartek, 2009). During bacterial infections, bacterial pathogens with defects in MMR, termed mutators or hypermutators, are overrepresented and are hypothesized to be advantageous for the establishment of chronic infections (Sundin and Weigand, 2007). DDR proteins also play important roles at normal telomeres and thus their defects cause telomere shortening and/or telomere dysfunction associated with chromosome fusions and instability (Jackson and Bartek, 2009). Telomeres are recognized by DDR proteins such as Mre11 (DSB repair), XPF/Ercc1 (NER), Ku70/Ku80 (NHEJ repair), Bloom and WRN RecQ helicases and Rad51D (HR repair) (Denchi, 2009). These factors are recruited to the telomeres through their direct interaction with protein of the shelterin complex, a complex of six telomere binding proteins that promote telomere homeostasis. Recent studies have also established a relationship between DDR and another physiological phenomenon, the circadian rhythm, a process controlled by light stimuli (Sancar et al., 2010). The circadian rhythm regulator clk-2 has been shown to affect radiation sensitivity in C.elegans and S phase checkpoint in response to replication stress in mammalian cells. NER has also been shown to be regulated by the circadian clock and there is strong evidence that the clock protein Cry participates in the maintenance of genomic integrity against DNA damage induced by UV and UV mimetics. It has been proposed that such linkages between light cycle and DNA repair can allow cells to respond appropriately to environmentally-induced DNA damage ((Jackson and Bartek, 2009)). Described in greater detail below are the physiological roles of DDR in the immune system, meiosis and in the maintenance of genome integrity of stem cells.

4.1 V(D)J recombination and class switch recombination

One of the cell types where programmed DSBs are generated are B and T lymphocytes. B and T cells are the main components of the adaptive immune system and responsible for the generation of B cell receptors (BCRs, also known as immunoglobulins) and T cell receptors (TCRs), which together recognize a large repertoire of antigens. During the development of antigen receptor genes, a large number of variable (V), diversity (D), joining (J) and constant (C) segments undergo rearrangement by processes termed as V(D)J recombination and class switch recombination (CSR) (Bassing and Alt, 2004; Stavnezer et al., 2008). Immunoglobulin (Ig) contains a heavy chain and either a κ or λ light chain. TCRs are composed of either αβ or γδ dimers. In humans, Ig heavy chain loci contain 51 V_H, 27 D_H, 6 J_H and 9 C_H segments and Ig light chain loci contain 40 Vκ, 31 Vλ, 5 Jκ and 4 Jλ segments; TCR loci consist of 54 Vα, 61 Jα, 67 Vβ, 14 Jβ, 2 Dβ, 14 Vγ, 5 Jγ, 3 Vδ, 3 Jδ and 3 Dδ segments. Roughly, 10^7 Igs and TCRs can be generated by V(D)J recombination. In response to antigens, antigen receptors are further diversified by CSR and somatic hypermutation (SHM). In the following section, V(D)J recombination and CSR during B cell development will be reviewed.

B cell development begins in the fetal liver during development and continues in the bone marrow shortly after birth. It is a highly ordered process, mediated by cytokines secreted by bone marrow stromal cells and lineage-specific transcription factors. In response to cytokines such as IL-7, common lymphoid progenitors are committed to B cell lineage. Subsequently, cells undergo D_H-J_H joining at the Ig heavy chain locus and begin expressing CD45 (B220) and class II MHC (major histocompatibility complex), which is followed by the joining of a V segment to the completed DJ_H. After successful V(D)J recombination, pro-B cells become pre-B cells, which undergo V-J joining on one L chain locus and further develop into mature B cells. V(D)J recombination is regulated at three levels: chromatin remodelling, DSB generation mediated by lymphoid-specific recombinases (Rag-1/2) and recombination via NHEJ and microhomology-mediated end joining (MMEJ, also called alternative NHEJ) machinery.

In eukaryotic cells, DNA is wrapped into a compact chromatic structure, which needs to be 'opened' to allow accessibility for further processing. Increasing evidence in genetically modified mouse models shows that covalent histone modifications, such as methylation on histone H3 at lysines 4, 9 and 27 (K4, K9 and K27) positions, mediate chromatin remodelling and subsequently V(D)J recombination. Enhancer of Zeste 2 (Ezh2) is a methyltransferase which trimethylates K27 of histone H3 (H3K27me3). Conditional deletion of Ezh2 in B lymphocytes leads to reduced H3K27me3 levels and defective V_H-DJ_H recombination at the most distal V segments (Su et al., 2003). Di- and tri-methylation of histone H3K4 are also found to be associated with the active segments in V(D)J recombination (Liu et al., 2007). Rag-2 binds to H3K4me3 via the PHD motif and mutations that abolish the interaction impair V(D)J recombination. In contrast, H3K9me2, a silent chromatin mark, inhibits distal V_H-DJ_H recombination (Osipovich et al., 2004), while Pax5, a transcriptional factor required for early B cell commitment, regulates the removal of H3K9me2 and promotes V_H-DJ_H recombination (Johnson et al., 2004).

The coding sequences of IgH are separated by recombination signal sequences (RSSs). RSSs are conserved heptamers (CACTGTG) and nonamers (GGTTTTTGT) flanking either 12 base pairs (bp) or 23±1 bp non-conserved DNA, called the spacer. The recombination of D_H to J_H, V_L to J_L or V_H to DJ_H occurs only between the 12 bp- and 23 bp-spacers, known as 12/23 spacer rule. Rag-1 and Rag-2 recognize RSSs and generate DSBs between the heptamers and its adjacent coding segment. Rag-1/2 first introduces a nick on one strand and then the nicked free coding end attacks the opposite strand, creating a closed hairpin structure. Disruption of either Rag-1 or Rag-2 in mice causes severely impaired V(D)J recombination, defective B cell development and immunodeficiency (Mombaerts et al., 1992; Shinkai et al., 1992).

The final step of V(D)J recombination involves NHEJ and MMEJ machineries where the two coding segments are ligated together. The proteins involved in NHEJ are not all known and new proteins are constantly being uncovered. Here, in this section we discuss those that are well-studied, including DNA-PK, Artemis endonuclease, and XLF (Xrcc4-like factor, also known as Cernunnos)-Xrcc4-DNA ligase IV complex. Deficiency in any of these proteins compromises B and/or T cell development. DNA-PK consists of catalytic subunit DNA-PKcs and regulatory subunits Ku70 and Ku80. As mentioned earlier, DNA-PKcs phosphorylates H2AX at DSB to transduce signalling, while Ku70 and Ku80 form a heterodimer to process the broken ends. DNA-PKcs deficiency is the main cause of murine severe combined immunodeficiency (SCID), where both B and T cells are depleted (Blunt et al., 1995). Any defects in Ku protein also impair V(D)J recombination (Gu et al., 1997; Taccioli et al., 1993). Artemis is thought to open the closed hairpin at the coding ends generated by Rag-1/2. Null mutants of Artemis also give rise to the severe combined immunodeficiency (SCID) phenotype (Li et al., 2005). Xrcc4 together with XLF and DNA ligase IV ligates the broken ends together. Cells deficient for either Xrcc4, XLF or DNA ligase IV are sensitive to γ-irradiation and compromised in V(D)J recombination (Ahnesorg et al., 2006; Gao et al., 1998).

Upon antigen or humoral stimulation, CSR further diversifies antibodies by switching their isotypes. Human BCR heavy chain gene contains 9 C_H segments: 1 μ (IgM), 1 δ (IgD), 4 γ (IgG), 1 ε (IgE) and 2 α (IgA). CSR occurs between two switch (S) regions located upstream of each C_H segment, except for Cδ; the switch between Cμ (IgM) and Cδ (IgD) is achieved by alternate splicing before complete maturation of B cells. Similar to V(D)J recombination, CSR also involves DSB generation and NHEJ. DSBs are created by dC deamination, BER and MMR machinery within or near S regions. In response to humoral stimulation, activation-induced cytidine deaminase (AID) deaminates dC resulting in dU bases on both strands of two transcriptionally active S regions (Chaudhuri et al., 2003). The dU is excised by the uracil DNA glycosylases (UNG) and the resultant abasic site is further cut by apurinic/apyrimidinic endonuclease 1/2 (APE-1/2), generating SSBs. Either two adjacent SSBs on opposite strands spontaneously lead to one DSB, or the MMR machinery is triggered to convert SSB to DSB (Schrader et al., 2007). Deficiency of AID, UNG, APE or any of the MMR components, including Msh2, Msh6, Mlh1, Pms2 and Exo1, leads to loss or reduction of CSR in B cells (Stavnezer et al., 2008). After DSB formation, NHEJ rather than HR pathway is activated. Components of classical NHEJ (C-NHEJ) pathway are important but not essential for CSR in B cells. Ku70-Ku80 heterodimers bind to the DNA ends and recruit necessary proteins to process the DNA ends to facilitate the ligation mediated by Xrcc4-DNA ligase IV complex (Nick McElhinny et al., 2000). CSR in *Ku70−/−* and *Ku80−/−* B cells is nearly ablated (Casellas et al., 1998; Manis et al., 1998). Either *Xrcc4* or *DNA ligase IV* deficiency causes significant reduction in CSR (Soulas-Sprauel et al., 2007; Yan et al., 2007). While compatible ends are joined rapidly by canonical NHEJ components, complex lesions need substantial processing and are re-ligated slowly. In the later case, ATM, 53BP1 and MRM complex cooperate with canonical NHEJ components to mediate end-joining recombination. Disruption of ATM (Bredemeyer et al., 2006; Reina-San-Martin et al., 2004), 53BP1 (Manis et al., 2004) or MRN complex (Kracker et al., 2005) in mice leads to defects in either V(D)J recombination or CSR or both. Recent studies in mouse models deficient for NHEJ core components revealed a robust alternative NHEJ pathway (A-NHEJ) that utilizes microhomology to mediate the end joining in CSR (Soulas-Sprauel et al., 2007; Yan et al., 2007). A-NHEJ leads to Ig locus deletion and translocation. The molecular mechanisms underlying A-NHEJ are not well elucidated so far.

4.2 Meiosis

Meiosis is a form of cell division occurring in sexually reproducing organisms by which maternal and paternal chromosomes are distributed between cells to generate genetic diversity. Prior to meiosis, each chromosome duplicates and creates two sister chromatids, which stay connected at the centromere. During meiosis, the homologous chromosomes align in parallel and chromosomal crossovers are induced by recombination. DSBs are generated by meiosis-specific topoisomerase-like enzyme Spo11 (Keeney et al., 1997), together with Mei1. Mice lacking *Spo11* or *Mei1* fail in the generation of DSBs, leading to absence of Rad51 foci, faulty synapsis, meiotic failure and eventually infertility (Baudat et al., 2000; Libby et al., 2003; Munroe et al., 2000; Romanienko and Camerini-Otero, 2000). The generation of DSB on meiotic chromosomes is not entirely random but occurs preferentially on specific chromosomal locations, known as hot spots. Recombination regulator 1 (RCR1) and double strand break control 1 (DSBC1) regulate the activities of recombination hot spots (Grey et al., 2009; Parvanov et al., 2009). Although the molecular mechanisms underlying the selection of hot spots for DSB induction are still under investigation, it has been found that high-order chromatin structure could be an important factor (Buard et al., 2009). Of particular interest is the methylation of histone H3K4me3 by the methyltransferase Prdm9 (also known as Meisetz), which is enriched at meiotic recombination hot spots (Baudat et al., 2010; Borde et al., 2009; Buard et al., 2009). *Prdm9* null mice are sterile owing to defective chromosome paring and impaired sex body formation (Hayashi et al., 2005; Mihola et al., 2009).

Many components of the HR pathway are of particular importance for proper strand exchange and meiosis. As mentioned earlier, MRN complex is recruited to the DSBs to remove Spo11 and degrade the 5′ of DNA, generating long 3′ ssDNA overhangs. ATM is activated by MRN and further amplifies the signaling via phosphorylation of many downstream transducers and effectors, such as H2AX and Chk2 (Shiloh, 2003). Finally, ubiquitously expressed Rad51 and meiosis-specific Dmc1 recognize and bind to the resected 3′ ssDNA overhangs and form nucleoprotein filaments, which mediate the search for homologous template and subsequent strand exchange. As they are all essential for development, disruption of either Rad51 or any component of MRN complex causes embryonic lethality (Buis et al., 2008; Luo et al., 1999; Zhu et al., 2001). Loss of ATM in mice causes general defects in DSB repair and mislocalization of Rad51 and Dmc1 in spermatocytes (Barlow et al., 1996; Barlow et al., 1998). During meiosis, *Dmc1*[-/-] germ cells arrest at the early zygotene stage due to the failure of homologous chromosome synapsis (Yoshida et al., 1998).

In contrast to mitotic recombination in which Rad51-mediated HR utilizes the identical sister chromatid as homologous template (reviewed earlier in Section 2.6), Rad51 and Dmc1-mediated strand invasion prefers the chromatids from the homologous chromosome in meiotic recombination. This preference is achieved with the help of other factors such as chromosome-associated kinase Mek1, which excludes identical sister chromatid from being selected as a homologous template for further meiotic recombination. As a byproduct, this generates a heteroduplex DNA (hDNA) if there are heterologies between the two homologous chromosomes (maternal and paternal). In this case, MMR pathway is activated to repair the hDNA, resulting in either gene conversion (GC) or restoration of original sequences (Kramer et al., 1989). Two recombination pathways are employed, i.e. cross-over (CO) and non-cross-over (NCO). CO occurs when double Holiday junctions (dHJs), which are visualized as chiasmata, are formed and subsequently cut by resolvases. NCO is also known as synthesis-dependent strand annealing (SDSA), leading to gene conversion. MMR pathways are not only restricted to resolving hDNA because $Mlh1^{-/-}$ mice exhibit defective gametogenesis due to reduction of chiasmata, recombination and COs, and deficiency in $Pms2$ leads to disrupted synapsis (Baker et al., 1995; Baker et al., 1996; Edelmann et al., 1996). Msh4 and Msh5 are two meiosis-specific homologues of MutS, which interact with Rad51 to stabilize the synaptonemal complex (SC) mediated chromosome paring. Targeted mutations of $Msh4$ and $Msh5$ in mice give rise to meiotic-specific phenotypes, including meiotic arrest at zygotene stage and defective synapsis (de Vries et al., 1999; Edelmann et al., 1999; Kneitz et al., 2000). $Mlh3$ and $Exo1$ null mice are also infertile, attributed to meiotic failure and apoptosis (Lipkin et al., 2002; Wei et al., 2003).

4.3 DNA damage signaling in stem cells

Recently, it has become apparent that tissue stem cells possess an elaborate DDR to maintain organ homeostasis, although the mechanistic details seem to vary greatly between different tissues. The DDR in response to radiation exposure has been studied in detail in at least four adult stem cell types: epidermal stem cells, hematopoietic stem cells, mammary stem cells and intestinal stem cells. By comparing the response of haematopoietic stem cells (HSCs) with their differentiated progeny at low doses of IR, it has become clear that different DNA repair and signalling mechanisms exist within the stem cell compartment. Using fetal human umbilical cord blood derived HSCs and by comparing them with their more mature progenitors, it was found that stem cells had greater level of apoptosis, due to the ASPP1 protein, and the phenotype could be rescued by the down regulation of p53 (Milyavsky et al., 2010). In contrast, when a similar experiment was performed using adult mouse HSCs, low doses of IR showed a greater degree of protection in stem cells as compared to their differentiated counterparts. The underlying mechanism was proposed to be the increased expression of anti-apoptotic Bcl2, Bcl-xl which inhibited p53-mediated cell death, while allowing p53-dependent increase in p21 expression (Mohrin et al., 2010). Interestingly, quiescent HSCs mostly preferred NHEJ pathway for DNA repair, and as a consequence their progeny often showed increased levels of genomic instability due to misrepaired DNA. Recent investigations using multipotent hair follicle bulge stem cells (BSC) also revealed that BSCs were more resistant to DNA damage-induced cell death as compared to other cells of the epidermis (Blanpain and Fuchs, 2009). The underlying mechanism was shown to be the increased expression levels of anti-apoptotic Bcl2 and the transient and reduced duration of p53 up regulation. BSCs also displayed accelerated repair by the error-prone NHEJ pathway and this result suggested that both HSCs and BSCs show short term survival in the wake of DNA damage at the expense of a compromise on their genomic integrity.

Irradiation experiments have also been performed on intestinal stem cells (ISC) to understand their DDR. The intestinal stem cells are localized at the bottom of the crypt, where they proliferate and generate the transit amplifying cells, which divide and migrate to the upper part of the crypt. At least two distinct stem cell populations have been isolated from the intestine corresponding to the +4 position from the bottom of the crypt, which are positive for the stem cell marker Bmi1+ and quiescent and the cycling Lgr5+ fraction located in between the paneth cells at the base of the intestinal crypt (Barker et al., 2010). Radiation sensitivity experiments have revealed that the quiescent stem cells at the +4 position are extremely radiosensitive, followed by the more active Lgr5+ve cells, whereas the rapidly cycling transit amplifying cells were the most radioresistant. Different mechanisms have been proposed for the extreme sensitivity of the Bmi1+ve ISCs to DNA damage, such as enhanced activation of the p53 pathway, lower expression of anti-apoptotic protein Bcl2. However, based on the observation that IR-induced stem cell apoptosis is blocked in PUMA-deficient mice, it is accepted that Puma is the main mediator of DDR in ISCs (Qiu et al., 2008). The DDR has also been studied in germ stem cells (GSC) since the inability to repair DNA damage in the germ line can be extremely dangerous and can directly lead to infertility or the transmission of genetic diseases. The main source of DNA damage in the germ-line could be from teratogenic chemicals or from normal metabolic activity and ROS production. In studies using human male GSCs, it was found that these cells are mostly kept in the G0/G1 phase of the cell cycle, and preferentially use NHEJ as their repair of choice. On the other hand, the female GSCs are located in the oogonia where the homologous chromosomes are close to each other and hence HR is the preferred pathway for DNA repair (Forand et al., 2009). Interestingly, in contrast to other stem cell populations, the female GSCs do not depend on p53 for their genomic integrity. Instead, TAp63, an isoform of the p63 gene, is constitutively expressed in oocytes and is the primary mediator of DDR. Consistently, TAp63 deletion in mice results in an increase in oocyte radioresistance (Suh et al., 2006). The study of DNA repair in another stem cell type, namely the mammary stem cells (MSCs), is clinically very relevant because, mutations in Brca1 and Brca2 are found in a majority of patients with hereditary breast cancers, demonstrating the importance of HR in preventing the onset of mammary tumors. The MSCs are responsible for the homeostasis of the breast tissue, and represent multipotent stem cells that self-renew and differentiate into the various lineages. Mouse MSCs are more radioresistant than their differentiated progeny. MSCs present less DNA damage and following IR exposure, activate the Wnt/beta-catenin pathway and increase the survival of MSCs through the upregulation of survivin, a direct Wnt target gene (Woodward et al., 2007).

5. DNA damage response and human diseases

Congenital or acquired defects in genes involved in the DDR give rise to disease phenotypes such as neurodegeneration, infertility, immune deficiencies, growth retardation, cancer and premature aging. In the following sections, human diseases caused due to impaired DDR are described in greater detail and summarized in Figure 3 and Table 1.

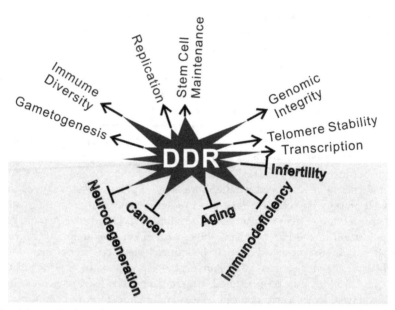

Fig. 3. Physiological roles of DDR and disease phenotypes caused by defective DNA repair

5.1 Neurodegeneration

The mammalian nervous system is generated through consecutive cycles of proliferation, differentiation and maturation that eventually give rise to the various cell types of the brain. Two main classes of cells make up the nervous system: the glia and the neurons, and these contain many specialized sub-types. These cells exit the cell cycle, migrate and differentiate to form the nervous system. In general, neurons display high rates of transcription and translation which are associated with high rates of mitochondrial and metabolic activity. Thus, the neural cells are more susceptible to DNA damage than other adult tissue cell types because they face high levels of oxidative and metabolic stress during their life time. The DNA damage takes the form of both SSBs and DSBs that have to be efficiently repaired to maintain neural homeostasis. Indeed, one of the most commonly observed symptoms in both DNA repair-deficient mice and in humans is that of neurodegeneration. This is mainly because individuals possessing mutations in DNA repair pathways are incapable of handling DNA damage in the neurons, resulting in neuronal cell death that is manifested as neurodegeneration (Katyal and McKinnon, 2008).

The DNA strand breaks in the nervous system may arise due to reactive oxygen species (ROS) that arise as a by-product of cellular metabolism. ROS, in turn carries out nucleophilic attack on DNA to generate single strand breaks. Due to the high levels of oxygen consumption in the brain, ROS levels are very high in the neurons compared to other adult cell types. In fact, tens to thousands of SSBs are generated by ROS in neuronal cells, and these constitute the single largest source of DNA damage in the nervous system (Katyal and McKinnon, 2008). As discussed earlier (Section 3.1), SSBs are efficiently detected by PARP which recruits the scaffolding protein XRCC1 so that the DNA lesions can be resolved by enzymes involved in DNA processing. Unrepaired SSBs can cause a block in transcription, or replication forks can collide with SSBs resulting in DSBs that have to be then repaired by the DSB repair pathway.

Human monogenic neurodegenerative defects associated with DDR defects can be broadly classified as those associated with DSB repair or SSB repair. Defective DSB repair associated neuropathologies include A-T, Nijmegen breakage syndrome (NBS), ATLD (A-T like disorder), Seckel syndrome, Primary microcephaly (PM), and the Lig4 syndrome. In most DNA repair-associated syndromes, cerebellum is often the primary target of neurodegeneration which then spreads to the remaining parts of the brain. A-T syndrome arises as a result of mutations in ATM. Since cerebellum is mainly responsible for sensory motor coordination, individuals with A-T often present with profound ataxia (defective motor coordination) and are wheelchair-bound within the first decade of life. The DDR pathway in A-T strongly affects the cerebellum and widespread loss of cerebellar purkinje cells and granule neurons is seen in A-T brains and is later accompanied by widespread cerebral and spinal defects. Additionally, A-T patients develop other neurological defects such as defective eye movement, speech defects (dysarthria) and non-neurological symptoms such as the absence or the rudimentary appearance of a thymus, immunodeficiency, insulin-resistant diabetes, clinical and cellular radiosensitivity, cell cycle checkpoint defects, chromosomal instability and predisposition to lymphoid malignancies (Biton et al., 2008). Because of the central role of the MRN complex in the ATM-dependent DDR, human syndromes caused by defects in the MRN complex have been regarded as AT-like disorders. Very similar to AT, NBS is characterized by growth retardation, frequent infections, microcephaly (described below), ovarian dysgenesis (defective development), primary amenorrhoea and lymphoma predisposition. However, NBS cells also appear to be defective in some aspects of the ATR pathway and exhibit phenotypes like microcephaly (described below), not usually seen in A-T patients. Patients suffering from ATLD (A-T like disorder) have hypomorphic mutations of MRE11 and show neurological symptoms very similar to A-T such as dysarthria, oculomotor apraxia and ataxia. Interestingly, a cancer predisposition phenotype has not been observed with ATLD. Also, in contrast to NBS patients, ATLD subjects do not have microcephaly (Katyal and McKinnon, 2008).

In addition to neurodegeneration, defective DSB repair can cause developmental defects in the brain, resulting in the development of a smaller brain, called microcephaly where the brain size is at least two standard deviations smaller than the normal brain. This phenotype probably arises as a result of brain cell loss due to the inability to cope with DNA damage in the developing brain. For example, patients harbouring germ-line mutations in ATR, suffer from the Seckel syndrome, an autosomal recessive disorder characterized by severe intrauterine growth retardation, profound microcephaly, a 'bird-like' facial profile, mental retardation and isolated skeletal abnormalities (O'Driscoll et al., 2009). Patients harbouring mutations in the centrosomal protein pericentrin also show pronounced microcephaly as a result of DNA replication fork defects and defective DNA repair. Patients bearing hypomorphic mutations in Lig4, the DNA ligase in the NHEJ pathway also present with microcephaly, developmental and growth delay, immunodeficiency and lymphoid malignancies. Mutation in another NHEJ protein XLF, causes a disorder called as HIM (Human immunodeficiency and microcephaly), primarily characterised by growth delay, recurrent infections, autoimmunity and microcephaly (Katyal and McKinnon, 2008).

Unlike defective DSB pathway, where the associated defects are more wide spread across tissues, defective SSB repair pathway often results in phenotypes restricted to the nervous system. For example, defective SSB repair pathway result in spinocerebellar ataxia and axonal neuropathy (SCAN1) and ataxia with oculomotor apraxia (AOA1), which are caused by mutations in the 3'-endprocessing enzyme tyrosyl DNA phosphodiesterase 1 (TDP1) and the 5'-end-processing enzyme aprataxin (APTX), respectively (McKinnon, 2009). As mentioned earlier, TDP1 is an enzyme involved in the processing of damaged DNA ends, such as 3'-phosphoglycolate and 3' Top1 and other non-ligatable termini generated after DNA oxidation, DNA replication and other types of genotoxic stress. APTX, on the other hand, is a nucleotide hydrolase that cleaves the 5' adenylate intermediate prior to sealing the nick after the generation of SSB. Similar to A-T patients, SCAN1 and AOA1 patients show ataxia, oculomotor apraxia, cerebellar atrophy and dysarthria. Cockayne's syndrome and XP/CS are associated with defects in CSA, CSB, XPB, XPD and is associated with neurological symptoms such as microcephaly, progressive neurodegeneration, cerebral and cerebellar atrophy and sensorineural deafness (Weidenheim et al., 2009). In another SSR-associated syndrome called as trichothiodystrophy (TTD), the proteins XPB, XPD, TTDA are found defective (Stefanini et al., 2010). This syndrome is associated with cerebral cortex microcephaly, hypomyelination and psychomotoric abnormalities.

Recent studies have also highlighted the role of defective DNA repair in late-onset chronic neuropathologies such as Alzheimer's disease and Parkinson's disease. For instance, decreased levels of NHEJ factor DNA-PKcs and of MRN proteins and reduced BER capacity has been documented in Alzheimer's disease patients, whereas increased DNA damage accumulation has been observed in the substantia nigra neurons, a population of neurons often depleted in Parkinson's disease patients (Katyal and McKinnon, 2008).

5.2 Infertility

Human infertility is primarily defined as the inability to conceive after 12 months' intercourse and is often underdiagnosed (Thonneau et al., 1991). However the investigation of human infertility is hampered by the fact that defective meiotic recombination usually leads to either germ cell arrest or abnormal gametes. Some candidate genes such as PRDM9 and MEI1 have been found to contain mutations/polymorphisms in patients suffering from infertility (Miyamoto et al., 2008; Sato et al., 2006). MSH4 and DMC1 mutations have also been found in patients suffering from testis vanishing syndrome and premature ovarian failure (Mandon-Pepin et al., 2002).

5.3 Immune deficiency

As reviewed earlier in this chapter (Section 4.1), NHEJ machinery is used for V(D)J recombination, CSR and SHM in order to generate antigen receptor diversity. Defects in DSB generation and NHEJ components usually compromise V(D)J recombination, CSR and/or SHM, thereby leading to primary inherited immunodeficiency. Severe combined immunodeficiency (SCID) is a severe form of inheritable immunodeficiency. In SCID, both B and T adaptive immune systems are impaired and the patients are extremely vulnerable to various infectious diseases. Defects in V(D)J recombination usually lead to SCID in humans because it is required for both B and T antigen receptor generation. During V(D)J recombination, RAG-1 and RAG-2 are responsible for DSB generation and mutations of either of them in humans are reported in some cases of SCID (Schwarz et al., 1996; Villa et al., 1998; Villa et al., 2001). Recently the first missense mutation of DNA-PKcs was reported in a human patient suffering from pronounced immunodeficiency. Strikingly, the mutation doesn't affect the kinase activity of DNA-PKcs but rather compromises the activity of Artemis (van der Burg et al., 2009). After DSB generation, Artemis processes the hairpin intermediates for end-joining. Mutations in Artermis arrest B and T cells at very early stage in some cases of SCID, owing to the defective V(D)J recombination (Ege et al., 2005; Moshous et al., 2001). Hypomorphic mutations of DNA ligase IV have been identified in individuals with SCID or combined immunodeficiency (CID) displaying microcephaly and delayed growth (Enders et al., 2006; O'Driscoll et al., 2001; Riballo et al., 1999; van der Burg et al., 2006). Similarly, patients with XLF mutations develop severe B-T lymphocytopenia, microcephaly and growth retardation (Ahnesorg et al., 2006; Buck et al., 2006).

In addition to the essential components of V(D)J recombination, mutations in other DSB repair factors also cause a less profound immunodeficiency characterized by defective lymphocyte development and IgG CSR defects. As described earlier (Section 5.1), Ataxia telangiectasia (AT) is a progressive genetic disorder caused by mutated ATM and is characterized with cerebellar ataxia, oculocutaneous telangiectasia, growth retardation, infertility, immunodeficiency and increased carcinogenesis mainly lymphoid tumours (Chun and Gatti, 2004). In AT patients, V(D)J recombination is not affected, but both B and T lymphocytes are restricted and skewed by diffused oligoclonal expansions (Giovannetti et al., 2002). While dispensable for SHM, ATM-deficient cells are compromised in diversifying IgM to other classes (Reina-San-Martin et al., 2004). Immunodeficiency is also manifested in NBS patients who are found more susceptible to infectious diseases (Digweed and Sperling, 2004). Similar to ATM, deficiency of either NBS1 or MRE11 doesn't affect normal V(D)J recombination although CSR is impaired (Lahdesmaki et al., 2004; van Engelen et al., 2001).

5.4 Cancer

Loss of genomic integrity and accumulation of mutations is a fundamental property of cancerous cells. In that context, the DDR influences cancer progression in multiple ways, as discussed below.

5.4.1 DNA repair defect and familial cancers

The concept that cancers could be acquired by DNA repair defects was first obtained by the study of patients suffering from familial hereditary cancers. Xeroderma pigmentosa (XP) was one of the first of many human cancers discovered to be acquired due to defective DNA repair (Cleaver, 2005). XP patients are defective in the NER of UV-induced DNA damage and have a 1000-fold greater risk of developing skin cancers and a 100,000 fold greater risk for developing squamous cell carcinoma of the tip of the tongue when compared to the general population. HNPCC (Hereditary non-polyposis colon cancer, also called as Lynch syndrome) is another inherited cancer syndrome where patients show an increased susceptibility to colon cancers. While the adenoma to carcinoma progression requires 8-10 years in the general population, this process is accelerated to 2-3 years in HNPCC patients. The majority of HNPCC cases result from germ-line mutations in genes encoding for the MMR proteins MSH2 and MLH1 (Fishel et al., 1993; Leach et al., 1993). Mutations in two other MMR genes MSH6 and PMS2 were also detected in a small proportion of cases. The resulting inability to detect and repair mismatches can lead to mutations of genes possessing microsatellite repeats in their sequences, causing a phenotype referred to as microsatellite instability. In addition to hereditary cases, MMR defects have also been detected in about 15% of sporadic gastric, endometrial and colon tumors owing to promoter hypermethylation and the consequent silencing of MLH1. In many of the tumors showing MMR defects and microsatellite instability, it is likely that hundreds of genes are concomitantly mutated and some of them such as the commonly studied type II TGF-β receptor may confer a proliferative advantage to incipient cancer cells and drive tumor progression. Another example is hereditary MYH-associated polyposis, in which biallelic germ-line mutations in *MYH*, a BER gene, result in increased GC to TA transversion and predisposition to colon cancer (Al-Tassan et al., 2002). Defective DSB repair attributed to germ-line transmission of mutant *BRCA1* and *BRCA2* alleles also confer enhanced susceptibility to breast and ovarian cancers. It is estimated that about 70-80% of all familial ovarian cancers is due to germ-line transmission of *BRCA1* or *BRCA2* (Scully and Livingston, 2000). Germ-line mutations in DNA repair genes *NBS1*, *ATM*, Werner syndrome helicase (*WRN*), Bloom syndrome helicase (*BLM*), RecQ protein-like 4 helicase (*RECQL4*) has also been linked to increased tumor susceptibility. Mutations in *p53* are present in cancer-prone families with Li-Fraumeni syndrome (Brown et al., 2009). As discussed in section 2.5, mutations in 14 FANC genes have been identified in Fanconi anaemia, which is an autosomal recessive hereditary disorder characterized by progressive bone marrow failure, congenital developmental abnormalities, and early onset of cancers such as acute myelogenous leukemia (AML) and squamous cell carcinomas of the head and neck. Together, these observations support the 'mutator hypothesis' which postulates that inherited defects in DDR contribute to the 'mutator' phenotype and increased mutation rate in many malignancies which might allow tumor cell survival and proliferation.

5.4.2 DDR and sporadic cancers

Apart from inherited mutations in proteins involved in DNA repair, recent large scale genome sequencing of cancer genomes have also identified mutational inactivation of components of the DDR machinery in sporadic cancers. Of these, mutations that perturb p53 functions, often in its DNA binding domain, or defects in p53's upstream or downstream regulatory network have been identified in more than half of all human cancer samples. Recently, coding sequences of about 20,000 genes in carcinomas of the colon, breast, pancreas and glioblastomas were sequenced. In these sequencing studies representing 68 cancers in the discovery screen and 221 cancers in the follow-up validation screen, one of the most frequently mutated gene was Cockayne syndrome B (*CSB*), found mutated in 6 cancers (Sequencing data compiled by Negrini et al, 2010 (Negrini et al., 2010)). Four genes involved in the DSB repair pathway, *BRCA1*, *BRCA2*, *MRE11* and *PRDKC* (gene encoding DNA-PKcs) were each mutated in two cancers and one mutation each in the genes encoding *FANCA*, *FANCG* and *FANCM*, *PABL2*, *WRN*, *XRCC 1*, *XPB*, *XPF*. *XPG*, *RAD23A* was identified. In a more controlled study involving the analysis of a limited set of DNA repair and cell cycle checkpoint genes in 188 lung adenocarcinomas and 91 glioblastomas, the NHEJ mutation in *PRDKC* and mismatch repair gene *MSH6* were each mutated in six and four cases respectively. The HR repair genes *BRCA2*, *BAP1* and *BARD1* were mutated in two cases each. Mutations in *ATM* were also identified in a few cases of lung adenocarcinomas. Notably, although large scale genome sequencing projects identified mutations in the genes involved in DNA repair, such mutations were detected only in a small proportion of human cancers (Negrini et al., 2010).

5.4.3 DDR and oncogene-induced senescence

An alternative model has been proposed that postulates that DDR, in fact, acts as a barrier to cellular transformation in the early stages of tumor progression by preventing the accumulation of mutations in the face of activated oncogenes (Bartek et al., 2007). According to this idea, the first hallmark to be acquired in sporadic cancer might be activated growth factor signalling owing to mutations in oncogenes and loss of tumor suppressor genes (Negrini et al., 2010). This results in an increased cell proliferation rate which generates a DNA replication stress, as shown for several oncogenes like Ras, Myc, Stat3 and E2FF1 (Bartkova et al., 2006). DNA replication stress, in turn, creates a high level of DNA damage, which results in the persistent activation of the DDR in the form of activated ATM/ATR signalling cascade causing cell death or senescence of incipient cancer cells. The senescence pathway evoked by oncogenes upon hyper-activation is now commonly referred to as the oncogene-induced senescence and is recognised as an important barrier to tumor progression (Gorgoulis and Halazonetis, 2010). Consistent with this idea, human lung, skin and colon precancerous lesions, show both apoptosis and senescence at the early stages of tumor development, whereas these processes are actively suppressed during cancer progression. Endogenous oncogenic K-Ras (K-Ras G12V) was shown to trigger senescence during the early stages of lung and pancreatic tumorigenesis. Melanocyte senescence has also been associated with the presence of oncogenic BRAFV60E, an oncogenic form of BRAF, *in vivo* (Michaloglou et al., 2005). Similarly, human prostate intraepithelial neoplasia (PIN) lesions and premalignant human colon adenomas display features of cellular senescence. Loss of the tumor suppressor neurofibromin 1 (NF 1), a Ras GTPase-activating protein that negatively regulates Ras, also leads to cellular senescence. By sharp contrast, senescence was absent in the corresponding malignant stages of human lung adenocarcinomas, pancreatic ductal adenocarcinomas, prostate adenocarcinoma and melanomas, suggesting that senescence acts as a barrier to tumor development. It is proposed that breaches to this anti-cancer barrier, arising due to mutational or epigenetic inactivation of DDR components help in the evasion of senescence and are subsequently selected for during tumor development.

5.4.4 DDR in cancer stem cells

Gaining a better understanding of the role of DDR in cancer cells is also important from a standpoint of therapy, since most chemotherapeutic compounds are DNA damaging agents. Many human cancers including leukemia, glioblastoma, breast and skin cancers contain a small proportion of cells which are functionally similar to tissue-stem cells, but have aberrant self-renewal and differentiation characteristics and these have been called as cancer stem cells (CSCs) (Clarke and Fuller, 2006). Recent studies have suggested that CSCs are responsible for disease progression and tumor relapse after therapy, since they may take advantage of the DNA repair systems used by tissue-stem cells to achieve resistance to chemotherapy/radiotherapy (Blanpain et al., 2011). Here, we discuss three instances where the DDR been demonstrated to have an effect on the outcome of cancer therapy. In the first case, the CSCs of leukemias, which exist in both acute myeloid leukemia (AML) and chronic myelogenous leukemia (CML) have been shown to be more resistant to cancer therapies as compared to the bulk of the leukemia cells. Leukemia CSCs have been shown to use protective mechanisms similar to HSCs, such as cell cycle quiescence, and DDR mechanisms to escape chemotherapy. For example, p53-dependent induction of p21 and the resulting growth arrest has been found to be critical in protecting adult HSCs from IR (Mohrin et al., 2010) and CSCs from leukemia co-opt similar protective mechanisms to evade apoptosis and during chemotherapy (Viale et al., 2009). There is also evidence that CSCs isolated from breast cancers (CD44 high, CD24 low cells) show resistance to chemo/and or radiotherapy. Transcriptional profiling of murine mammary CSCs also showed increased expression of several DDR and DNA repair genes (Zhang et al., 2008), suggesting that mammary gland CSCs may also be more resistant to therapy. Indeed, a comparison of tumor biopsies before and after neoadjuvant chemotherapy showed increased proportion of CSCs following chemotherapy. One possible mechanism seems to be that like normal mammary stem cells, CSCs from mammary gland have increased levels of genes regulating free radical scavenging systems, like those of glutathione metabolism (Diehn et al., 2009). Lastly, glioblastoma multiforme (GBM) represents the most aggressive form of brain tumor and CSCs are isolated from these tumors based on the expression of prominin (CD133-positive cells).   Upon irradiation, the proportion of CD133+ cells increased, suggesting that CSCs may be responsible for tumor relapse after radiotherapy (Bao et al., 2006). It was found that CSCs from GBM exhibited a more robust activation of DNA damage checkpoint and increased phosphorylation of ATM, Chk1 and Chk2 were observed in the CSCs as compared to the non-CSC counterparts. Consistently, treatment with Chk1/Chk2 inhibitors sensitized the CSC to IR-induced cell death.

6. DNA repair and aging

Aging involves a gradual deterioration of several physiological functions, resulting in the reduced capacity to repair injured organs, increased propensity to infections, cancer predisposition and decreased fecundity (DiGiovanna, 2000; Partridge and Mangel, 1999). Many hypotheses have been proposed to understand the underlying mechanisms of the aging process, and these include the disease theory, free radical theory and DNA damage accumulation theory. In this section, we only discuss evidences that support the relationship between DNA damage accumulation and aging, a concept proposed more than half century ago by Leo Szilard (Szilard, 1959). Throughout the life-span, cells are constantly exposed to different endogenous or exogenous conditions that lead to DNA lesions which trigger DNA damage checkpoint response and DNA repair signalling. The accumulation of unrepaired/unrepairable DNA damage within cells leads to a sustained DNA damage checkpoint response and induces a state called cellular senescence, wherein cells permanently exit from the cell cycle. Consistent with this idea, it has been documented that DNA damage in the form of DSB-specific foci containing γ-H2AX accumulate in senescent human cells, germ and somatic cells of aged mice, and in dermal fibroblasts from aged primates (Maslov and Vijg, 2009). Mouse models harbouring deficiency in DNA repair proteins, such as ATM, Ku70, Ku80, DNA ligase IV or Ercc1 also show premature aging phenotypes, providing   evidence of a direct correlation between impaired DDR and premature aging (Hasty, 2005; Hoeijmakers, 2009).

So far, the relationship between DNA damage accumulation and aging has gained maximum credibility through studies conducted on various human progeria syndromes. Progeria syndromes are genetic disorders where patients precociously develop features resembling natural aging. Interestingly, most of the reported progeria syndromes, including Werner syndrome (WS), Bloom's syndrome (BS), Rothmund-Thomson syndrome (RTS), Cockayne syndrome type A and type B (CSA and CSB), Xeroderma pigmentosum (XP), Trichothiodystrophy (TTD) and Hutchinson-Gilford progeria syndrome (HGPS) were caused by mutations of genes that were directly or indirectly involved in DNA repair pathways. WS, BS and RTS are associated with defects in RecQ helicases, i.e. RECQL2 (WRN), RECQL3 (BLM) and RECQL4 respectively, whereas CS, XP and TTD shared similar defects in NER pathway. RecQ helicases are a group of highly conserved proteins from bacteria to humans. The roles of RecQ helicases in DNA metabolism, including DNA replication (Lebel et al., 1999), transcription (Balajee et al., 1999), repair (Cooper et al., 2000; Li and Comai, 2000) and recombination, have been extensively investigated and are demonstrated to be the underlying pathological basis of WS, BS and RTS. Most recently, delayed DNA damage checkpoint response and defective DNA repair were found to contribute to the progeria phenotypes in HGPS as well (Liu et al., 2005).

Since WS closely resembles physiological aging, WS cells have been the subject of intense investigation to understand the biology and molecular mechanism of normal aging. WS is an autosomal recessive genetic disorder of "progeria in adulthood", affecting about 10 in one million (Multani and Chang, 2007). Patients suffering from WS are usually born healthy, with obvious growth retardation from the second decade and other ageing-related features, including short stature, premature cataract, beaked nose, skin atrophy and alopecia, loss of adipose tissues, type II diabetes, osteoporosis, arteriosclerosis, hypogonadism and predisposition to cancer. WS patients typically die of early onset cardiovascular diseases or neoplasia in the fourth decade of life and have an average life expectancy of 47 years. Skin fibroblasts cultured from affected individuals develop accelerated senescence with increased chromosome aberrations (Melcher et al., 2000; Salk et al., 1981). By positional cloning, WRN was firstly linked to WS (Yu et al., 1996). Before the identification of *LMNA* mutations (see below) in atypical WS, WRN was the only protein implicated in WS. WRN belongs to the family of RecQ helicases, and is the only member with a specific exonuclease domain within the N-terminus (Gray et al., 1997; Huang et al., 1998). Physiological and functional interactions between WRN and other proteins suggest that it has crucial roles in DNA replication and repair. WRN interacts with proteins required for DNA replication, such as RPA (Brosh et al., 1999), PCNA (Lebel et al., 1999), FEN1 (Brosh et al., 2001) and DNA polymerase (Polδ) (Kamath-Loeb et al., 2001). Studies from Lebel and colleagues (1999) indicated that WRN was involved in restoration of stalled replication forks. WRN also interacts with heterodimer of Ku70-Ku80, which is involved in NHEJ pathway, indicating its potential role in regulating DSB repair (Cooper et al., 2000; Li and Comai, 2000). WRN also plays an important role in maintaining telomere integrity. It has been reported that WRN associates with three of the six members of telomere complex, including telomeric repeat binding factor 1/2 (TRF1/2) and POT1, to modulate exonuclease and helicase activities of WRN during telomeric metabolism (Machwe et al., 2004; Multani and Chang, 2007). Recently, lamin A/C mutations (A57P, R133L, L140R, and E578V) were also reported in autosomal dominant atypical WS where patients presented with more severe phenotypes compared to those associated with WRN (Chen et al., 2003; Csoka et al., 2004; Fukuchi et al., 2004).

Bloom's syndrome is another rare genetic disease characterized by dwarfism, sun-induced erythaema, type II diabetes, narrow face and prominent ears, infertility, benign and malignant tumors. Deaths usually result from neoplasia before the age of 30. RecQ helicase BLM is associated with BS, which is shown to be capable of regulating HR. Upon DNA damage, BLM forms discrete nucleoplasmic foci that co-localize with RAD51 as well as BRCA1-associated genome surveillance complex (BASC) containing BRCA1, MLH1, MRN complex and ATM in mammalian cells (Hickson, 2003). BLM is also involved in the correct localization and activation of topoisomerase IIIα (Wu et al., 2000). Deletion of Blm in mice results in early embryonic death by E13.5. Blm mutant embryos show growth retardation and *Blm−/−* ES cells have an elevated HR between sister chromatids (Chester et al., 1998; Guo et al., 2004). Goss et al (Goss et al., 2002) showed that haploinsufficiency of Blm caused early development of lymphoma. In another example involving the XPF-XRCC1 endonuclease, a patient bearing a severe XPF mutation presented with dramatic progeroid symptoms. A mouse model for this mutation was generated and expression data from this mouse indicated a shift towards reduced growth hormone/insulin-like growth factor 1 (IGF1) signalling, a known regulator of lifespan. It was proposed that DNA damage accumulation re-allocates resources from growth to life extension by suppressing the somatotroph axis (Niedernhofer et al., 2006).

Hutchinson-Gilford progeria syndrome (HGPS) is an extremely rare severe genetic disorder of early onset premature aging, also referred to as "progeria in childhood". The prevalence is one out of 8 million. So far only about 100 patients have been reported, mainly in western world. Patients with HGPS can only survive for 12-16 years with a mean age of 13.4 years and are clinically characterized with early growth retardation, short stature, lipodystrophy, alopecia, stiff joints, osteolysis, dilated cardiomyopathy and atherosclerosis (Hennekam, 2006; Pollex and Hegele, 2004). A recurrent, *de novo*, dominant point mutation (1824 C→T) of *LMNA* gene was identified to be responsible for about 76% reported cases of HGPS. This mutation (G608G) activates a cryptic splicing donor signal in exon 11, leading to 150 nucleotides deletion in mutant transcript and a 50-residue truncation in lamin A protein (Eriksson et al., 2003; Reddel and Weiss, 2004). The 50-residue truncation in lamin A removes the second proteolytic cleavage site of ZMPSTE24 but leaving the CAAX motif unaffected. A detailed study demonstrated that the mutant allele only expressed about 80% transcripts of total lamin A from the same allele and ~40% of total lamin A from both alleles (Reddel and Weiss, 2004). Studies in HGPS cells and mice lacking Zmpste24, a metalloprotease processing prelamin A to its mature form, reveal that accumulation of progerin and unprocessed prelamin A leads to either delayed or reduced recruitment of necessary DNA repair proteins, such as 53BP1 and Rad51 to sites of double strand breaks (Liu et al., 2005).

Cockayne syndrome is an autosomal recessive disorder with growth retardation, skin atrophy, sparse hair, cataract, neural system deterioration, but without cancer susceptibility. As described earlier (section 3.3), Cockayne syndrome proteins are involved in TCR.

Human Syndrome	Mutated Gene	Phenotypes	Disrupted DNA repair pathway
Ataxia Telangiectasia (AT)	ATM	Cerebellar ataxia, telangiectases, oculomotor apraxia, predisposition to lymphoid malignancies, leukemias, immune defects, dilated blood vessel, infertility, metabolic defects, growth defects	DSB repair, DNA damage signalling
Ataxia Telangiectasia-like disorder (A-TLD)	MRE11	Ataxia, oculomotor apraxia, immunodeficiency	DSB repair, DNA damage signalling
Nijmegan break syndrome (NBS)	NBS1	Microcephaly, immunodeficiency, growth defects, mental retardation, B cell lymphoma, facial dysmorphism	DSB repair, DNA damage signalling
NBS-like syndrome	RAD50	Microcephaly, facial dysmorphism, growth defects	DSB repair, DNA damage signalling

Human Syndrome	Mutated Gene	Phenotypes	Disrupted DNA repair pathway
RIDDLE syndrome	RNF168	Radiosensitivity, immunodeficiency, dysmorphic features and learning difficulties	DSB repair, DNA damage signalling
Primary microcephaly 1	MCPH1/BRIT1	Microcephaly and mental retardation	DSB repair, DNA damage signalling
Seckel Syndrome	ATR, PCTN, SCKL2, SCKL3	Severe intrauterine growth retardation, profound microcephaly, a 'bird-like' facial profile, mental retardation and isolated skeletal abnormalities dysmorphic facial features	DSB repair, DNA damage signalling
Restrictive dermopathy (RD)	LMNA, ZMPSTE24	Tight adherent skin, joint contractures and respiratory insufficiency, features of progeroid syndromes and premature death during gestation	DSB repair
Hutchinson-Gilford progeria syndrome	LMNA	Progeria (early growth retardation, short stature, lipodystrophy, alopecia, stiff joints, osteolysis, dilated cardiomyopathy and atherosclerosis)	DSB repair, DNA damage signalling
Li-Fraumeni syndrome	TP53	Brain, breast cancer, sarcomas, leukemias, melanomas and gastrointestinal cancers	DNA damage signalling
Xeroderma pigmentosum	XPA-XPG, POL H	Skin cancer, photosensitivity, neurodegeneration and microcephaly	NER
Trichothiodystrophy	XPB, XPD, TTDA	Neurodegeneration, hypomyelination, progeria (cachexia, cataracts, osteoporosis), microcephaly, and psychomotoric abnormalities.	NER
Cockayne syndrome	CSA, CSB, XPB, XPD, XPG	Microcephaly, neurodegeneration, neuronal demyelination, microcephaly, progeria (skin atrophy, sparse hair cachexia, cataracts, hearing loss, retinopathy), photosensitivity, growth defects	NER
Cerebro-oculo-facio-skeletal (COFS) syndrome	XPD, XPG, CSB, ERCC1	Neuronal demyelination and dysmyelination, brain calcification, microcephaly, neurodegeneration, progeria (cataracts, hearing loss, retinopathy), photosensitivity, growth defects and facial dysmorphism	NER
Ataxia with oculomotor apraxia 1 (AOA1)	APTX	Ataxia, neurodegeneration, oculomotor apraxia, hypercolesterolemia and dysarthria	SSB repair
Spinocerebeller ataxia with axonal neuropathy (SCAN1)	TDP1	Ataxia, oculomotor apraxia, cerebellar atrophy, dysarthria, hypercholesterolemia, muscle weakness, sensory neuropathy	SSB repair
Immunodeficiency with microcephaly	XLF	Growth delay, recurrent infections, autoimmunity, hypoglobulinemia, lymphopenia and microcephaly	NHEJ

Human Syndrome	Mutated Gene	Phenotypes	Disrupted DNA repair pathway
Ligase IV syndrome	*LIG4*	Microcephaly, developmental and growth delay, immunodeficiency (Aggamaglobulinemia, lymphopenia) and lymphoid malignancies	NHEJ
Radiosensitive severe combined immunodeficiency (RS-SCID)	*ARTEMIS*	Aggamaglobulinemia, lymphopenia, growth defects	NHEJ
Severe combined immunodeficiency (SCID)	*RAG1, RAG2*	Aggamaglobulinemia, lymphopenia, growth defects	NHEJ
Bloom syndrome	*BLM*	Microcephaly, short stature, dysmorphic feature, elevated predisposition to all cancers, mild/moderate mental retardation, immunoglobulin deficiency, infertility, growth defects	HR
Werner syndrome	*WRN*	Premature aging (short stature, premature cataract, beaked nose, skin atrophy and alopecia, loss of adipose tissues) type II diabetes, osteoporosis, arteriosclerosis, hypogonadism and predisposition to cancer	HR, BER, telomere maintenance
Rothmund Thomson syndrome (RTS)	*RECQL4*	Stunted growth, premature aging (cataracts, grey hair), osteosarcomas, skin cancers, skin and skeletal abnormalities	BER
Early onset breast cancer	*BRCA1*	Breast and ovarian cancer	HR
Early onset breast cancer	*BRCA2*	Breast and ovarian cancer, increased predisposition to prostrate, gastric, pancreatic cancers and melanoma	HR
Fanconi anemia	*FANCA-FANCL, BRCA2 (FANCD1)*	Congenital abnormalities, pancytopenia, microcephaly, AML, myelodysplasia, squamous cell carcinoma of head and neck, abnormal skin pigmentation, infertility, limb deformities, renal dysfunction	ICL repair and HR
Hereditary non-polyposis colorectal cancer (HNPCC)	*MSH2, MSH3, MSH6, MLH1, PMS2*	Colon and gynaecological cancers	MMR
Dyskeratosis congenita (DKC)	*DKC1, TERC*	Progeria (progressive bone marrow failure, pancytopenia, growth defects, osteoporosis), abnormal skin pigmentation, microcephaly, mental retardation carcinomas	Telomere maintenance

Table 1. Human diseases and syndromes caused by defective DNA repair

7. Conclusions and future directions

Much of our current understanding of mammalian DNA damage signalling, checkpoint and repair is based on elegant experiments done using yeast and Xenopus as models. During the past decade, greater insights into the mechanism/regulation of the DDR were obtained using mouse models and human congenital disorders. It is now clear that the DDR pathway is critical for both repairing DNA lesions arising from genotoxic stress, as well as for several developmental processes like VDJ recombination, CSR, SHM and meiosis. Through extensive studies conducted in mouse models and human syndromes, it is now known that the principle phenotypes manifested in diseases associated with defective DNA repair are immunodeficiency, infertility, growth retardation, neurodegeneration, microcephaly, increased cancer predisposition and premature aging. Even so, some caveats in our knowledge exist that need further research. The molecular basis for certain phenotypes associated with DNA repair-related human diseases are not clear. For example, the learning difficulty in RIDDLE patients harbouring mutations in RNF168, skeletal abnormalities in ATR-defective Seckel syndrome and Fanconi anemia patients or insulin resistance and glucose intolerance in ATM-defective patients are some of the phenotypes not fully understood. Perhaps, some of these outcomes are related to tissue-specific novel effectors of the DDR pathway, and future studies are required in this direction. In this regard, it is really interesting that some unexpected substrates of the ATM/ATR pathway were uncovered in an unbiased genome-wide proteomic screen and studies on these substrates are likely to shed light on how the DRR can profoundly influence certain tissue-specific phenotypes. Likewise, recent studies have revealed an amazing complexity in the DDR pathway of stem cells and it seems the mechanistic details of how tissue stem cells respond to DNA damage vary between different stem cells populations. Since tissue stem cells have a critical role in the maintenance of organ homeostasis, any disruption in the genomic integrity of stem cells is likely to elicit diseased states such neurodegeneration, cancer or premature aging, or other specific phenotypes depending on the stem cell from the tissue of origin. In this context, further studies are clearly required to gain a total understanding of the genome maintenance pathways in stem cells.

Apart from providing an in-depth understanding of human diseases, understanding the complexity of the DDR pathway has been harnessed for therapeutic benefit against certain cancer subtypes. The proposed rationale is that the DNA repair pathways and their downstream cellular components have undergone genetic alterations in cancer cells resulting in drug resistance. Hence abrogating or modulating the DDR through the use of DDR inhibitors can sensitize cancer cells to chemotherapy (Al-Ejeh et al., 2010). The most successful example in support of this concept has been the use of PARP inhibitors to sensitize Brca-deficient tumors to chemotherapy by about 1000 fold due to excessive DSBs generated as a result of compromised HR (Bryant et al., 2005). The idea being that the enzyme PARP-1 binds SSBs and BER intermediates to facilitate these repair processes. But in HR-defective Brca1 or Brca2 tumors, PARP inhibitors become particularly toxic due to the accumulation of unrepaired DSBs, while PARP inhibition remains nontoxic to normal cells, due to availability of backup mechanisms. PARP inhibitors are currently undergoing clinical trials in Brca-deficient breast and ovarian cancers. Along similar lines, Chk1 inhibition sensitizes p53-deficient tumors to DNA damaging agents better than p53-wild type cells. Thus, both DNA damaging therapies and DDR-inhibitor therapies can be tailored to the needs of each patient, based on the genetic alteration detected in their tumors.

In conclusion, great strides have been made towards understanding the DDR and its regulation in the past decade. We now have a detailed understanding of how exactly normal cells maintain their genomic integrity when faced with DNA damaging agents. It is now known that the DDR network is critical for several important physiological processes and for human health as evident by the growing list of human syndromes known to be associated with defective DNA repair. The real future challenge lies in developing a more thorough understanding of the functioning and regulation of DDR across various cell/tissue types and then harnessing this knowledge to develop therapeutics for the better management of human health or, perhaps, even extend life span.

8. Acknowledgment

This work was supported by Research Grant Council of Hong Kong (HKU7698/05M, HKU7655/06M, HKU7817/07M, CRF HKU3/07C), Innovation and Technology Fund of Hong Kong (ITS/102/07), Progeria Research Foundation, Natural Science Foundation of China (30672205, 30871440, 30971620), Ministry of Science and Technology of CHINA (973 Projects 2007CB50740).

9. References

Ahnesorg, P., P. Smith, and S.P. Jackson. 2006. XLF interacts with the XRCC4-DNA ligase IV complex to promote DNA nonhomologous end-joining. *Cell* 124:301-313.

Al-Ejeh, F., R. Kumar, A. Wiegmans, S.R. Lakhani, M.P. Brown, and K.K. Khanna. 2010. Harnessing the complexity of DNA-damage response pathways to improve cancer treatment outcomes. *Oncogene* 29:6085-6098.

Al-Hakim, A., C. Escribano-Diaz, M.C. Landry, L. O'Donnell, S. Panier, R.K. Szilard, and D. Durocher. 2010. The ubiquitous role of ubiquitin in the DNA damage response. *DNA Repair (Amst)* 9:1229-1240.

Al-Tassan, N., N.H. Chmiel, J. Maynard, N. Fleming, A.L. Livingston, G.T. Williams, A.K. Hodges, D.R. Davies, S.S. David, J.R. Sampson, and J.P. Cheadle. 2002. Inherited variants of MYH associated with somatic G:C-->T:A mutations in colorectal tumors. *Nature genetics* 30:227-232.

Arias EE, Walter JC. Strength in numbers: preventing rereplication via multiple mechanisms in eukaryotic cells. Genes Dev. 2007 Mar 1;21(5):497-518

Baker, S.M., C.E. Bronner, L. Zhang, A.W. Plug, M. Robatzek, G. Warren, E.A. Elliott, J. Yu, T. Ashley, N. Arnheim, R.A. Flavell, and R.M. Liskay. 1995. Male mice defective in the DNA mismatch repair gene PMS2 exhibit abnormal chromosome synapsis in meiosis. *Cell* 82:309-319.

Baker, S.M., A.W. Plug, T.A. Prolla, C.E. Bronner, A.C. Harris, X. Yao, D.M. Christie, C. Monell, N. Arnheim, A. Bradley, T. Ashley, and R.M. Liskay. 1996. Involvement of mouse Mlh1 in DNA mismatch repair and meiotic crossing over. *Nat Genet* 13:336-342.

Bakkenist, C.J., and M.B. Kastan. 2003. DNA damage activates ATM through intermolecular autophosphorylation and dimer dissociation. *Nature* 421:499-506.

Balajee, A.S., A. Machwe, A. May, M.D. Gray, J. Oshima, G.M. Martin, J.O. Nehlin, R. Brosh, D.K. Orren, and V.A. Bohr. 1999. The Werner syndrome protein is involved in RNA polymerase II transcription. *Mol Biol Cell* 10:2655-2668.

Bao, S., Q. Wu, R.E. McLendon, Y. Hao, Q. Shi, A.B. Hjelmeland, M.W. Dewhirst, D.D. Bigner, and J.N. Rich. 2006. Glioma stem cells promote radioresistance by preferential activation of the DNA damage response. *Nature* 444:756-760.

Barker, N., S. Bartfeld, and H. Clevers. 2010. Tissue-resident adult stem cell populations of rapidly self-renewing organs. *Cell Stem Cell* 7:656-670.

Barlow, C., S. Hirotsune, R. Paylor, M. Liyanage, M. Eckhaus, F. Collins, Y. Shiloh, J.N. Crawley, T. Ried, D. Tagle, and A. Wynshaw-Boris. 1996. Atm-deficient mice: a paradigm of ataxia telangiectasia. *Cell* 86:159-171.

Barlow, C., M. Liyanage, P.B. Moens, M. Tarsounas, K. Nagashima, K. Brown, S. Rottinghaus, S.P. Jackson, D. Tagle, T. Ried, and A. Wynshaw-Boris. 1998. Atm deficiency results in severe meiotic disruption as early as leptonema of prophase I. *Development* 125:4007-4017.

Bartek, J., J. Bartkova, and J. Lukas. 2007. DNA damage signalling guards against activated oncogenes and tumour progression. *Oncogene* 26:7773-7779.

Bartek, J., and J. Lukas. 2007. DNA damage checkpoints: from initiation to recovery or adaptation. *Curr Opin Cell Biol* 19:238-245.

Bartkova, J., N. Rezaei, M. Liontos, P. Karakaidos, D. Kletsas, N. Issaeva, L.V. Vassiliou, E. Kolettas, K. Niforou, V.C. Zoumpourlis, M. Takaoka, H. Nakagawa, F. Tort, K. Fugger, F. Johansson, M. Sehested, C.L. Andersen, L. Dyrskjot, T. Orntoft, J. Lukas, C. Kittas, T. Helleday, T.D. Halazonetis, J. Bartek, and V.G. Gorgoulis. 2006. Oncogene-induced senescence is part of the tumorigenesis barrier imposed by DNA damage checkpoints. *Nature* 444:633-637.

Bassing, C.H., and F.W. Alt. 2004. The cellular response to general and programmed DNA double strand breaks. *DNA Repair (Amst)* 3:781-796.

Baudat, F., J. Buard, C. Grey, A. Fledel-Alon, C. Ober, M. Przeworski, G. Coop, and B. de Massy. 2010. PRDM9 is a major determinant of meiotic recombination hotspots in humans and mice. *Science* 327:836-840.

Baudat, F., K. Manova, J.P. Yuen, M. Jasin, and S. Keeney. 2000. Chromosome synapsis defects and sexually dimorphic meiotic progression in mice lacking Spo11. *Mol Cell* 6:989-998.

Bekker-Jensen, S., C. Lukas, R. Kitagawa, F. Melander, M.B. Kastan, J. Bartek, and J. Lukas. 2006. Spatial organization of the mammalian genome surveillance machinery in response to DNA strand breaks. *J Cell Biol* 173:195-206.

Bekker-Jensen, S., and N. Mailand. 2010. Assembly and function of DNA double-strand break repair foci in mammalian cells. *DNA Repair (Amst)* 9:1219-1228.

Biton, S., A. Barzilai, and Y. Shiloh. 2008. The neurological phenotype of ataxia-telangiectasia: solving a persistent puzzle. *DNA repair* 7:1028-1038.

Blanpain, C., and E. Fuchs. 2009. Epidermal homeostasis: a balancing act of stem cells in the skin. *Nature reviews. Molecular cell biology* 10:207-217.

Blanpain, C., M. Mohrin, P.A. Sotiropoulou, and E. Passegue. 2011. DNA-damage response in tissue-specific and cancer stem cells. *Cell Stem Cell* 8:16-29.

Blunt, T., N.J. Finnie, G.E. Taccioli, G.C. Smith, J. Demengeot, T.M. Gottlieb, R. Mizuta, A.J. Varghese, F.W. Alt, P.A. Jeggo, and et al. 1995. Defective DNA-dependent protein kinase activity is linked to V(D)J recombination and DNA repair defects associated with the murine scid mutation. *Cell* 80:813-823.

Borde, V., N. Robine, W. Lin, S. Bonfils, V. Geli, and A. Nicolas. 2009. Histone H3 lysine 4 trimethylation marks meiotic recombination initiation sites. *EMBO J* 28:99-111.

Bredemeyer, A.L., G.G. Sharma, C.Y. Huang, B.A. Helmink, L.M. Walker, K.C. Khor, B. Nuskey, K.E. Sullivan, T.K. Pandita, C.H. Bassing, and B.P. Sleckman. 2006. ATM stabilizes DNA double-strand-break complexes during V(D)J recombination. *Nature* 442:466-470.

Brosh, R.M., Jr., D.K. Orren, J.O. Nehlin, P.H. Ravn, M.K. Kenny, A. Machwe, and V.A. Bohr. 1999. Functional and physical interaction between WRN helicase and human replication protein A. *J Biol Chem* 274:18341-18350.

Brosh, R.M., Jr., C. von Kobbe, J.A. Sommers, P. Karmakar, P.L. Opresko, J. Piotrowski, I. Dianova, G.L. Dianov, and V.A. Bohr. 2001. Werner syndrome protein interacts with human flap endonuclease 1 and stimulates its cleavage activity. *Embo J* 20:5791-5801.

Brown, C.J., S. Lain, C.S. Verma, A.R. Fersht, and D.P. Lane. 2009. Awakening guardian angels: drugging the p53 pathway. *Nature reviews. Cancer* 9:862-873.

Bryant, H.E., N. Schultz, H.D. Thomas, K.M. Parker, D. Flower, E. Lopez, S. Kyle, M. Meuth, N.J. Curtin, and T. Helleday. 2005. Specific killing of BRCA2-deficient tumours with inhibitors of poly(ADP-ribose) polymerase. *Nature* 434:913-917.

Buard, J., P. Barthes, C. Grey, and B. de Massy. 2009. Distinct histone modifications define initiation and repair of meiotic recombination in the mouse. *EMBO J* 28:2616-2624.

Buck, D., L. Malivert, R. de Chasseval, A. Barraud, M.C. Fondaneche, O. Sanal, A. Plebani, J.L. Stephan, M. Hufnagel, F. le Deist, A. Fischer, A. Durandy, J.P. de Villartay, and P. Revy. 2006. Cernunnos, a novel nonhomologous end-joining factor, is mutated in human immunodeficiency with microcephaly. *Cell* 124:287-299.

Buis, J., Y. Wu, Y. Deng, J. Leddon, G. Westfield, M. Eckersdorff, J.M. Sekiguchi, S. Chang, and D.O. Ferguson. 2008. Mre11 nuclease activity has essential roles in DNA repair and genomic stability distinct from ATM activation. *Cell* 135:85-96.

Bunting, S.F., E. Callen, N. Wong, H.T. Chen, F. Polato, A. Gunn, A. Bothmer, N. Feldhahn, O. Fernandez-Capetillo, L. Cao, X. Xu, C.X. Deng, T. Finkel, M. Nussenzweig, J.M. Stark, and A. Nussenzweig. 2010. 53BP1 inhibits homologous recombination in Brca1-deficient cells by blocking resection of DNA breaks. *Cell* 141:243-254.

Caldecott, K.W. 2008. Single-strand break repair and genetic disease. *Nat Rev Genet* 9:619-631.

Casellas, R., A. Nussenzweig, R. Wuerffel, R. Pelanda, A. Reichlin, H. Suh, X.F. Qin, E. Besmer, A. Kenter, K. Rajewsky, and M.C. Nussenzweig. 1998. Ku80 is required for immunoglobulin isotype switching. *EMBO J* 17:2404-2411.

Celeste, A., S. Petersen, P.J. Romanienko, O. Fernandez-Capetillo, H.T. Chen, O.A. Sedelnikova, B. Reina-San-Martin, V. Coppola, E. Meffre, M.J. Difilippantonio, C. Redon, D.R. Pilch, A. Olaru, M. Eckhaus, R.D. Camerini-Otero, L. Tessarollo, F. Livak, K. Manova, W.M. Bonner, M.C. Nussenzweig, and A. Nussenzweig. 2002. Genomic instability in mice lacking histone H2AX. *Science* 296:922-927.

Chaudhuri, J., M. Tian, C. Khuong, K. Chua, E. Pinaud, and F.W. Alt. 2003. Transcription-targeted DNA deamination by the AID antibody diversification enzyme. *Nature* 422:726-730.

Chen, L., L. Lee, B.A. Kudlow, H.G. Dos Santos, O. Sletvold, Y. Shafeghati, E.G. Botha, A. Garg, N.B. Hanson, G.M. Martin, I.S. Mian, B.K. Kennedy, and J. Oshima. 2003. LMNA mutations in atypical Werner's syndrome. *Lancet* 362:440-445.

Chester, N., F. Kuo, C. Kozak, C.D. O'Hara, and P. Leder. 1998. Stage-specific apoptosis, developmental delay, and embryonic lethality in mice homozygous for a targeted disruption in the murine Bloom's syndrome gene. *Genes Dev* 12:3382-3393.

Chun, H.H., and R.A. Gatti. 2004. Ataxia-telangiectasia, an evolving phenotype. *DNA Repair (Amst)* 3:1187-1196.

Ciccia, A., and S.J. Elledge. 2010. The DNA damage response: making it safe to play with knives. *Mol Cell* 40:179-204.

Clarke, M.F., and M. Fuller. 2006. Stem cells and cancer: two faces of eve. *Cell* 124:1111-1115.

Cleaver, J.E. 2005. Cancer in xeroderma pigmentosum and related disorders of DNA repair. *Nature reviews. Cancer* 5:564-573.

Cooper, M.P., A. Machwe, D.K. Orren, R.M. Brosh, D. Ramsden, and V.A. Bohr. 2000. Ku complex interacts with and stimulates the Werner protein. *Genes Dev* 14:907-912.

Csoka, A.B., H. Cao, P.J. Sammak, D. Constantinescu, G.P. Schatten, and R.A. Hegele. 2004. Novel lamin A/C gene (LMNA) mutations in atypical progeroid syndromes. *J Med Genet* 41:304-308.

Cui, X., Y. Yu, S. Gupta, Y.M. Cho, S.P. Lees-Miller, and K. Meek. 2005. Autophosphorylation of DNA-dependent protein kinase regulates DNA end processing and may also alter double-strand break repair pathway choice. *Mol Cell Biol* 25:10842-10852.

Daniel, J.A., M. Pellegrini, J.H. Lee, T.T. Paull, L. Feigenbaum, and A. Nussenzweig. 2008. Multiple autophosphorylation sites are dispensable for murine ATM activation in vivo. *J Cell Biol* 183:777-783.

de Vries, S.S., E.B. Baart, M. Dekker, A. Siezen, D.G. de Rooij, P. de Boer, and H. te Riele. 1999. Mouse MutS-like protein Msh5 is required for proper chromosome synapsis in male and female meiosis. *Genes Dev* 13:523-531.

Denchi, E.L. 2009. Give me a break: how telomeres suppress the DNA damage response. *DNA repair* 8:1118-1126.

Di Noia, J.M., and M.S. Neuberger. 2007. Molecular mechanisms of antibody somatic hypermutation. *Annual review of biochemistry* 76:1-22.

Diehn, M., R.W. Cho, N.A. Lobo, T. Kalisky, M.J. Dorie, A.N. Kulp, D. Qian, J.S. Lam, L.E. Ailles, M. Wong, B. Joshua, M.J. Kaplan, I. Wapnir, F.M. Dirbas, G. Somlo, C. Garberoglio, B. Paz, J. Shen, S.K. Lau, S.R. Quake, J.M. Brown, I.L. Weissman, and M.F. Clarke. 2009. Association of reactive oxygen species levels and radioresistance in cancer stem cells. *Nature* 458:780-783.

DiGiovanna, A.G. 2000. Human Aging: Biological Perspectives. McGraw-Hill, New York.

Digweed, M., and K. Sperling. 2004. Nijmegen breakage syndrome: clinical manifestation of defective response to DNA double-strand breaks. *DNA Repair (Amst)* 3:1207-1217.

Dillon, L.W., A.A. Burrow, and Y.H. Wang. 2010. DNA instability at chromosomal fragile sites in cancer. *Curr Genomics* 11:326-337.

Edelmann, W., P.E. Cohen, M. Kane, K. Lau, B. Morrow, S. Bennett, A. Umar, T. Kunkel, G. Cattoretti, R. Chaganti, J.W. Pollard, R.D. Kolodner, and R. Kucherlapati. 1996. Meiotic pachytene arrest in MLH1-deficient mice. *Cell* 85:1125-1134.

Edelmann, W., P.E. Cohen, B. Kneitz, N. Winand, M. Lia, J. Heyer, R. Kolodner, J.W. Pollard, and R. Kucherlapati. 1999. Mammalian MutS homologue 5 is required for chromosome pairing in meiosis. *Nat Genet* 21:123-127.

Ege, M., Y. Ma, B. Manfras, K. Kalwak, H. Lu, M.R. Lieber, K. Schwarz, and U. Pannicke. 2005. Omenn syndrome due to ARTEMIS mutations. *Blood* 105:4179-4186.

Enders, A., P. Fisch, K. Schwarz, U. Duffner, U. Pannicke, E. Nikolopoulos, A. Peters, M. Orlowska-Volk, D. Schindler, W. Friedrich, B. Selle, C. Niemeyer, and S. Ehl. 2006. A severe form of human combined immunodeficiency due to mutations in DNA ligase IV. *J Immunol* 176:5060-5068.

Eriksson, M., W.T. Brown, L.B. Gordon, M.W. Glynn, J. Singer, L. Scott, M.R. Erdos, C.M. Robbins, T.Y. Moses, P. Berglund, A. Dutra, E. Pak, S. Durkin, A.B. Csoka, M. Boehnke, T.W. Glover, and F.S. Collins. 2003. Recurrent de novo point mutations in lamin A cause Hutchinson-Gilford progeria syndrome. *Nature* 423:293-298.

Fishel, R., M.K. Lescoe, M.R. Rao, N.G. Copeland, N.A. Jenkins, J. Garber, M. Kane, and R. Kolodner. 1993. The human mutator gene homolog MSH2 and its association with hereditary nonpolyposis colon cancer. *Cell* 75:1027-1038.

Forand, A., P. Fouchet, J.B. Lahaye, A. Chicheportiche, R. Habert, and J. Bernardino-Sgherri. 2009. Similarities and differences in the in vivo response of mouse neonatal gonocytes and spermatogonia to genotoxic stress. *Biol Reprod* 80:860-873.

Friedel, A.M., B.L. Pike, and S.M. Gasser. 2009. ATR/Mec1: coordinating fork stability and repair. *Curr Opin Cell Biol* 21:237-244.

Fukuchi, K., T. Katsuya, K. Sugimoto, M. Kuremura, H.D. Kim, L. Li, and T. Ogihara. 2004. LMNA mutation in a 45 year old Japanese subject with Hutchinson-Gilford progeria syndrome. *J Med Genet* 41:e67.

Fukui, K. 2010. DNA mismatch repair in eukaryotes and bacteria. *J Nucleic Acids* 2010:

Gao, Y., Y. Sun, K.M. Frank, P. Dikkes, Y. Fujiwara, K.J. Seidl, J.M. Sekiguchi, G.A. Rathbun, W. Swat, J. Wang, R.T. Bronson, B.A. Malynn, M. Bryans, C. Zhu, J. Chaudhuri, L. Davidson, R. Ferrini, T. Stamato, S.H. Orkin, M.E. Greenberg, and F.W. Alt. 1998. A critical role for DNA end-joining proteins in both lymphogenesis and neurogenesis. *Cell* 95:891-902.

Giovannetti, A., F. Mazzetta, E. Caprini, A. Aiuti, M. Marziali, M. Pierdominici, A. Cossarizza, L. Chessa, E. Scala, I. Quinti, G. Russo, and M. Fiorilli. 2002. Skewed T-cell receptor repertoire, decreased thymic output, and predominance of terminally differentiated T cells in ataxia telangiectasia. *Blood* 100:4082-4089.

Goodarzi, A.A., Y. Yu, E. Riballo, P. Douglas, S.A. Walker, R. Ye, C. Harer, C. Marchetti, N. Morrice, P.A. Jeggo, and S.P. Lees-Miller. 2006. DNA-PK autophosphorylation facilitates Artemis endonuclease activity. *EMBO J* 25:3880-3889.

Gorgoulis, V.G., and T.D. Halazonetis. 2010. Oncogene-induced senescence: the bright and dark side of the response. *Current opinion in cell biology* 22:816-827.

Goss, K.H., M.A. Risinger, J.J. Kordich, M.M. Sanz, J.E. Straughen, L.E. Slovek, A.J. Capobianco, J. German, G.P. Boivin, and J. Groden. 2002. Enhanced tumor formation in mice heterozygous for Blm mutation. *Science* 297:2051-2053.

Gray, M.D., J.C. Shen, A.S. Kamath-Loeb, A. Blank, B.L. Sopher, G.M. Martin, J. Oshima, and L.A. Loeb. 1997. The Werner syndrome protein is a DNA helicase. *Nat Genet* 17:100-103.

Grey, C., F. Baudat, and B. de Massy. 2009. Genome-wide control of the distribution of meiotic recombination. *PLoS Biol* 7:e35.

Gu, Y., S. Jin, Y. Gao, D.T. Weaver, and F.W. Alt. 1997. Ku70-deficient embryonic stem cells have increased ionizing radiosensitivity, defective DNA end-binding activity, and inability to support V(D)J recombination. *Proc Natl Acad Sci U S A* 94:8076-8081.

Guardavaccaro, D., and M. Pagano. 2006. Stabilizers and destabilizers controlling cell cycle oscillators. *Mol Cell* 22:1-4.

Guo, C., T.S. Tang, and E.C. Friedberg. 2010. SnapShot: nucleotide excision repair. *Cell* 140:754-754 e751.

Guo, G., W. Wang, and A. Bradley. 2004. Mismatch repair genes identified using genetic screens in Blm-deficient embryonic stem cells. *Nature* 429:891-895.

Hanawalt, P.C., and G. Spivak. 2008. Transcription-coupled DNA repair: two decades of progress and surprises. *Nat Rev Mol Cell Biol* 9:958-970.

Harper, J.W., and S.J. Elledge. 2007. The DNA damage response: ten years after. *Mol Cell* 28:739-745.

Hartlerode, A.J., and R. Scully. 2009. Mechanisms of double-strand break repair in somatic mammalian cells. *The Biochemical journal* 423:157-168.

Hasty, P. 2005. The impact of DNA damage, genetic mutation and cellular responses on cancer prevention, longevity and aging: observations in humans and mice. *Mech Ageing Dev* 126:71-77.

Hayashi, K., K. Yoshida, and Y. Matsui. 2005. A histone H3 methyltransferase controls epigenetic events required for meiotic prophase. *Nature* 438:374-378.

Hennekam, R.C. 2006. Hutchinson-Gilford progeria syndrome: review of the phenotype. *Am J Med Genet A* 140:2603-2624.

Hickson, I.D. 2003. RecQ helicases: caretakers of the genome. *Nat Rev Cancer* 3:169-178.

Hoeijmakers, J.H. 2009. DNA damage, aging, and cancer. *The New England journal of medicine* 361:1475-1485.

Huang, S., B. Li, M.D. Gray, J. Oshima, I.S. Mian, and J. Campisi. 1998. The premature ageing syndrome protein, WRN, is a 3'-->5' exonuclease. *Nat Genet* 20:114-116.

Huen, M.S., and J. Chen. 2010. Assembly of checkpoint and repair machineries at DNA damage sites. *Trends Biochem Sci* 35:101-108.

Huen, M.S., S.M. Sy, and J. Chen. 2010. BRCA1 and its toolbox for the maintenance of genome integrity. *Nat Rev Mol Cell Biol* 11:138-148.

Jackson, S.P., and J. Bartek. 2009. The DNA-damage response in human biology and disease. *Nature* 461:1071-1078.

Johnson, K., D.L. Pflugh, D. Yu, D.G. Hesslein, K.I. Lin, A.L. Bothwell, A. Thomas-Tikhonenko, D.G. Schatz, and K. Calame. 2004. B cell-specific loss of histone 3 lysine 9 methylation in the V(H) locus depends on Pax5. *Nat Immunol* 5:853-861.

Kamath-Loeb, A.S., L.A. Loeb, E. Johansson, P.M. Burgers, and M. Fry. 2001. Interactions between the Werner syndrome helicase and DNA polymerase delta specifically facilitate copying of tetraplex and hairpin structures of the d(CGG)n trinucleotide repeat sequence. *J Biol Chem* 276:16439-16446.

Katyal, S., and P.J. McKinnon. 2008. DNA strand breaks, neurodegeneration and aging in the brain. *Mech Ageing Dev* 129:483-491.

Keeney, S., C.N. Giroux, and N. Kleckner. 1997. Meiosis-specific DNA double-strand breaks are catalyzed by Spo11, a member of a widely conserved protein family. *Cell* 88:375-384.

Kitao, H., and M. Takata. 2011. Fanconi anemia: a disorder defective in the DNA damage response. *Int J Hematol* 93:417-424.

Kneitz, B., P.E. Cohen, E. Avdievich, L. Zhu, M.F. Kane, H. Hou, Jr., R.D. Kolodner, R. Kucherlapati, J.W. Pollard, and W. Edelmann. 2000. MutS homolog 4 localization to meiotic chromosomes is required for chromosome pairing during meiosis in male and female mice. *Genes Dev* 14:1085-1097.

Kolodner, R.D., and G.T. Marsischky. 1999. Eukaryotic DNA mismatch repair. *Curr Opin Genet Dev* 9:89-96.

Kracker, S., Y. Bergmann, I. Demuth, P.O. Frappart, G. Hildebrand, R. Christine, Z.Q. Wang, K. Sperling, M. Digweed, and A. Radbruch. 2005. Nibrin functions in Ig class-switch recombination. *Proc Natl Acad Sci U S A* 102:1584-1589.

Kramer, B., W. Kramer, M.S. Williamson, and S. Fogel. 1989. Heteroduplex DNA correction in Saccharomyces cerevisiae is mismatch specific and requires functional PMS genes. *Mol Cell Biol* 9:4432-4440.

Kunkel, T.A., and D.A. Erie. 2005. DNA mismatch repair. *Annu Rev Biochem* 74:681-710.

Lahdesmaki, A., A.M. Taylor, K.H. Chrzanowska, and Q. Pan-Hammarstrom. 2004. Delineation of the role of the Mre11 complex in class switch recombination. *J Biol Chem* 279:16479-16487.

Larrea, A.A., S.A. Lujan, and T.A. Kunkel. 2010. SnapShot: DNA mismatch repair. *Cell* 141:730 e731.

Leach, F.S., N.C. Nicolaides, N. Papadopoulos, B. Liu, J. Jen, R. Parsons, P. Peltomaki, P. Sistonen, L.A. Aaltonen, M. Nystrom-Lahti, and et al. 1993. Mutations of a mutS homolog in hereditary nonpolyposis colorectal cancer. *Cell* 75:1215-1225.

Lebel, M., E.A. Spillare, C.C. Harris, and P. Leder. 1999. The Werner syndrome gene product co-purifies with the DNA replication complex and interacts with PCNA and topoisomerase I. *J Biol Chem* 274:37795-37799.

Lee, J.H., and T.T. Paull. 2004. Direct activation of the ATM protein kinase by the Mre11/Rad50/Nbs1 complex. *Science* 304:93-96.

Li, B., and L. Comai. 2000. Functional interaction between Ku and the werner syndrome protein in DNA end processing. *J Biol Chem* 275:28349-28352.

Li, L., E. Salido, Y. Zhou, S. Bhattacharyya, S.M. Yannone, E. Dunn, J. Meneses, A.J. Feeney, and M.J. Cowan. 2005. Targeted disruption of the Artemis murine counterpart results in SCID and defective V(D)J recombination that is partially corrected with bone marrow transplantation. *J Immunol* 174:2420-2428.

Libby, B.J., L.G. Reinholdt, and J.C. Schimenti. 2003. Positional cloning and characterization of Mei1, a vertebrate-specific gene required for normal meiotic chromosome synapsis in mice. *Proc Natl Acad Sci U S A* 100:15706-15711.

Lieber, M.R. 2010. The mechanism of double-strand DNA break repair by the nonhomologous DNA end-joining pathway. *Annu Rev Biochem* 79:181-211.

Lieber, M.R., and T.E. Wilson. 2010. SnapShot: Nonhomologous DNA end joining (NHEJ). *Cell* 142:496-496 e491.

Lindahl, T. 1993. Instability and decay of the primary structure of DNA. *Nature* 362:709-715.

Lipkin, S.M., P.B. Moens, V. Wang, M. Lenzi, D. Shanmugarajah, A. Gilgeous, J. Thomas, J. Cheng, J.W. Touchman, E.D. Green, P. Schwartzberg, F.S. Collins, and P.E. Cohen. 2002. Meiotic arrest and aneuploidy in MLH3-deficient mice. *Nat Genet* 31:385-390.

Liu, B., J. Wang, K.M. Chan, W.M. Tjia, W. Deng, X. Guan, J.D. Huang, K.M. Li, P.Y. Chau, D.J. Chen, D. Pei, A.M. Pendas, J. Cadinanos, C. Lopez-Otin, H.F. Tse, C. Hutchison, J. Chen, Y. Cao, K.S. Cheah, K. Tryggvason, and Z. Zhou. 2005. Genomic instability in laminopathy-based premature aging. *Nat Med* 11:780-785.

Liu, Y., R. Subrahmanyam, T. Chakraborty, R. Sen, and S. Desiderio. 2007. A plant homeodomain in RAG-2 that binds Hypermethylated lysine 4 of histone H3 is necessary for efficient antigen-receptor-gene rearrangement. *Immunity* 27:561-571.

Lopez-Contreras, A.J., and O. Fernandez-Capetillo. 2010. The ATR barrier to replication-born DNA damage. *DNA Repair (Amst)* 9:1249-1255.

Lukas, J., C. Lukas, and J. Bartek. 2004. Mammalian cell cycle checkpoints: signalling pathways and their organization in space and time. *DNA Repair (Amst)* 3:997-1007.

Luo, G., M.S. Yao, C.F. Bender, M. Mills, A.R. Bladl, A. Bradley, and J.H. Petrini. 1999. Disruption of mRad50 causes embryonic stem cell lethality, abnormal embryonic development, and sensitivity to ionizing radiation. *Proc Natl Acad Sci U S A* 96:7376-7381.

Machwe, A., L. Xiao, and D.K. Orren. 2004. TRF2 recruits the Werner syndrome (WRN) exonuclease for processing of telomeric DNA. *Oncogene* 23:149-156.

Mahaney, B.L., K. Meek, and S.P. Lees-Miller. 2009. Repair of ionizing radiation-induced DNA double-strand breaks by non-homologous end-joining. *Biochem J* 417:639-650.

Mailand, N., S. Bekker-Jensen, H. Faustrup, F. Melander, J. Bartek, C. Lukas, and J. Lukas. 2007. RNF8 ubiquitylates histones at DNA double-strand breaks and promotes assembly of repair proteins. *Cell* 131:887-900.

Mandon-Pepin, B., C. Derbois, F. Matsuda, C. Cotinot, D.J. Wolgemuth, K. Smith, K. McElreavey, A. Nicolas, and M. Fellous. 2002. [Human infertility: meiotic genes as potential candidates]. *Gynecol Obstet Fertil* 30:817-821.

Manis, J.P., Y. Gu, R. Lansford, E. Sonoda, R. Ferrini, L. Davidson, K. Rajewsky, and F.W. Alt. 1998. Ku70 is required for late B cell development and immunoglobulin heavy chain class switching. *J Exp Med* 187:2081-2089.

Manis, J.P., J.C. Morales, Z. Xia, J.L. Kutok, F.W. Alt, and P.B. Carpenter. 2004. 53BP1 links DNA damage-response pathways to immunoglobulin heavy chain class-switch recombination. *Nat Immunol* 5:481-487.

Maslov, A.Y., and J. Vijg. 2009. Genome instability, cancer and aging. *Biochimica et biophysica acta* 1790:963-969.

Matsuoka, S., B.A. Ballif, A. Smogorzewska, E.R. McDonald, 3rd, K.E. Hurov, J. Luo, C.E. Bakalarski, Z. Zhao, N. Solimini, Y. Lerenthal, Y. Shiloh, S.P. Gygi, and S.J. Elledge. 2007. ATM and ATR substrate analysis reveals extensive protein networks responsive to DNA damage. *Science* 316:1160-1166.

Maynard, S., S.H. Schurman, C. Harboe, N.C. de Souza-Pinto, and V.A. Bohr. 2009. Base excision repair of oxidative DNA damage and association with cancer and aging. *Carcinogenesis* 30:2-10.

McKinnon, P.J. 2009. DNA repair deficiency and neurological disease. *Nat Rev Neurosci* 10:100-112.

Melcher, R., R. von Golitschek, C. Steinlein, D. Schindler, H. Neitzel, K. Kainer, M. Schmid, and H. Hoehn. 2000. Spectral karyotyping of Werner syndrome fibroblast cultures. *Cytogenet Cell Genet* 91:180-185.

Michaloglou, C., L.C. Vredeveld, M.S. Soengas, C. Denoyelle, T. Kuilman, C.M. van der Horst, D.M. Majoor, J.W. Shay, W.J. Mooi, and D.S. Peeper. 2005. BRAFE600-associated senescence-like cell cycle arrest of human naevi. *Nature* 436:720-724.

Mihola, O., Z. Trachtulec, C. Vlcek, J.C. Schimenti, and J. Forejt. 2009. A mouse speciation gene encodes a meiotic histone H3 methyltransferase. *Science* 323:373-375.

Milyavsky, M., O.I. Gan, M. Trottier, M. Komosa, O. Tabach, F. Notta, E. Lechman, K.G. Hermans, K. Eppert, Z. Konovalova, O. Ornatsky, E. Domany, M.S. Meyn, and J.E. Dick. 2010. A distinctive DNA damage response in human hematopoietic stem cells reveals an apoptosis-independent role for p53 in self-renewal. *Cell Stem Cell* 7:186-197.

Miyamoto, T., E. Koh, N. Sakugawa, H. Sato, H. Hayashi, M. Namiki, and K. Sengoku. 2008. Two single nucleotide polymorphisms in PRDM9 (MEISETZ) gene may be a genetic risk factor for Japanese patients with azoospermia by meiotic arrest. *J Assist Reprod Genet* 25:553-557.

Mohrin, M., E. Bourke, D. Alexander, M.R. Warr, K. Barry-Holson, M.M. Le Beau, C.G. Morrison, and E. Passegue. 2010. Hematopoietic stem cell quiescence promotes error-prone DNA repair and mutagenesis. *Cell Stem Cell* 7:174-185.

Moldovan, G.L., and A.D. D'Andrea. 2009. FANCD2 hurdles the DNA interstrand crosslink. *Cell* 139:1222-1224.

Mombaerts, P., J. Iacomini, R.S. Johnson, K. Herrup, S. Tonegawa, and V.E. Papaioannou. 1992. RAG-1-deficient mice have no mature B and T lymphocytes. *Cell* 68:869-877.

Moshous, D., I. Callebaut, R. de Chasseval, B. Corneo, M. Cavazzana-Calvo, F. Le Deist, I. Tezcan, O. Sanal, Y. Bertrand, N. Philippe, A. Fischer, and J.P. de Villartay. 2001. Artemis, a novel DNA double-strand break repair/V(D)J recombination protein, is mutated in human severe combined immune deficiency. *Cell* 105:177-186.

Moynahan, M.E., and M. Jasin. 2010. Mitotic homologous recombination maintains genomic stability and suppresses tumorigenesis. *Nat Rev Mol Cell Biol* 11:196-207.

Multani, A.S., and S. Chang. 2007. WRN at telomeres: implications for aging and cancer. *J Cell Sci* 120:713-721.

Munroe, R.J., R.A. Bergstrom, Q.Y. Zheng, B. Libby, R. Smith, S.W. John, K.J. Schimenti, V.L. Browning, and J.C. Schimenti. 2000. Mouse mutants from chemically mutagenized embryonic stem cells. *Nat Genet* 24:318-321.

Negrini, S., V.G. Gorgoulis, and T.D. Halazonetis. 2010. Genomic instability--an evolving hallmark of cancer. *Nature reviews. Molecular cell biology* 11:220-228.

Nick McElhinny, S.A., C.M. Snowden, J. McCarville, and D.A. Ramsden. 2000. Ku recruits the XRCC4-ligase IV complex to DNA ends. *Mol Cell Biol* 20:2996-3003.

Niedernhofer, L.J., G.A. Garinis, A. Raams, A.S. Lalai, A.R. Robinson, E. Appeldoorn, H. Odijk, R. Oostendorp, A. Ahmad, W. van Leeuwen, A.F. Theil, W. Vermeulen, G.T. van der Horst, P. Meinecke, W.J. Kleijer, J. Vijg, N.G. Jaspers, and J.H. Hoeijmakers. 2006. A new progeroid syndrome reveals that genotoxic stress suppresses the somatotroph axis. *Nature* 444:1038-1043.

Nouspikel, T. 2009. DNA repair in mammalian cells : Nucleotide excision repair: variations on versatility. *Cell Mol Life Sci* 66:994-1009.

O'Connell, B.C., and J.W. Harper. 2007. Ubiquitin proteasome system (UPS): what can chromatin do for you? *Curr Opin Cell Biol* 19:206-214.

O'Driscoll, M., K.M. Cerosaletti, P.M. Girard, Y. Dai, M. Stumm, B. Kysela, B. Hirsch, A. Gennery, S.E. Palmer, J. Seidel, R.A. Gatti, R. Varon, M.A. Oettinger, H. Neitzel, P.A. Jeggo, and P. Concannon. 2001. DNA ligase IV mutations identified in patients exhibiting developmental delay and immunodeficiency. *Mol Cell* 8:1175-1185.

O'Driscoll, M.F., P.A. Smith, and C.M. Magnusson. 2009. Evaluation of a part-time adult diploma nursing programme - 'Tailor-made' provision? *Nurse Educ Today* 29:208-216.

Osipovich, O., R. Milley, A. Meade, M. Tachibana, Y. Shinkai, M.S. Krangel, and E.M. Oltz. 2004. Targeted inhibition of V(D)J recombination by a histone methyltransferase. *Nat Immunol* 5:309-316.

Partridge, L., and M. Mangel. 1999. Messages from mortality: the evolution of death rates in the old. *Trends in Ecology and Evolution* 14:438-442.

Parvanov, E.D., S.H. Ng, P.M. Petkov, and K. Paigen. 2009. Trans-regulation of mouse meiotic recombination hotspots by Rcr1. *PLoS Biol* 7:e36.

Pei, H., L. Zhang, K. Luo, Y. Qin, M. Chesi, F. Fei, P.L. Bergsagel, L. Wang, Z. You, and Z. Lou. 2011. MMSET regulates histone H4K20 methylation and 53BP1 accumulation at DNA damage sites. *Nature* 470:124-128.

Peng, A., and J.L. Maller. 2010. Serine/threonine phosphatases in the DNA damage response and cancer. *Oncogene* 29:5977-5988.

Pollex, R.L., and R.A. Hegele. 2004. Hutchinson-Gilford progeria syndrome. *Clin Genet* 66:375-381.

Qiu, W., E.B. Carson-Walter, H. Liu, M. Epperly, J.S. Greenberger, G.P. Zambetti, L. Zhang, and J. Yu. 2008. PUMA regulates intestinal progenitor cell radiosensitivity and gastrointestinal syndrome. *Cell Stem Cell* 2:576-583.

Rastogi, R.P., Richa, A. Kumar, M.B. Tyagi, and R.P. Sinha. 2010. Molecular mechanisms of ultraviolet radiation-induced DNA damage and repair. *J Nucleic Acids* 2010:592980.

Reddel, C.J., and A.S. Weiss. 2004. Lamin A expression levels are unperturbed at the normal and mutant alleles but display partial splice site selection in Hutchinson-Gilford progeria syndrome. *J Med Genet* 41:715-717.

Reina-San-Martin, B., H.T. Chen, A. Nussenzweig, and M.C. Nussenzweig. 2004. ATM is required for efficient recombination between immunoglobulin switch regions. *J Exp Med* 200:1103-1110.

Riballo, E., S.E. Critchlow, S.H. Teo, A.J. Doherty, A. Priestley, B. Broughton, B. Kysela, H. Beamish, N. Plowman, C.F. Arlett, A.R. Lehmann, S.P. Jackson, and P.A. Jeggo. 1999. Identification of a defect in DNA ligase IV in a radiosensitive leukaemia patient. *Curr Biol* 9:699-702.

Richard, D.J., E. Bolderson, L. Cubeddu, R.I. Wadsworth, K. Savage, G.G. Sharma, M.L. Nicolette, S. Tsvetanov, M.J. McIlwraith, R.K. Pandita, S. Takeda, R.T. Hay, J. Gautier, S.C. West, T.T. Paull, T.K. Pandita, M.F. White, and K.K. Khanna. 2008. Single-stranded DNA-binding protein hSSB1 is critical for genomic stability. *Nature* 453:677-681.

Richardson, C., N. Horikoshi, and T.K. Pandita. 2004. The role of the DNA double-strand break response network in meiosis. *DNA Repair (Amst)* 3:1149-1164.

Rogakou, E.P., D.R. Pilch, A.H. Orr, V.S. Ivanova, and W.M. Bonner. 1998. DNA double-stranded breaks induce histone H2AX phosphorylation on serine 139. *J Biol Chem* 273:5858-5868.

Romanienko, P.J., and R.D. Camerini-Otero. 2000. The mouse Spo11 gene is required for meiotic chromosome synapsis. *Mol Cell* 6:975-987.

Salk, D., K. Au, H. Hoehn, and G.M. Martin. 1981. Cytogenetics of Werner's syndrome cultured skin fibroblasts: variegated translocation mosaicism. *Cytogenet Cell Genet* 30:92-107.

San Filippo, J., P. Sung, and H. Klein. 2008. Mechanism of eukaryotic homologous recombination. *Annual review of biochemistry* 77:229-257.

Sancar, A., L.A. Lindsey-Boltz, T.H. Kang, J.T. Reardon, J.H. Lee, and N. Ozturk. 2010. Circadian clock control of the cellular response to DNA damage. *FEBS letters* 584:2618-2625.

Sato, H., T. Miyamoto, L. Yogev, M. Namiki, E. Koh, H. Hayashi, Y. Sasaki, M. Ishikawa, D.J. Lamb, N. Matsumoto, O.S. Birk, N. Niikawa, and K. Sengoku. 2006. Polymorphic alleles of the human MEI1 gene are associated with human azoospermia by meiotic arrest. *J Hum Genet* 51:533-540.

Schrader, C.E., J.E. Guikema, E.K. Linehan, E. Selsing, and J. Stavnezer. 2007. Activation-induced cytidine deaminase-dependent DNA breaks in class switch recombination occur during G1 phase of the cell cycle and depend upon mismatch repair. *J Immunol* 179:6064-6071.

Schreiber, V., F. Dantzer, J.C. Ame, and G. de Murcia. 2006. Poly(ADP-ribose): novel functions for an old molecule. *Nat Rev Mol Cell Biol* 7:517-528.

Schwarz, K., G.H. Gauss, L. Ludwig, U. Pannicke, Z. Li, D. Lindner, W. Friedrich, R.A. Seger, T.E. Hansen-Hagge, S. Desiderio, M.R. Lieber, and C.R. Bartram. 1996. RAG mutations in human B cell-negative SCID. *Science* 274:97-99.

Scully, R., and D.M. Livingston. 2000. In search of the tumour-suppressor functions of BRCA1 and BRCA2. *Nature* 408:429-432.

Shiloh, Y. 2003. ATM and related protein kinases: safeguarding genome integrity. *Nat Rev Cancer* 3:155-168.

Shinkai, Y., G. Rathbun, K.P. Lam, E.M. Oltz, V. Stewart, M. Mendelsohn, J. Charron, M. Datta, F. Young, A.M. Stall, and et al. 1992. RAG-2-deficient mice lack mature lymphocytes owing to inability to initiate V(D)J rearrangement. *Cell* 68:855-867.

Simsek, D., and M. Jasin. 2010. Alternative end-joining is suppressed by the canonical NHEJ component Xrcc4-ligase IV during chromosomal translocation formation. *Nature structural & molecular biology* 17:410-416.

So, S., A.J. Davis, and D.J. Chen. 2009. Autophosphorylation at serine 1981 stabilizes ATM at DNA damage sites. *J Cell Biol* 187:977-990.

Soulas-Sprauel, P., G. Le Guyader, P. Rivera-Munoz, V. Abramowski, C. Olivier-Martin, C. Goujet-Zalc, P. Charneau, and J.P. de Villartay. 2007. Role for DNA repair factor XRCC4 in immunoglobulin class switch recombination. *J Exp Med* 204:1717-1727.

Soutoglou, E., and T. Misteli. 2008. Activation of the cellular DNA damage response in the absence of DNA lesions. *Science* 320:1507-1510.

Starcevic, D., S. Dalal, and J.B. Sweasy. 2004. Is there a link between DNA polymerase beta and cancer? *Cell Cycle* 3:998-1001.

Stavnezer, J., J.E. Guikema, and C.E. Schrader. 2008. Mechanism and regulation of class switch recombination. *Annu Rev Immunol* 26:261-292.

Stefanini, M., E. Botta, M. Lanzafame, and D. Orioli. 2010. Trichothiodystrophy: from basic mechanisms to clinical implications. *DNA repair* 9:2-10.

Stewart, G.S., S. Panier, K. Townsend, A.K. Al-Hakim, N.K. Kolas, E.S. Miller, S. Nakada, J. Ylanko, S. Olivarius, M. Mendez, C. Oldreive, J. Wildenhain, A. Tagliaferro, L. Pelletier, N. Taubenheim, A. Durandy, P.J. Byrd, T. Stankovic, A.M. Taylor, and D. Durocher. 2009. The RIDDLE syndrome protein mediates a ubiquitin-dependent signaling cascade at sites of DNA damage. *Cell* 136:420-434.

Stracker, T.H., and J.H. Petrini. 2011. The MRE11 complex: starting from the ends. *Nat Rev Mol Cell Biol* 12:90-103.

Su, I.H., A. Basavaraj, A.N. Krutchinsky, O. Hobert, A. Ullrich, B.T. Chait, and A. Tarakhovsky. 2003. Ezh2 controls B cell development through histone H3 methylation and Igh rearrangement. *Nat Immunol* 4:124-131.

Sugasawa, K., Y. Okuda, M. Saijo, R. Nishi, N. Matsuda, G. Chu, T. Mori, S. Iwai, K. Tanaka, and F. Hanaoka. 2005. UV-induced ubiquitylation of XPC protein mediated by UV-DDB-ubiquitin ligase complex. *Cell* 121:387-400.

Suh, E.K., A. Yang, A. Kettenbach, C. Bamberger, A.H. Michaelis, Z. Zhu, J.A. Elvin, R.T. Bronson, C.P. Crum, and F. McKeon. 2006. p63 protects the female germ line during meiotic arrest. *Nature* 444:624-628.

Sundin, G.W., and M.R. Weigand. 2007. The microbiology of mutability. *FEMS Microbiol Lett* 277:11-20.

Szilard, L. 1959. On the Nature of the Aging Process. *Proc Natl Acad Sci U S A* 45:30-45.

Taccioli, G.E., G. Rathbun, E. Oltz, T. Stamato, P.A. Jeggo, and F.W. Alt. 1993. Impairment of V(D)J recombination in double-strand break repair mutants. *Science* 260:207-210.

Tang, J.B., and R.A. Greenberg. 2010. Connecting the Dots: Interplay Between Ubiquitylation and SUMOylation at DNA Double Strand Breaks. *Genes Cancer* 1:787-796.

Thonneau, P., S. Marchand, A. Tallec, M.L. Ferial, B. Ducot, J. Lansac, P. Lopes, J.M. Tabaste, and A. Spira. 1991. Incidence and main causes of infertility in a resident population (1,850,000) of three French regions (1988-1989). *Hum Reprod* 6:811-816.

van der Burg, M., H. Ijspeert, N.S. Verkaik, T. Turul, W.W. Wiegant, K. Morotomi-Yano, P.O. Mari, I. Tezcan, D.J. Chen, M.Z. Zdzienicka, J.J. van Dongen, and D.C. van Gent. 2009. A DNA-PKcs mutation in a radiosensitive T-B- SCID patient inhibits Artemis activation and nonhomologous end-joining. *J Clin Invest* 119:91-98.

van der Burg, M., L.R. van Veelen, N.S. Verkaik, W.W. Wiegant, N.G. Hartwig, B.H. Barendregt, L. Brugmans, A. Raams, N.G. Jaspers, M.Z. Zdzienicka, J.J. van Dongen, and D.C. van Gent. 2006. A new type of radiosensitive T-B-NK+ severe combined immunodeficiency caused by a LIG4 mutation. *J Clin Invest* 116:137-145.

van Engelen, B.G., J.A. Hiel, F.J. Gabreels, L.P. van den Heuvel, D.C. van Gent, and C.M. Weemaes. 2001. Decreased immunoglobulin class switching in Nijmegen Breakage syndrome due to the DNA repair defect. *Hum Immunol* 62:1324-1327.

Venkatesan, R.N., J.H. Bielas, and L.A. Loeb. 2006. Generation of mutator mutants during carcinogenesis. *DNA Repair (Amst)* 5:294-302.

Viale, A., F. De Franco, A. Orleth, V. Cambiaghi, V. Giuliani, D. Bossi, C. Ronchini, S. Ronzoni, I. Muradore, S. Monestiroli, A. Gobbi, M. Alcalay, S. Minucci, and P.G. Pelicci. 2009. Cell-cycle restriction limits DNA damage and maintains self-renewal of leukaemia stem cells. *Nature* 457:51-56.

Villa, A., S. Santagata, F. Bozzi, S. Giliani, A. Frattini, L. Imberti, L.B. Gatta, H.D. Ochs, K. Schwarz, L.D. Notarangelo, P. Vezzoni, and E. Spanopoulou. 1998. Partial V(D)J recombination activity leads to Omenn syndrome. *Cell* 93:885-896.

Villa, A., C. Sobacchi, L.D. Notarangelo, F. Bozzi, M. Abinun, T.G. Abrahamsen, P.D. Arkwright, M. Baniyash, E.G. Brooks, M.E. Conley, P. Cortes, M. Duse, A. Fasth, A.M. Filipovich, A.J. Infante, A. Jones, E. Mazzolari, S.M. Muller, S. Pasic, G. Rechavi, M.G. Sacco, S. Santagata, M.L. Schroeder, R. Seger, D. Strina, A. Ugazio, J. Valiaho, M. Vihinen, L.B. Vogler, H. Ochs, P. Vezzoni, W. Friedrich, and K. Schwarz. 2001. V(D)J recombination defects in lymphocytes due to RAG mutations: severe immunodeficiency with a spectrum of clinical presentations. *Blood* 97:81-88.

Wei, K., A.B. Clark, E. Wong, M.F. Kane, D.J. Mazur, T. Parris, N.K. Kolas, R. Russell, H. Hou, Jr., B. Kneitz, G. Yang, T.A. Kunkel, R.D. Kolodner, P.E. Cohen, and W. Edelmann. 2003. Inactivation of Exonuclease 1 in mice results in DNA mismatch repair defects, increased cancer susceptibility, and male and female sterility. *Genes Dev* 17:603-614.

Weidenheim, K.M., D.W. Dickson, and I. Rapin. 2009. Neuropathology of Cockayne syndrome: Evidence for impaired development, premature aging, and neurodegeneration. *Mech Ageing Dev* 130:619-636.

Wilson, D.M., 3rd, and V.A. Bohr. 2007. The mechanics of base excision repair, and its relationship to aging and disease. *DNA Repair (Amst)* 6:544-559.

Woodward, W.A., M.S. Chen, F. Behbod, M.P. Alfaro, T.A. Buchholz, and J.M. Rosen. 2007. WNT/beta-catenin mediates radiation resistance of mouse mammary progenitor cells. *Proceedings of the National Academy of Sciences of the United States of America* 104:618-623.

Wu, L., S.L. Davies, P.S. North, H. Goulaouic, J.F. Riou, H. Turley, K.C. Gatter, and I.D. Hickson. 2000. The Bloom's syndrome gene product interacts with topoisomerase III. *J Biol Chem* 275:9636-9644.

Yan, C.T., C. Boboila, E.K. Souza, S. Franco, T.R. Hickernell, M. Murphy, S. Gumaste, M. Geyer, A.A. Zarrin, J.P. Manis, K. Rajewsky, and F.W. Alt. 2007. IgH class switching and translocations use a robust non-classical end-joining pathway. *Nature* 449:478-482.

Yoshida, K., G. Kondoh, Y. Matsuda, T. Habu, Y. Nishimune, and T. Morita. 1998. The mouse RecA-like gene Dmc1 is required for homologous chromosome synapsis during meiosis. *Mol Cell* 1:707-718.

Yu, C.E., J. Oshima, Y.H. Fu, E.M. Wijsman, F. Hisama, R. Alisch, S. Matthews, J. Nakura, T. Miki, S. Ouais, G.M. Martin, J. Mulligan, and G.D. Schellenberg. 1996. Positional cloning of the Werner's syndrome gene. *Science* 272:258-262.

Zhang, M., F. Behbod, R.L. Atkinson, M.D. Landis, F. Kittrell, D. Edwards, D. Medina, A. Tsimelzon, S. Hilsenbeck, J.E. Green, A.M. Michalowska, and J.M. Rosen. 2008. Identification of tumor-initiating cells in a p53-null mouse model of breast cancer. *Cancer research* 68:4674-4682.

Zhang, Y., and M. Jasin. 2011. An essential role for CtIP in chromosomal translocation formation through an alternative end-joining pathway. *Nature structural & molecular biology* 18:80-84.

Zhu, J., S. Petersen, L. Tessarollo, and A. Nussenzweig. 2001. Targeted disruption of the Nijmegen breakage syndrome gene NBS1 leads to early embryonic lethality in mice. *Curr Biol* 11:105-109.

DNA Damage Repair and Cancer: The Role of RAD51 Protein and Its Genetic Variants

Augusto Nogueira[1,4], Raquel Catarino[1] and Rui Medeiros[1,2,3,4]
[1]Molecular Oncology & Virology - Portuguese Institute of Oncology
[2]CEBIMED, Faculty of Health Sciences of Fernando Pessoa University
[3]ICBAS, Abel Salazar Institute for the Biomedical Sciences
[4]Portuguese League Against Cancer (LPCC-NRNorte)
Portugal

1. Introduction

Genomes are continually attacked by both endogenous and exogenous agents that damage DNA. DNA damage in the form of DNA breaks can lead to chromosome translocations, cell cycle arrest, and apoptosis. Homologous recombination is an essential biological process that ensures the accurate repair of DNA breaks and thereby contributes to genomic integrity (Kuzminov 1999; Paques and Haber 1999).

DNA double-strand breaks (DSBs) are considered the principal lethal DNA damage resulting from ionizing radiation and cross-linking drugs. In addition, DSB can arise from endogenous processes, such as replication fork stalling during attempted replication over a single strand-break and topoisomerase poisons that are common therapies in the treatment of human cancers (Arnaudeau, Lundin et al. 2001).

It is of great importance that cells recognise DSBs and act upon them rapidly and efficiently, because cell death or impaired cell function can occur if these are left unrepaired or are repaired inaccurately. In addition to DNA repair mechanisms, cell cycle checkpoint activation processes are initiated in response to DNA damage. More specifically, DNA damage signals to arrest cell cycle progression, giving the cell more time to repair what might otherwise be a fatal lesion (Henning and Sturzbecher 2003).

2. DNA damage – repair pathways

Faithful genome transmission requires the co-ordination of a network of pathways such as cell cycle checkpoint, DNA replication, DNA repair/recombination and programmed cell death. In response to DNA damage, cells arrest their cell cycle progression, thus providing time for repair, or activate programmed cell death – both responses preventing transmission of genetic instability (Khanna and Jackson 2001). Thus, maintenance of the genomic integrity by DNA repair genes is an essential step in normal cellular growth and differentiation (Hoeijmakers 2001).

Failure to repair DNA lesions such as DSBs can lead to mutations, genomic instability, and cell death. Due to the severe consequences of DSBs, cells have developed two major repair pathways: homologous recombination (HR) and non-homolgous end joining (NHEJ) (Helleday, Lo et al. 2007).

HR takes advantage of large sequence homologies to repair DSBs. These homologous sequences can be found on homologous chromosome or in DNA repeats. HR refers to several processes, the two most documented in mammalian cells being single-strand annealing (SSA) and gene conversion associated or not with crossing over (Lin, Sperle et al. 1984). SSA process occurs between direct repeat sequences (Lin, Sperle et al. 1984) and is initiated by homologous pairing, except that — unlike HR — the homology is between short stretches of single-stranded DNA at staggered DSBs, and pairing precedes re-ligation, not strand exchange. It is a non-conservative process and error-prone because sequence information can be lost or rearranged when ends overlapping by as little as 30 bp are unsuitably joined (Henning and Sturzbecher 2003). Homologous recombination requires a homologous intact sequence and results in gene conversion associated or not with crossing over (Szostak, Orr-Weaver et al. 1983). Gene conversion is a conservative, generally error-free process, although it can also generate genetic variability. Gene conversion is involved in meiosis and molecular evolution (Daboussi, Dumay et al. 2002).

The mitotic cell cycle is an important determinant in the choice of the right repair pathway for a given physiological situation. Repair by HR predominates during S/G phases of the cell cycle, when sister chromatids, the preferred substrate for error-free exchange, are present (Henning and Sturzbecher 2003).

Non-homologous end joining (NHEJ) ligates the two broken DNA ends and does not require extensive sequence homologies between the two recombining DNA molecules. During the process, limited degradation of the DNA ends or DNA capture can lead to deletion or insertion of nucleotides or DNA fragments. It is thus a potentially error-prone process (Smith and Jackson 1999).

3. Role of mammalian protein RAD51

Mammalian RAD51 protein is a structural, biochemical and genetic homologue of the bacterial RecA and of the yeast RAD51 recombination proteins. Interestingly, overexpression of RAD51 alone is sufficient to stimulate gene conversion in mammalian cells (Vispe, Cazaux et al. 1998; Arnaudeau, Helleday et al. 1999; Lambert and Lopez 2000). In contrast, expression of dominant negative forms of RAD51 is enough to abolish almost totally gene conversion between tandem repeat sequences (Lambert and Lopez 2000). These data suggest that RAD51 plays a pivotal role in gene conversion regulation.

In vitro, RAD51 protein promotes DNA homologous pairing and strand exchange, in association with other proteins of the gene conversion complex (Benson, Baumann et al. 1998). In cultured mammalian cells, RAD51 is involved in spontaneous gene conversion as well as in HR induced by γ-rays (Lambert and Lopez 2000) , alkylating agents, UV-C and replication elongation inhibitors (Saintigny, Delacote et al. 2001). More precisely, RAD51 controls DSB repair via gene conversion leading to gene conversion associated or not with crossing over (Lambert and Lopez 2000).

Finally, RAD51 partly participates in induced sister chromatid exchange in mammalian cells (Lambert and Lopez 2001). These roles of mammalian RAD51 in gene conversion are very similar to the roles of yeast RAD51. However, there are important differences between yeast and vertebrate RAD51 (Daboussi, Dumay et al. 2002).

The RAD51 gene consists of 10 exons and spans at least 30 kb. All exon-intron boundaries follow the GT-AC rule. Further sequencing of the region 5′ of the first exon revealed that nonconding exon 1 contained a CpG island that was approximately 900 bp in size. This putative promoter region contains several recognition sites for Sp1 transcription factors but lacks a TATA box (Schmutte, Tombline et al. 1999). The presence of several putative Sp1 promoter binding sites is consistent with the observed cell cycle-dependent expression of *RAD51* (Johnson 1992). The translation start codon is located in exon 2, and the average size of the coding exons is 112 bp (Schmutte, Tombline et al. 1999).

RAD51 gene encodes a highly conserved well-characterized DNA repair protein (Liu, Lamerdin et al. 1998) (Table 1). *RAD51* gene is located at chromosome position 15q15.1 (Takahashi, Matsuda et al. 1994), a region that exhibits loss of heterozygosity in a large of cancers, including those of the lung, the colorectum and the breast (Wick, Petersen et al. 1996).

RAD51	
Gene symbol	*hRAD51*
Molecular Weight (Da)	36966
Gene type	Protein coding (RAD51)
Function	Involved in the homologous recombination and repair of DNA
Gene Map Locus	15q15.1
Localization primary	Nucleus
Protein interactions	BRCA1, RAD51C, ABL, P53, BRCA2, RAD54-like protein, RAD54B, RAD52, ERCC2, Cell cycle checkpoint kinase (CHEK1/CHK1), ATM, RAD51C, XRCC3, XRCC2, RAD51B
Described polymorphisms	5′ UTR G135C and 5′ UTR G172T

Table 1. Characteristics of the gene *RAD51*.

When cells are exposed to genotoxic agents or irradiation, such as mitomycin C, UV, and ionizing radiation, RAD51 protein is recruited to sites of DNA damage where it mediates the search for a homologous sequence during homologous recombination (Buchhop, Gibson et al. 1997; Vispe, Cazaux et al. 1998). It has been revealed that the RAD51 nuclear foci are the sites of repair of DNA damage (Tashiro, Kotomura et al. 1996).

This protein is therefore required for meiotic and mitotic recombination and plays a central role in homology-dependent recombinational repair of DSBs (Levy-Lahad, Lahad et al. 2001). Upon its regulated recruitment to sites of DNA breaks, RAD51 forms a nucleoprotein filament by polymerizing onto single-stranded DNA at the processed break. This filament catalyses DNA strand exchange with an undamaged sister chromatid or homologous chromosome, which serve as templates for the restoration of missing genetic information (Li and Heyer 2008; San Filippo, Sung et al. 2008).

So when HR is used for repair, in eukaryotes it is promoted by the recombinase RAD51, which binds to 3′-tailed single strands at the end of DSBs in a helical fashion and promotes pairing with homologous DNA sequences as a prelude to strand invasion and repair of the DSBs (Sung and Klein 2006) (Figure 1).

In response to DNA damage, RAD51 is translocated from the cytosol to the nucleus (Haaf, Golub et al. 1995). In the nucleus, RAD51 sequesters into foci together with other proteins involved in homologous recombination, e. g., RAD52 (Liu and Maizels 2000).

RAD51 is required for the resistance to ionising radiation (Ohnishi, Taki et al. 1998), and high levels of RAD51 have been correlated with resistance to chemotherapeutics agents

(Maacke, Jost et al. 2000; Slupianek, Hoser et al. 2002). Importantly, RAD51 is also essential for embryonic survival in the absence of exogenous DNA damaging agents and has a role in the repair of spontaneously occurring chromosome breaks in proliferating cells of higher eukaryotes (Sonoda, Sasaki et al. 1998). This protein has been shown to be involved in the repair of different kinds of DNA lesions during replication (Lundin, Schultz et al. 2003). Thus, RAD51 is likely to promote genomic stability in eukaryotic cells (Orre, Falt et al. 2006). However, despite its role in maintaining genomic integrity, it has been proposed that the aberrant increase in RAD51 expression found in tumour cells may contribute to genomic instability by stimulating aberrant recombination between short repetitive elements and homologous sequences (Xia, Shammas et al. 1997; Flygare, Falt et al. 2001).

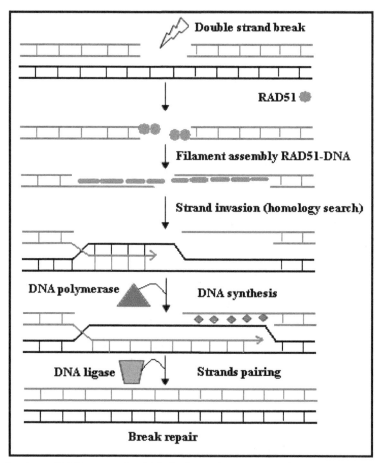

Fig. 1. Mechanism of DNA repair by RAD51 (homologous recombination).

The regulation of RAD51 appears to occur through at least two ways: (a) transcriptionally, by genes that confer a proliferative potential, as well as by checkpoint signaling pathways that regulate DNA damage responses; and (b) at the protein level, where interactions with other molecules leads to distinct cellular localization in RAD51 nuclear foci. It is possible that RAD51 regulation may occur at the transcriptional level in a cell type-, cell cycle-, or damage response-coordinated manner.

RAD51 gene expression is controlled by a variety of transcriptional activators and repressors (Hasselbach, Haase et al. 2005; Arias-Lopez, Lazaro-Trueba et al. 2006), but is not affected by DNA damage (Henson, Tsai et al. 2006).

The accurate functioning of the DNA-repair proteins is a crucial step in maintaining genomic homeostasis and preventing carcinogenesis.

4. Levels of RAD51 protein expression

RAD51 expression is cell cycle-regulated, being lowest in resting cells. In proliferating cells, RAD51 expression peaks in the S/G2 phases of the cell cycle (Flygare, Benson et al. 1996; Yamamoto, Taki et al. 1996), indicating a role of the protein in intrachromosomal recombinational repair (Flygare, Falt et al. 2001).

Several studies have shown RAD51 protein expression levels to be elevated in immortalized cells and a wide variety of human cancer cell lines (Xia, Shammas et al. 1997; Raderschall, Stout et al. 2002). Given this high RAD51 expression, it is possible that RAD51 overexpression followed by hyperrecombination may contribute to genomic instability and malignant transformation (Vispe, Cazaux et al. 1998; Yanez and Porter 1999). Moreover, a growing body of literature suggests that RAD51 overexpression can increase cellular resistance to radiation and some chemotherapeutic drugs (Maacke, Jost et al. 2000; Henning and Sturzbecher 2003; Qiao, Wu et al. 2005). This could be of clinical importance for the treatment of cancer patients with radio- and/or chemotherapy (Flygare, Falt et al. 2001).

Aberrant overexpression of RAD51 protein could confer several advantages to tumor cells. First, the DNA repair function of RAD51 may protect cells from DNA damage and apoptosis. Secondly, overstimulation of homologous recombination and chromatid exchange mechanisms by RAD51 protein (Xia, Shammas et al. 1997; Arnaudeau, Helleday et al. 1999) may contribute to genomic instability and genetic diversity of tumour cells (Raderschall, Stout et al. 2002).

Hasselbach and co-workers (Hasselbach, Haase et al. 2005) identified three separate cis-acting sequence elements within the RAD51 transcriptional promoter, one ensuring basal levels of expression and two elements limiting expression to relatively low levels. The characterisation of transcription factor binding might help to explain high-level expression of RAD51 in a variety of solid tumours.

The mechanisms underlying the observed radioresistance accompanying RAD51 overexpression are poorly understood. It is possible that an increased DSB repair capacity following RAD51 upregulation is responsible for the increased radioresistance. Alternatively, the overexpression of RAD51 might affect other cellular processes influencing cell survival, e.g., cell cycle progression (Flygare, Falt et al. 2001). The tumour suppressors p53 (Buchhop, Gibson et al. 1997) and BRCA2 (Patel, Yu et al. 1998; Yuan, Lee et al. 1999) associate with RAD51 and play roles in DNA repair and cell cycle checkpoint pathways (Dasika, Lin et al. 1999).

The reasons for RAD51 overexpression in cancer cells are not entirely understood. It is not the result of gene duplication or protein stability, but is thought to occur at the level of transcriptional regulation in the promoter region (Raderschall, Stout et al. 2002).

Since many tumours exhibit resistance to therapeutic drugs that damage DNA, it is important to understand the molecular mechanisms causing this DNA damage resistance. In several cases it appears that the resistance is from enhanced RAD51 expression, due to oncogene-induced expression of RAD51 and inhibition of pathways that limit RAD51 protein levels. Cells that express the oncogenes BCR/ABL have increased levels of RAD51 protein (Slupianek, Schmutte et al. 2001). This occurs through STAT5-dependent transcription of RAD51 and inhibition of RAD51 protein cleavage by caspase-3. These cells have increased resistance to cisplatin and mitomycin C, drugs whose damage requires RAD51 for repair. Additionally, double strand break-induced homologous recombination is elevated in these cells (Klein 2008).

Therefore, another level of regulation of RAD51 activity occurs through protein modification. RAD51 is a target of the BCR/ABL kinase and is phosphorylated on tyrosine 315. Mutation of this tyrosine residue to phenylalanine resulted in increased sensitivity to cisplatin and mitomycin C, suggesting that RAD51 recombinational repair of DNA crosslink damage is controlled trough RAD51 tyrosine 315 (Klein 2008).

Thus, upon DNA damage, RAD51 is phosphorylated by c-Abl. In addition, RAD51 is cleaved by capase-3 during apoptosis (Slupianek, Schmutte et al. 2001; Klein 2008). Together, these findings suggest that the cellular level of the RAD51 protein is important for the control of homologous recombination and survival after DNA damage (Hansen, Lundin et al. 2003).

A study demonstrated that RAD51 expression levels in human cell lines were modulated by introducing various fusion tyrosine kinase (FTK) proteins. All of the FTK's, except one, elevated RAD51 expression levels (5- to 8-fold) relative to the parental cell line. The RAD51 expression levels correlated with cellular resistance to cisplatin, and this resistance was partially reversed by blocking RAD51 expression with an anti-sense strategy (Slupianek, Hoser et al. 2002).

Earlier studies found that due to its central role in recombination, RAD51 was likely to be a target for regulatory factors that coordinate DNA repair, transcription, replication and cell-cycle progression. The tumour-suppressor protein p53 is one of several factors that could interact directly with human RAD51 (Buchhop, Gibson et al. 1997). The p53 protein has a well-established role in linking progression through the cell cycle with genome integrity. This function is likely to require contact with the DNA-repair machinery, and RAD51 is therefore a potential target. There are some indications that the presence of TP53 affects the activities of RAD51 (Levine 1997). Overexpression of the c-myc, β-catenin or human papilloma virus E7 oncogenes results in induction of RAD51 and increased protein levels (Pauklin, Kristjuhan et al. 2005). RAD51 induction is dependent on the ATM and ATR kinases acting on p53 phosphorylation and downregulation of RAD51 levels. Increased RAD51 levels are correlated with an induction of the DNA damage response when oncogenes are overexpressed, using formation of γ-H2AX foci as a marker of DNA damage. Further studies suggested that the ARF tumor suppressor pathway also regulated RAD51 levels through p53 activation (Klein 2008).

Therefore, the tumor suppressor protein p53, which is frequently mutated in cancer, interacts with the RAD51 core promoter and RAD51 protein to inhibit both its expression and activity (Linke, Sengupta et al. 2003; Arias-Lopez, Lazaro-Trueba et al. 2006), while the transcription factor STAT5 has been shown to stimulate the expression of RAD51 (Slupianek, Schmutte et al. 2001; Slupianek, Hoser et al. 2002).

There are only a few studies that have investigated RAD51 expression levels in human tumors. Since increased levels of RAD51 have been correlated with elevated recombination rates (Xia, Shammas et al. 1997; Vispe, Cazaux et al. 1998), but also increased genomic instability, the consequences of increased RAD51 expression were studied in human cells. Elevated RAD51 protein levels have been detected in human pancreatic adenocarcinoma cell lines (Maacke, Jost et al. 2000) and in cells derived from a patient with Bloom's syndrome (Magnusson, Sandstrom et al. 2000), a disorder that confers pronounced genomic instability. It has also been shown that elevated levels of RAD51 correlate with increased invasiveness of breast cancer (Maacke, Opitz et al. 2000) and can be used as an independent prognostic marker for mean survival time in patients with non-small cell lung cancer (Qiao, Wu et al. 2005).

It has already been demonstrated that increased RAD51 protein expression leads to a perturbation of the cellular state of equilibrium, reflected in alterations of gene expression patterns detectable at the mRNA level. Up-regulation of p53 and auto-regulated decrease of RAD51 protein indicate that high RAD51 protein levels may have induced stress responses in our system (Orre, Falt et al. 2006). However, the resulting RAD51 protein level remained higher than that observed in cells expressing RAD51 and was similar to the degree of RAD51 up-regulation observed in many cancer cell lines (Raderschall, Stout et al. 2002).

However, additional studies will be required to determine at which point during the multistage process of tumorigenesis RAD51 up-regulation occurs and to understand its clinical significance. Raderschall and co-workers (Raderschall, Stout et al. 2002) showed possible diagnostic and therapeutic applications. Firstly, RAD51 could serve as a diagnostic/prognostic marker to improve tumour classification. More importantly, down-regulation of RAD51 protein by RAD51 antisense oligonucleotides (Ohnishi, Taki et al. 1998) or RAD51-inhibitory drugs could be used to sensitize tumours to radiation or chemotherapy.

Therefore, various studies of DNA damage and repair in cancer are important, because they can give not only deeper insight into molecular mechanisms of carcinogenesis, but may also yield information on risk markers for cancer and help to improve cancer therapy as well as fight its hindrances (Synowiec, Stefanska et al. 2008).

5. Genetic variants and cancer

In the process of generating a draft sequence of the human genome, it has become clear that the extent of genetic variation is much larger than previously estimated (Lander, Linton et al. 2001; Venter, Adams et al. 2001). The most common variations in human genome are single nucleotide polymorphisms (SNPs), which are polymorphisms with only one nucleotide substitution. By definition, SNPs are single base pair positions in genomic DNA at which different sequence alternatives (alleles) exist in normal individuals in some population(s), wherein the least frequent allele has an abundance of 1% or greater (Brookes 1999; Risch 2000).

These genetic variants are defined as low penetrance susceptibility alleles, providing an altered risk for cancer development. This risk appears to be influenced by individual SNPs profile in key genes for cancer susceptibility (Brookes 1999).

The association between exposure factor (polymorphism) and the disease is evaluated by relative risk (RR) estimation, indicating the probability of disease development in the group of polymorphic variant carriers. The great majority of molecular epidemiology studies on cancer are of case-control type; therefore RR is evaluated through Odds Ratio (OR). OR represents an association magnitude and supplies helpful information on causality and definition of attributable risk, which is the proportion of all cases that is attributed to the risk factor (Knudsen, Loft et al. 2001).

SNPs and haplotype analysis in cancer research may contribute to the determination of high risk groups and help cancer prevention and development of new therapeutic orientations.

Several studies have reported that variations in genes involved in DNA repair and in the maintenance of genome integrity may be responsible in the increase of cancer risk (Jara, Acevedo et al. 2007). Thus, there is increasing volume of data supporting the hypothesis that genetic polymorphisms in various DNA repair genes result in reduced DNA repair capacity, in this way, being associated with increased susceptibility to various human solid tumours (Qiao, Spitz et al. 2002; Au, Salama et al. 2003; Hung, Hall et al. 2005).

Presence of polymorphisms in DNA repair genes could change the DNA-repair capacity and subsequently modulate the response to DNA-damaging agents and alter an individual's susceptibility to cancer (Hu, Mohrenweiser et al. 2002).

5.1 *RAD51* gene polymorphisms (G135C and G172T)

Two single-nucleotide polymorphisms (SNPs) polymorphisms have been described in the 5'- untranslated region (5'-UTR) of *RAD51* gene , a G to C substitution at position +135 bp, and a G to T substitution at position +172 bp from the start of the cDNA sequence (Levy-Lahad, Lahad et al. 2001; Wang, Spurdle et al. 2001; Rollinson, Smith et al. 2007). Promoter activity is significantly enhanced by substituting G at the polymorphic positions +135 and +172 for C and T, respectively (Hasselbach, Haase et al. 2005).

The biological effect of these polymorphisms is yet to be elucidated and will be important to investigate (Blasiak, Przybylowska et al. 2003). However, *RAD51* G135C polymorphism could affect mRNA splicing, regulation of transcription, translation efficiency or mRNA stability by association of 5'UTR region with regulatory elements (Gray 1998), leading to altered polypeptide product levels, which could affect the function of the final product – the RAD51 protein (Poplawski, Arabski et al. 2006). Because a guanine-to-cytosine substitution at position +135 of the *RAD51* is a gain-of-function mutation, it is expected to result in increased activity of RAD51. This effect is opposite to those found for most of the other genetic variations in DNA repair genes, which result in the decrease of function (Chistiakov, Voronova et al. 2008).

Human *RAD51*, known to function in DNA repair, interacts with a number of proteins implicated in breast cancer, including *BRCA1* and *BRCA2*. Few studies have investigated the role of *RAD51* gene variations in familial breast cancer (Jara, Acevedo et al. 2007). However, some authors hypothesize that several polymorphisms of DNA repair genes could modify either DNA capacity or fidelity, which may contribute to familial and sporadic breast cancer susceptibility (Costa, Pinto et al. 2007). These genes involved in DNA repair, especially those that interact with the product of the *BRCA1* or *BRCA2* genes, are of particular interest as cancer risk modifiers in *BRCA1/2* mutation carriers. Both *BRCA1* and *BRCA2* participate in DNA double-strand break repair through homologous recombination (Venkitaraman 2002). Therefore, the problem of genetic variability of the *RAD51* gene in breast cancer is worth studying for at least two reasons: (1) the involvement of *RAD51* in the stability of the genome and (2) its potential to modify the penetrance of *BRCA1/BRCA2* mutations, which can increase susceptibility for breast cancer (Blasiak, Przybylowska et al. 2003).

It was reported that the G135C polymorphism of the *RAD51* gene is a clinically significant modifier of *BRCA2* penetrance, specifically in raising breast cancer risk at younger ages (Levy-Lahad, Lahad et al. 2001).

Previous studies have linked the *RAD51* 135C allele with altered susceptibility to both breast cancer and ovarian cancer. In breast cancer, although a study found no association for the genetic variant (Kuschel, Auranen et al. 2002), Wang *et al.* (Wang, Spurdle et al. 2001) reported an increased risk of breast cancer and a lower risk of ovarian cancer amongst cases also possessing a *BRCA2* mutation, however, no association was seen for individuals known to have a *BRCA1* mutation. Apparently conflicting results have been reported by Jakubowska *et al.* (Jakubowska, Gronwald et al. 2007). These researchers investigated the role of the *RAD51 G135C* polymorphism in breast and ovarian cancer in case-control populations of Polish women matched for *BRCA1* mutation and age. The results revealed that women who harboured the C allele had almost two times reduced risk of breast and ovarian cancer risk compared with women who harboured only the G allele. Moreover, it was shown in this study that the site of the *BRCA1* mutation did not influence the effect of the *RAD51* C allele, indicating that this polymorphism contributes to prevention of the disease among *BRCA1* carriers.

These differences in associated risk among for *BRCA1* mutation carriers may be due to chance, but also could be explained by the nature of the *BRCA1* mutations reported in the two studies. The most common mutation seen in the Jakubowska study was the 5382insC, which results in a truncated protein but which retains an intact RAD51 binding site (Jakubowska, Narod et al. 2003). The primary mutation reported in the Wang study was the 185delAG, which also results in a truncated protein but abolishes the *BRCA1-RAD51* binding site. This suggests that for a protective effect to be seen in *BRCA1* mutation carriers, the RAD51 interaction site must be present, enabling the *RAD51* 135C allele to enhance the activity of mutant BRCA1 (Jakubowska, Narod et al. 2003).

Another study showed an elevated breast cancer risk associated with the *RAD51* 135C allele in *BRCA2* mutation carriers, but not in *BRCA1* mutation carriers (Levy-Lahad, Lahad et al. 2001; Wang, Spurdle et al. 2001).

Synowiec *et al.* (Synowiec, Stefanska et al. 2008) showed previously that the G135C polymorphism was not an independent marker in breast cancer, but it could be associated with an increased breast cancer risk in BRCA2 mutation carriers (Blasiak, Przybylowska et al. 2003; Sliwinski, Krupa et al. 2005), confirming similar results from other studies (Levy-Lahad, Lahad et al. 2001; Antoniou, Sinilnikova et al. 2007). They also observed a protective effect against breast cancer occurrence for the G/C genotype of this polymorphism (OR 0.25; 95% CI 0.10-0.63). The results from a combined analysis of 19 studies revealed an increased risk of breast cancer in the C/C homozygotes with *BRCA2* mutation [41].

Jara *et al.* (Jara, Acevedo et al. 2007) proposed that *RAD51 G135C* polymorphism presents an increased risk of familial breast cancer in women with age < 50 years at diagnosis, and this polymorphism may be a breast cancer risk variant. This finding should be confirmed in other populations.

BRCA2 is required for the orderly assembly of *RAD51* on single stranded DNA ends. In the absence of *BRCA2*, initiation of accurate HR is impaired and repair errors will rapidly accumulate (Powell, Willers et al. 2002). The increased risk associated with the *RAD51* 135C allele suggests an increase in repair errors. The biological explanation for this is uncertain but may reflect the use of an alternative pathway such as NHEJ (Moynahan, Pierce et al. 2001), or may be a result of error prone HR (Tutt, Bertwistle et al. 2001).

Costa *et al.* (Costa, Pinto et al. 2007) in a case–control study, showed an association of *RAD51* 135C allele and increased breast cancer risk only among women with family history of breast cancer, suggesting that this polymorphism contributed to the familial breast cancer in the Portuguese population, in opposition to reported results in a Brazilian population (Dufloth, Costa et al. 2005). Concerning sporadic breast cancer risk, similar results to Costa and co-workers findings were obtained by other studies in Australian women (Webb, Hopper et al. 2005) and in the Anglo-Saxon population (Kuschel, Auranen et al. 2002), where no association was obtained.

In order to confirm these results, Kadouri *et al.* (Kadouri, Easton et al. 2001) evaluated the effect of the *RAD51 G135C* polymorphism on breast cancer risk in *BRCA1/2* mutation carriers and in non-carrier breast cancer cases, mainly of Ashkenazi origin. These researchers reported a modifying effect for the *RAD51 G135C* polymorphism in *BRCA2* carriers, similar to the effect shown in two previous studies. This is the first modifier gene identified in *BRCA2* carriers. The clinical implication of these findings is still limited; however, it hints at differences in molecular mechanisms involved in tumour development in *BRCA1* and *BRCA2* carriers. The study of polymorphisms in other DNA repair genes could further elucidate the mechanism of tumorigenesis in *BRCA1* and *BRCA2* carriers.

Recent structural studies suggest a mechanism for the regulation of *RAD51* activity by *BRCA2*, and cancer-associated mutations affecting the domain where *RAD51* binds to *BRCA2* or reduced level of the protein itself disrupt this interaction leading to impaired DNA repair via HR (Galkin, Esashi et al. 2005; Martin, Winkelmann et al. 2005). Because mutations in the *BRCA2* gene may be associated with breast and ovarian cancer and results from multi-site cancer phenotype, genetic variation in the *RAD51* gene may contribute to cancer (Martinez, Herzog et al. 2004). Some studies suggest that the G135C polymorphism of the *RAD51* gene may have a phenotypic effect, manifested in the changes in the extent of oxidative DNA damage. Recently, HR has been implicated in the repair of stalled replication forks (Michel, Grompone et al. 2004). This type of cellular events can occur as a consequence of oxidation of DNA. DNA double strand breaks (DSBs), which are the main substrate for HR, can arise directly from reactive oxygen species (ROS) (Galli, Piroddi et al. 2005).

A study in gastric cancer suggested that that the G135C polymorphism of the *RAD51* gene may be linked with gastric cancer by the modulation of the cellular response to oxidative stress. In this work, the authors correlated the genetic constitution expressed by genotypes of the G135C polymorphism with susceptibility to DNA damage and efficacy of DNA repair in human lymphocytes of gastric cancer patients (Poplawski, Arabski et al. 2006). The results of this study suggest that the variants of the G135C polymorphism of the *RAD51* gene can be associated with the occurrence of gastric cancer in individuals with a high level of oxidative DNA damage or impaired repair of such damage, which can be a consequence of another genetic variation or/and environmental factor(s). Therefore, this polymorphism can be considered as an additional marker in gastric cancer. However, this study had mainly preliminary character and further research, performed on a larger group, is needed to establish a correlation between gastric cancer and the G/C polymorphism of the *RAD51* gene (Poplawski, Arabski et al. 2006).

It is known that in humans, inherited defects in HR pathways are known to predispose to acute myeloid leukaemia (AML), an example of this, Fanconi anemia (FA) (Bogliolo, Cabre et al. 2002) is characterized by spontaneous and mutagen-induced chromosome instability. Recently BRCA2, was identified as an FA protein, linking this pathway to HR through the interaction of BRCA2 with *RAD51* (Godthelp, Artwert et al. 2002). There is a study that highlights the importance of the link between *RAD51*, BRCA1, BRCA2 and a risk for AML. An increased risk for AML has been noted in patients previously diagnosed with breast cancer (Pagano, Pulsoni et al. 2001) . Rollinson *et al.* (Rollinson, Smith et al. 2007) observed a protective effect for the *RAD51 135–172 C–G* haplotype suggesting that it may be associated with increased RAD51 expression, modulating HR and protecting the cells against aberrant DNA repair events, thus reducing the risk of AML.

Therapy-related acute myeloid leukemia (t-AML) is a devastating complication of chemotherapy and/or radiotherapy for a primary cancer. The risk of the development of t-AML was found to be associated with the G-to-C polymorphism at –135 of the 5' untranslated region (135G/C-5'UTR) of *RAD51* (Seedhouse and Russell 2007). The promoter activity of the *RAD51* gene is enhanced by the G-to-C substitution (135G/C-5'UTR), resulting in high levels of RAD51 expression in individuals with the variation. *RAD51's* role in t-AML was also supported by an indirect finding that *RAD51* was upregulated in mismatch repair-deficient murine embryonic stem cells. This process can be recapitulated by treatment with alkylating agents. Mismatch repair deficiency has been proposed to play an early role in therapy-related carcinogenesis. These data indicate that high levels of RAD51 not only confer resistance to DNA-damaging agents but also contribute to the development of therapy-related cancers (Miyagawa 2008).

We previously reported a study evaluating the prognostic and predictive role of *RAD51* G135C polymorphism in non-small lung cancer (NSCLC) patients treated with combined platinum taxanes/gemcitabine first line chemotherapy (Nogueira, Catarino et al. 2009). In this study, our results demonstrated that the C allele is associated with a higher survival time, conferring a better prognosis than the GG genotype carrier patients. Thus, individuals carrying the C allele showed a longer overall survival after chemotherapy, compared with individuals carrying the allele G. This study also indicates that the influence of *RAD51* G135C polymorphism in treatment response of NSCLC patients seems to be modulated by smoking history. Our results demonstrate that smoker or ex-smoker patients carriers of *RAD51 135*C allele present a higher mean overall survival time (Nogueira, Catarino et al. 2009). According to the results obtained, we believe that *RAD51* genotypes could be useful molecular markers for predicting the clinical outcome of NSCLC patients.

The following table shows the main characteristics of some association studies between polymorphisms in the *RAD51* gene and risk for cancer (table 2).

6. Conclusion

New factors and pathways with the ability to recognize and repair DSBs are being discovered and studied. DSB production is now recognized as a general occurrence in cells, and these lesions frequently arise through endogenous and exogenous events. As a consequence of evolution from prokaryotes to eukaryotes, cells have developed complex mechanisms which can recognize and repair this type of severe damage rapidly and correctly. Cells have been exposed to many types of environmental stresses, and these stresses can sometimes lead to sub-lethal damage. In order to survive and function under adverse conditions, it is necessary to repair or eliminate DNA damage, and as a consequence, cells have developed a number of complex repair systems to enable their survival and functioning. Knowledge and understanding of these complex systems will make contributions to biology and medicine (Ohnishi, Mori et al. 2009).

A recent series of findings established a connection between apoptosis, HR regulation and tumorigenesis. Regulation of RAD51 activity appears to be essential in these regulation networks. It is questionable whether other kinases or signalling processes can affect RAD51 regulation. These data should enhance understanding of the general mechanisms

Authors	RAD51 SNP	Tumoral model	Population (case/control)	Ethnicity	Genotyping methods	Results
Synowiec et al. (2008)	5' UTR G135C	Breast cancer	41/48	European	PCR-RFLP	Polymorphism was not an independent marker in breast cancer, but it could be associated with an increased breast cancer risk in BRCA2 mutation carriers
Costa et al. (2007)	5' UTR G135C	Breast cancer	285/442	European	PCR-RFLP	Association of RAD51 135C allele and increased breast cancer risk only among women with family history of breast cancer. No association for sporadic breast cancer risk
Kadouri et al. (2001)	5' UTR G135C	Breast cancer	309/152	Jewish	PCR-RFLP	Elevated risk for breast cancer in carriers of BRCA2 mutations who also carry a 135 C allele. No association for BRCA1 carriers. No association for BRCA1 non-carriers
Jara et al. (2007)	5' UTR G135C	Breast cancer	143/ 247	South American	PCR-RFLP	Increased risk of familial breast cancer in women with age < 50 years at diagnosis
Blasiak et al. (2003)	5' UTR G135C	Breast cancer	46/60	European	PCR-RFLP	No association between the polymorphism and appearance and progression of breast cancer

Jakubowska et al. (2007)	5′ UTR G135C	Breast and ovarian cancer	485/485	European	PCR-RFLP	Women who harbour the C allele have almost twice the reduction in breast cancer risk and ovarian cancer risk compared with women who harbour the G allele
Wang et al. (2001)	5′ UTR G135C	Breast and ovarian cancer	317/263	Mixed	PCR-RFLP	Increased risk of breast cancer and a lower risk of ovarian cancer for cases with a BRCA2 mutation. No association in cases with a BRCA1 mutation
Nogueira et al. (2009)	5′ UTR G135C	Non-small lung cancer	234/-	European	PCR-RFLP	C allele associated with a higher survival time. Smoker or ex-smoker patients carrying RAD51 135C allele presented a higher mean overall survival time, but this association was not observed in non-smoker patients
Pagano et al. (2001)	5′ UTR G135C 5′ UTR G172T	Acute myeloid leukaemia	3934/-	European	PCR-RFLP	Increased risk for AML in patients previously diagnosed with breast cancer. Protective effect for the RAD51 135-172 C-G haplotype.

| Rollinson et al. (2007) | 5' UTR G135C 5' UTR G172T | Acute myeloid leukaemia | 479/952 | European | Real-Time PCR | Protective effect for the RAD51 135-172 C-G haplotype, reducing the risk of AML. |
| Poplawski et al.(2006) | 5' UTR G135C | Gastric cancer | 30/30 | European | PCR-RFLP | The variants of the G135C polymorphism can be associated with the occurrence of gastric cancer in individuals with a high level of oxidative DNA damage or impaired repair of such damage. |

Table 2. Main characteristics of some studies included in this review

controlling genome stability, their connections with cell cycle control, apoptosis regulation and more generally predisposition to tumour development (Daboussi, Dumay et al. 2002). Most of case-control studies searching for the contribution of genetic alterations within DNA repair genes to susceptibility to radiation-related cancer have been focused on genes involved in HR. Additional efforts are needed to find novel genetic variants of DNA repair genes involved in HR that confer susceptibility to radiation-induced cancer as well as to confirm already discovered disease-associated variants. To date, significant advances have been achieved in evaluating the role of genetic variations within DNA repair genes in clinical radiosensitivity in cancer. RAD51 gene polymorphisms have been suggested to be associated with radiosensitivity in cancer (Chistiakov, Voronova et al. 2008).

Recently, several national and international clinical research projects have been initiated to find markers of genetic predisposition to radiation-induced cancer and clinical radiosensitivity in tumour tissues. However, over the next few years, a considerable molecular characterization of large-scale cohorts of individuals who show therapeutic radiation sensitivity is likely to be achieved. The construction and use of genetic-risk profiles may provide significant improvements in the efficacy of population-based programs of intervention for cancers. This also should help in predicting radiosensitivity that will eventually allow individual tailoring of treatment and reduce the risk of developing acute reactions in anticancer radiotherapy (Kuhne, Riballo et al. 2004; Chistiakov, Voronova et al. 2008).

7. Acknowledgment

The authors thank the Portuguese League Against Cancer (LPCC-NRNorte) for their support.

8. References

Antoniou, A. C., O. M. Sinilnikova, et al. (2007). "RAD51 135G-->C modifies breast cancer risk among BRCA2 mutation carriers: results from a combined analysis of 19 studies." *Am J Hum Genet* 81(6): 1186-200.

Arias-Lopez, C., I. Lazaro-Trueba, et al. (2006). "p53 modulates homologous recombination by transcriptional regulation of the RAD51 gene." *EMBO Rep* 7(2): 219-24.

Arnaudeau, C., T. Helleday, et al. (1999). "The RAD51 protein supports homologous recombination by an exchange mechanism in mammalian cells." *J Mol Biol* 289(5): 1231-8.

Arnaudeau, C., C. Lundin, et al. (2001). "DNA double-strand breaks associated with replication forks are predominantly repaired by homologous recombination involving an exchange mechanism in mammalian cells." *J Mol Biol* 307(5): 1235-45.

Au, W. W., S. A. Salama, et al. (2003). "Functional characterization of polymorphisms in DNA repair genes using cytogenetic challenge assays." *Environ Health Perspect* 111(15): 1843-50.

Benson, F. E., P. Baumann, et al. (1998). "Synergistic actions of Rad51 and Rad52 in recombination and DNA repair." *Nature* 391(6665): 401-4.

Blasiak, J., K. Przybylowska, et al. (2003). "Analysis of the G/C polymorphism in the 5'-untranslated region of the RAD51 gene in breast cancer." *Acta Biochim Pol* 50(1): 249-53.

Bogliolo, M., O. Cabre, et al. (2002). "The Fanconi anaemia genome stability and tumour suppressor network." *Mutagenesis* 17(6): 529-38.

Brookes, A. J. (1999). "The essence of SNPs." *Gene* 234(2): 177-86.

Buchhop, S., M. K. Gibson, et al. (1997). "Interaction of p53 with the human Rad51 protein." *Nucleic Acids Res* 25(19): 3868-74.

Chistiakov, D. A., N. V. Voronova, et al. (2008). "Genetic variations in DNA repair genes, radiosensitivity to cancer and susceptibility to acute tissue reactions in radiotherapy-treated cancer patients." *Acta Oncol* 47(5): 809-24.

Costa, S., D. Pinto, et al. (2007). "DNA repair polymorphisms might contribute differentially on familial and sporadic breast cancer susceptibility: a study on a Portuguese population." *Breast Cancer Res Treat* 103(2): 209-17.

Daboussi, F., A. Dumay, et al. (2002). "DNA double-strand break repair signalling: the case of RAD51 post-translational regulation." *Cell Signal* 14(12): 969-75.

Dasika, G. K., S. C. Lin, et al. (1999). "DNA damage-induced cell cycle checkpoints and DNA strand break repair in development and tumorigenesis." *Oncogene* 18(55): 7883-99.

Dufloth, R. M., S. Costa, et al. (2005). "DNA repair gene polymorphisms and susceptibility to familial breast cancer in a group of patients from Campinas, Brazil." *Genet Mol Res* 4(4): 771-82.

Flygare, J., F. Benson, et al. (1996). "Expression of the human RAD51 gene during the cell cycle in primary human peripheral blood lymphocytes." *Biochim Biophys Acta* 1312(3): 231-6.

Flygare, J., S. Falt, et al. (2001). "Effects of HsRad51 overexpression on cell proliferation, cell cycle progression, and apoptosis." *Exp Cell Res* 268(1): 61-9.

Galkin, V. E., F. Esashi, et al. (2005). "BRCA2 BRC motifs bind RAD51-DNA filaments." *Proc Natl Acad Sci U S A* 102(24): 8537-42.

Galli, F., M. Piroddi, et al. (2005). "Oxidative stress and reactive oxygen species." *Contrib Nephrol* 149: 240-60.

Godthelp, B. C., F. Artwert, et al. (2002). "Impaired DNA damage-induced nuclear Rad51 foci formation uniquely characterizes Fanconi anemia group D1." *Oncogene* 21(32): 5002-5.

Gray, N. K. (1998). "Translational control by repressor proteins binding to the 5'UTR of mRNAs." *Methods Mol Biol* 77: 379-97.

Haaf, T., E. I. Golub, et al. (1995). "Nuclear foci of mammalian Rad51 recombination protein in somatic cells after DNA damage and its localization in synaptonemal complexes." *Proc Natl Acad Sci U S A* 92(6): 2298-302.

Hansen, L. T., C. Lundin, et al. (2003). "The role of RAD51 in etoposide (VP16) resistance in small cell lung cancer." *Int J Cancer* 105(4): 472-9.

Hasselbach, L., S. Haase, et al. (2005). "Characterisation of the promoter region of the human DNA-repair gene Rad51." *Eur J Gynaecol Oncol* 26(6): 589-98.

Helleday, T., J. Lo, et al. (2007). "DNA double-strand break repair: from mechanistic understanding to cancer treatment." *DNA Repair (Amst)* 6(7): 923-35.

Henning, W. and H. W. Sturzbecher (2003). "Homologous recombination and cell cycle checkpoints: Rad51 in tumour progression and therapy resistance." *Toxicology* 193(1-2): 91-109.

Henson, S. E., S. C. Tsai, et al. (2006). "Pir51, a Rad51-interacting protein with high expression in aggressive lymphoma, controls mitomycin C sensitivity and prevents chromosomal breaks." *Mutat Res* 601(1-2): 113-24.

Hoeijmakers, J. H. (2001). "Genome maintenance mechanisms for preventing cancer." *Nature* 411(6835): 366-74.

Hu, J. J., H. W. Mohrenweiser, et al. (2002). "Symposium overview: genetic polymorphisms in DNA repair and cancer risk." *Toxicol Appl Pharmacol* 185(1): 64-73.

Hung, R. J., J. Hall, et al. (2005). "Genetic polymorphisms in the base excision repair pathway and cancer risk: a HuGE review." *Am J Epidemiol* 162(10): 925-42.

Jakubowska, A., J. Gronwald, et al. (2007). "The RAD51 135 G>C polymorphism modifies breast cancer and ovarian cancer risk in Polish BRCA1 mutation carriers." *Cancer Epidemiol Biomarkers Prev* 16(2): 270-5.

Jakubowska, A., S. A. Narod, et al. (2003). "Breast cancer risk reduction associated with the RAD51 polymorphism among carriers of the BRCA1 5382insC mutation in Poland." *Cancer Epidemiol Biomarkers Prev* 12(5): 457-9.

Jara, L., M. L. Acevedo, et al. (2007). "RAD51 135G>C polymorphism and risk of familial breast cancer in a South American population." *Cancer Genet Cytogenet* 178(1): 65-9.

Johnson, L. F. (1992). "G1 events and the regulation of genes for S-phase enzymes." *Curr Opin Cell Biol* 4(2): 149-54.

Kadouri, L., D. F. Easton, et al. (2001). "CAG and GGC repeat polymorphisms in the androgen receptor gene and breast cancer susceptibility in BRCA1/2 carriers and non-carriers." *Br J Cancer* 85(1): 36-40.

Khanna, K. K. and S. P. Jackson (2001). "DNA double-strand breaks: signaling, repair and the cancer connection." *Nat Genet* 27(3): 247-54.

Klein, H. L. (2008). "The consequences of Rad51 overexpression for normal and tumor cells." *DNA Repair (Amst)* 7(5): 686-93.

Knudsen, L. E., S. H. Loft, et al. (2001). "Risk assessment: the importance of genetic polymorphisms in man." *Mutat Res* 482(1-2): 83-8.

Kuhne, M., E. Riballo, et al. (2004). "A double-strand break repair defect in ATM-deficient cells contributes to radiosensitivity." *Cancer Res* 64(2): 500-8.

Kuschel, B., A. Auranen, et al. (2002). "Variants in DNA double-strand break repair genes and breast cancer susceptibility." *Hum Mol Genet* 11(12): 1399-407.

Kuzminov, A. (1999). "Recombinational repair of DNA damage in Escherichia coli and bacteriophage lambda." *Microbiol Mol Biol Rev* 63(4): 751-813, table of contents.

Lambert, S. and B. S. Lopez (2000). "Characterization of mammalian RAD51 double strand break repair using non-lethal dominant-negative forms." *Embo J* 19(12): 3090-9.

Lambert, S. and B. S. Lopez (2001). "Role of RAD51 in sister-chromatid exchanges in mammalian cells." *Oncogene* 20(45): 6627-31.

Lander, E. S., L. M. Linton, et al. (2001). "Initial sequencing and analysis of the human genome." *Nature* 409(6822): 860-921.

Levine, A. J. (1997). "p53, the cellular gatekeeper for growth and division." *Cell* 88(3): 323-31.

Levy-Lahad, E., A. Lahad, et al. (2001). "A single nucleotide polymorphism in the RAD51 gene modifies cancer risk in BRCA2 but not BRCA1 carriers." *Proc Natl Acad Sci U S A* 98(6): 3232-6.

Li, X. and W. D. Heyer (2008). "Homologous recombination in DNA repair and DNA damage tolerance." *Cell Res* 18(1): 99-113.

Lin, F. L., K. Sperle, et al. (1984). "Homologous recombination in mouse L cells." *Cold Spring Harb Symp Quant Biol* 49: 139-49.

Lin, F. L., K. Sperle, et al. (1984). "Model for homologous recombination during transfer of DNA into mouse L cells: role for DNA ends in the recombination process." *Mol Cell Biol* 4(6): 1020-34.

Linke, S. P., S. Sengupta, et al. (2003). "p53 interacts with hRAD51 and hRAD54, and directly modulates homologous recombination." *Cancer Res* 63(10): 2596-605.

Liu, N., J. E. Lamerdin, et al. (1998). "XRCC2 and XRCC3, new human Rad51-family members, promote chromosome stability and protect against DNA cross-links and other damages." *Mol Cell* 1(6): 783-93.

Liu, Y. and N. Maizels (2000). "Coordinated response of mammalian Rad51 and Rad52 to DNA damage." *EMBO Rep* 1(1): 85-90.

Lundin, C., N. Schultz, et al. (2003). "RAD51 is involved in repair of damage associated with DNA replication in mammalian cells." *J Mol Biol* 328(3): 521-35.

Maacke, H., K. Jost, et al. (2000). "DNA repair and recombination factor Rad51 is over-expressed in human pancreatic adenocarcinoma." *Oncogene* 19(23): 2791-5.

Maacke, H., S. Opitz, et al. (2000). "Over-expression of wild-type Rad51 correlates with histological grading of invasive ductal breast cancer." *Int J Cancer* 88(6): 907-13.

Magnusson, K. P., M. Sandstrom, et al. (2000). "p53 splice acceptor site mutation and increased HsRAD51 protein expression in Bloom's syndrome GM1492 fibroblasts." *Gene* 246(1-2): 247-54.

Martin, J. S., N. Winkelmann, et al. (2005). "RAD-51-dependent and -independent roles of a Caenorhabditis elegans BRCA2-related protein during DNA double-strand break repair." *Mol Cell Biol* 25(8): 3127-39.

Martinez, S. L., J. Herzog, et al. (2004). "Loss of five amino acids in BRCA2 is associated with ovarian cancer." *J Med Genet* 41(2): e18.

Michel, B., G. Grompone, et al. (2004). "Multiple pathways process stalled replication forks." *Proc Natl Acad Sci U S A* 101(35): 12783-8.

Miyagawa, K. (2008). "Clinical relevance of the homologous recombination machinery in cancer therapy." *Cancer Sci* 99(2): 187-94.

Moynahan, M. E., A. J. Pierce, et al. (2001). "BRCA2 is required for homology-directed repair of chromosomal breaks." *Mol Cell* 7(2): 263-72.

Nogueira, A., R. Catarino, et al. (2009). "Influence of DNA repair RAD51 gene variants in overall survival of non-small cell lung cancer patients treated with first line chemotherapy." *Cancer Chemother Pharmacol.*

Ohnishi, T., E. Mori, et al. (2009). "DNA double-strand breaks: their production, recognition, and repair in eukaryotes." *Mutat Res* 669(1-2): 8-12.

Ohnishi, T., T. Taki, et al. (1998). "In vitro and in vivo potentiation of radiosensitivity of malignant gliomas by antisense inhibition of the RAD51 gene." *Biochem Biophys Res Commun* 245(2): 319-24.

Orre, L. M., S. Falt, et al. (2006). "Rad51-related changes in global gene expression." *Biochem Biophys Res Commun* 341(2): 334-42.

Pagano, L., A. Pulsoni, et al. (2001). "Acute myeloid leukemia in patients previously diagnosed with breast cancer: experience of the GIMEMA group." *Ann Oncol* 12(2): 203-7.

Paques, F. and J. E. Haber (1999). "Multiple pathways of recombination induced by double-strand breaks in Saccharomyces cerevisiae." *Microbiol Mol Biol Rev* 63(2): 349-404.

Patel, K. J., V. P. Yu, et al. (1998). "Involvement of Brca2 in DNA repair." *Mol Cell* 1(3): 347-57.

Pauklin, S., A. Kristjuhan, et al. (2005). "ARF and ATM/ATR cooperate in p53-mediated apoptosis upon oncogenic stress." *Biochem Biophys Res Commun* 334(2): 386-94.

Poplawski, T., M. Arabski, et al. (2006). "DNA damage and repair in gastric cancer--a correlation with the hOGG1 and RAD51 genes polymorphisms." *Mutat Res* 601(1-2): 83-91.

Powell, S. N., H. Willers, et al. (2002). "BRCA2 keeps Rad51 in line. High-fidelity homologous recombination prevents breast and ovarian cancer?" *Mol Cell* 10(6): 1262-3.

Qiao, G. B., Y. L. Wu, et al. (2005). "High-level expression of Rad51 is an independent prognostic marker of survival in non-small-cell lung cancer patients." *Br J Cancer* 93(1): 137-43.

Qiao, Y., M. R. Spitz, et al. (2002). "Modulation of repair of ultraviolet damage in the host-cell reactivation assay by polymorphic XPC and XPD/ERCC2 genotypes." *Carcinogenesis* 23(2): 295-9.

Raderschall, E., K. Stout, et al. (2002). "Elevated levels of Rad51 recombination protein in tumor cells." *Cancer Res* 62(1): 219-25.

Risch, N. J. (2000). "Searching for genetic determinants in the new millennium." *Nature* 405(6788): 847-56.

Rollinson, S., A. G. Smith, et al. (2007). "RAD51 homologous recombination repair gene haplotypes and risk of acute myeloid leukaemia." *Leuk Res* 31(2): 169-74.

Saintigny, Y., F. Delacote, et al. (2001). "Characterization of homologous recombination induced by replication inhibition in mammalian cells." *Embo J* 20(14): 3861-70.

San Filippo, J., P. Sung, et al. (2008). "Mechanism of eukaryotic homologous recombination." *Annu Rev Biochem* 77: 229-57.

Schmutte, C., G. Tombline, et al. (1999). "Characterization of the human Rad51 genomic locus and examination of tumors with 15q14-15 loss of heterozygosity (LOH)." *Cancer Res* 59(18): 4564-9.

Seedhouse, C. and N. Russell (2007). "Advances in the understanding of susceptibility to treatment-related acute myeloid leukaemia." *Br J Haematol* 137(6): 513-29.

Sliwinski, T., R. Krupa, et al. (2005). "Polymorphisms of the BRCA2 and RAD51 genes in breast cancer." *Breast Cancer Res Treat* 94(2): 105-9.

Slupianek, A., G. Hoser, et al. (2002). "Fusion tyrosine kinases induce drug resistance by stimulation of homology-dependent recombination repair, prolongation of G(2)/M phase, and protection from apoptosis." *Mol Cell Biol* 22(12): 4189-201.

Slupianek, A., C. Schmutte, et al. (2001). "BCR/ABL regulates mammalian RecA homologs, resulting in drug resistance." *Mol Cell* 8(4): 795-806.

Smith, G. C. and S. P. Jackson (1999). "The DNA-dependent protein kinase." *Genes Dev* 13(8): 916-34.

Sonoda, E., M. S. Sasaki, et al. (1998). "Rad51-deficient vertebrate cells accumulate chromosomal breaks prior to cell death." *Embo J* 17(2): 598-608.

Sung, P. and H. Klein (2006). "Mechanism of homologous recombination: mediators and helicases take on regulatory functions." *Nat Rev Mol Cell Biol* 7(10): 739-50.

Synowiec, E., J. Stefanska, et al. (2008). "Association between DNA damage, DNA repair genes variability and clinical characteristics in breast cancer patients." *Mutat Res* 648(1-2): 65-72.

Szostak, J. W., T. L. Orr-Weaver, et al. (1983). "The double-strand-break repair model for recombination." *Cell* 33(1): 25-35.

Takahashi, E., Y. Matsuda, et al. (1994). "Chromosome mapping of the human (RECA) and mouse (Reca) homologs of the yeast RAD51 and Escherichia coli recA genes to human (15q15.1) and mouse (2F1) chromosomes by direct R-banding fluorescence in situ hybridization." *Genomics* 19(2): 376-8.

Tashiro, S., N. Kotomura, et al. (1996). "S phase specific formation of the human Rad51 protein nuclear foci in lymphocytes." *Oncogene* 12(10): 2165-70.

Tutt, A., D. Bertwistle, et al. (2001). "Mutation in Brca2 stimulates error-prone homology-directed repair of DNA double-strand breaks occurring between repeated sequences." *Embo J* 20(17): 4704-16.

Venkitaraman, A. R. (2002). "Cancer susceptibility and the functions of BRCA1 and BRCA2." *Cell* 108(2): 171-82.

Venter, J. C., M. D. Adams, et al. (2001). "The sequence of the human genome." *Science* 291(5507): 1304-51.

Vispe, S., C. Cazaux, et al. (1998). "Overexpression of Rad51 protein stimulates homologous recombination and increases resistance of mammalian cells to ionizing radiation." *Nucleic Acids Res* 26(12): 2859-64.

Wang, W. W., A. B. Spurdle, et al. (2001). "A single nucleotide polymorphism in the 5' untranslated region of RAD51 and risk of cancer among BRCA1/2 mutation carriers." *Cancer Epidemiol Biomarkers Prev* 10(9): 955-60.

Webb, P. M., J. L. Hopper, et al. (2005). "Double-strand break repair gene polymorphisms and risk of breast or ovarian cancer." *Cancer Epidemiol Biomarkers Prev* 14(2): 319-23.

Wick, W., I. Petersen, et al. (1996). "Evidence for a novel tumor suppressor gene on chromosome 15 associated with progression to a metastatic stage in breast cancer." *Oncogene* 12(5): 973-8.

Xia, S. J., M. A. Shammas, et al. (1997). "Elevated recombination in immortal human cells is mediated by HsRAD51 recombinase." *Mol Cell Biol* 17(12): 7151-8.

Yamamoto, A., T. Taki, et al. (1996). "Cell cycle-dependent expression of the mouse Rad51 gene in proliferating cells." *Mol Gen Genet* 251(1): 1-12.

Yanez, R. J. and A. C. Porter (1999). "Gene targeting is enhanced in human cells overexpressing hRAD51." *Gene Ther* 6(7): 1282-90.

Yuan, S. S., S. Y. Lee, et al. (1999). "BRCA2 is required for ionizing radiation-induced assembly of Rad51 complex in vivo." *Cancer Res* 59(15): 3547-51.

3

Double Strand Break Signaling in Health and Diseases

Marie-jo Halaby and Razqallah Hakem
The Ontario Cancer Institute
Canada

1. Introduction

Living organisms are constantly subjected to DNA damage whether it originates from intrinsic physiological processes or extrinsic stressors. Of the various types of DNA damage, double strand breaks (DSBs) are the most dangerous since if left unrepaired they can lead to either cell death or genomic instability. For this reason cells have evolved an arsenal of signaling and repair proteins involved in DNA double strand break sensing and repair as well as downstream physiological responses such as apoptosis or cell cycle arrest. DSBs can be generated by reactive oxygen species which are produced during normal metabolism. DSB formation and repair also occurs during the tightly regulated physiological processes of gametogenesis, V(D)J recombination of T- and B-cell receptors and antibody diversification during class switch recombination (CSR). In addition, DSBs can be caused by external agents such as ionizing radiation or chemotherapeutic agents such as etoposide. The importance of DSB signaling and repair is underscored by the many human diseases and syndromes caused by the mutation of genes coding for DNA damage response (DDR) proteins. The study of knockout mouse models for DDR genes has also furthered our understanding of the role of these proteins in DSB repair and in normal physiology. In this chapter, DSB signaling and repair are reviewed. In addition, an overview of the human diseases associated with mutations of DSB signaling and repair proteins is given. Finally, the impact of mouse models on our understanding of DSB signaling and repair and its physiological roles is discussed.

2. Signaling at DNA double strand breaks

2.1 Sensing the DNA double strand breaks

When DSBs are generated they are initially recognized by either the Ku70/Ku80 heterodimer, the Mre11-Rad50-NBS1 (MRN) complex or members of the PARP (PARP1/2) family of proteins (Ciccia & Elledge, 2010). The role of these protein sensors is to bind to and tether the DNA ends, thereby preventing further breakage as well as to recruit additional proteins that are required for DSB signaling and repair. The first group of proteins to be recruited to DSBs after initial sensing of the breaks belongs to the phosphatidylinositol-3-kinase-like protein kinases family. These include ATM (ataxia-telangiectasia mutated), ATR (ATM and Rad3-related) and the catalytic subunit of DNA-PK known as DNA-PKcs. While ATM and DNA-PK respond only to DSBs, ATR also responds to single strand DNA breaks.

Ku70/80 recruits DNA-PKcs to DSBs where it promotes DNA repair by non-homologous end joining whereas both PARP1/2 and the MRN complex lead to the recruitment of ATM which promotes homologous recombination. The MRN complex is recruited to DSBs in both a PARP1/2 dependent and independent manner (Ciccia & Elledge, 2010). ATM is a central component of the cellular response to DSBs and is predicted to have several hundred downstream targets many of which play a role in the DNA damage response (Matsuoka et al, 2007). Under normal conditions ATM is in a homodimeric form. Following DNA damage, it becomes autophosphorylated at Ser1981 and dissociates into its monomeric form and binds the damaged DNA (Bakkenist & Kastan, 2003). There, it leads to the phosphorylation of many downstream targets involved in the DSB response. The phosphorylation of ATM at Ser1981 and its initial binding to DSBs depend upon the MRN complex. MRN consists of three different proteins Mre11, NBS1 and Rad50. Mre11 is a DNA nuclease that interacts with both Rad50 and NBS1 as well as with other Mre11 molecules to form dimers. When paired with the other components of the MRN complex, Mre11 can have both double strand DNA exonuclease activity and single strand DNA endonuclease activity (D'Amours & Jackson, 2002). In addition, Mre11 has two DNA binding sites and intrinsic DNA binding activity. Rad50 is a protein that bears homology to the structural maintenance of chromosome (SMC) family. It is an ATPase and is needed for tethering of DNA ends together during the process of DNA repair. NBS1 has a fork-head-associated (FHA) domain and two BRCT (BRCA1-tandem repeats) domains at its N-terminus which are used to recognize phospho-threonine and phospho-serine residues respectively in Ser-X-Thr motifs. These domains allow RAD50 to interact with several DNA damage signaling proteins following DSB formation. NBS1 also contains a nuclear localization signal (NLS) that allows the translocation of the MRN complex into the nucleus following DNA damage (Lamarche et al, 2010). NBS1 interacts with ATM thereby leading to its recruitment to DSBs. There, ATM is involved in one of the very early response to the formation of DSBs, mainly the phosphorylation of histone variant H2AX on Ser139 to form γ-H2AX (Figure 1). This phosphorylation can extend over a megabase of DNA from the site of DSBs (Modesti & Kanaar, 2001). The formation of γ-H2AX at the sites of DSBs is key for the recruitment of many effector proteins to the break sites including the regulators of cell cycle checkpoint and DNA repair 53BP1, BRCA1 and Rad51 (Bohgaki et al, 2010). The accumulation of γ-H2AX and other DNA damage signaling and repair proteins at the sites of ionizing-radiation induced breaks leads to the formation of microscopically distinct foci known as IR-induced nuclear foci (IRIFs) which can be used experimentally to study IR-induced DNA damage signaling and repair. The ability of H2AX to recruit DNA damage proteins under normal physiological conditions is hampered by its constitutive phosphorylation at Tyr142 by William's syndrome transcription factor (WSTF). This phosphorylation suppresses the ability of H2AX to recruit downstream signaling and effectors of the DNA damage response to the breaks. However, following DNA damage Tyr142 residue is dephosphorylated by the EYA protein phosphatases (Cook et al, 2009). γ-H2AX recruits MDC1, a mediator of the DNA damage response that functions as an adaptor to recruit downstream effector proteins to the break sites. MDC1 has two BRCT domains at its C-terminus and one FHA domain at its N-terminus that allow it to recognize and interact with other DNA damage response proteins (Stewart et al, 2003). The BRCT domains of MDC1 can recognize phosphorylation sites and were shown to mediate MDC1 binding to γ-H2AX.

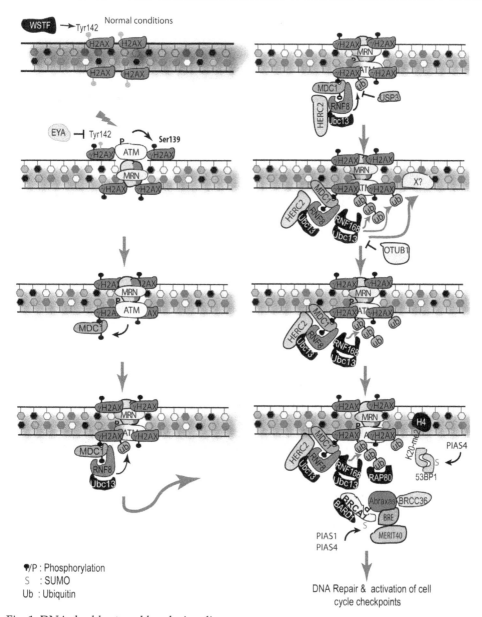

**/P : Phosphorylation
S : SUMO
Ub : Ubiquitin

Fig. 1. DNA double strand break signaling

This interaction occurs specifically between the BRCT domain of MDC1 and the Ser139 phosphoylation site of γ-H2AX located at the C-terminus of this protein. MDC1 also interacts with ATM and is phosphorylated by it at its FHA domain (Goldberg et al, 2003; Stewart et al, 2003). Four potential consensus TQFX sites for ATM phosphorylation have been found and two sites, T719 and T752, were confirmed to be phosphorylated by ATM

(Kolas et al, 2007; Matsuoka et al, 2007). MDC1 is thought to be dispensable for the initial binding of ATM to the DSBs and early H2AX phosphorylation but important for ATM and γ-H2AX retention at the damaged DNA sites. In fact, MDC1 acts in a positive feedback loop with γ-H2AX and ATM to amplify the signal at the breaks (Lou et al, 2006). MDC1 was also found to be important for the recruitment of other DNA damage response proteins such as 53BP1 and NBS1 to the break sites. Recent studies have provided us with greater insight about the mechanisms by which MDC1 leads to the recruitment of DNA damage proteins to the DSBs and have highlighted the role of posttranslational modifications such as ubiquitylation and sumoylation in the amplification of the DNA damage response.

2.2 Role of ubiquitylation in the DNA double strand break response
The important role ubiquitylation plays in DNA damage signaling and DNA repair has been recently highlighted (Bohgaki et al, 2010; Panier & Durocher, 2009). Ubiquitin is a small polypeptide of about 8 KDa that can be covalently attached through an isopeptide bond to substrate proteins. This requires the activity of three different enzymes, a ubiquitin-activating enzyme (E1), a ubiquitin conjugating enzyme (E2) and a ubiquitin ligase (E3). The combination of E2 and E3 enzymes used to ubiquitylate target proteins differ from one to the other thereby conferring substrate specificity to the enzyme. Ubiquitin chain attachment can occur through several lysine residues on the ubiquitin polypeptide. The best studied ones are lysine 48 (K48) and lysine 63 (K63). While K48-linked ubiquitin most often leads to proteasomal degradation, K63-linked ubiquitylation is involved in cellular signaling including DSB signaling and DNA repair. Using an siRNA screen for proteins whose absence lead to an impairment of 53BP1 foci formation it was found that knock-down of MDC1 and the E3 ubiquitin ligase RNF8 (Ring Finger protein 8) strongly inhibited 53BP1 recruitment to DSBs (Kolas et al, 2007). RNF8 has a RING domain which is required for its E3 ligase activity and is located at its C-terminus and an FHA domain located at its N-terminus. The FHA domain of RNF8 can recognize phosphorylated MDC1 thereby allowing binding of RNF8 to MDC1. Therefore, MDC1 phosphorylation is required for formation of RNF8 IRIFs. Furthermore, it was found that RNF8 partners up with the E2 ligase UBC13 to mediate K63-linked ubiquitylation of H2A, H2AX and H2B (Huen et al, 2007; Kolas et al, 2007; Mailand et al, 2007). This initial ubiquitylation of chromatin components leads to the recruitment of another ubiquitin ligase RNF168 (Doil et al, 2009; Stewart et al, 2009). RNF168 contains two motifs interacting with ubiquitin (MIUs) and is thought to interact with ubiquitylated chromatin components through its MIUs. At the DNA breaks, RNF168, in collaboration with the E2 ligase UBC13, adds K63-linked polybiquitin chains to H2A and H2AX. This ultimately results in the subsequent recruitment of other DDR proteins to the break sites. For example, RNF168 is required for the formation of 53BP1 IRIFs and the recruitment of BRCA1 to DSB site is severely reduced in the absence of this E3 ligase (Bohgaki et al, 2011; Doil et al, 2009; Stewart et al, 2009). HERC2 is a recently identified protein that leads to binding and stabilization of the RNF8-UBC13 complex to mediate K63-linked histone ubiquitylation (Bekker-Jensen et al, 2010). Additionally, HERC2 was also found to stabilize RNF168 and to promote recruitment of DSB signaling proteins including 53BP1 and BRCA1 to the break sites. The mechanisms through which chromatin component ubiquitylation leads to the recruitment of 53BP1 and BRCA1 are only partially understood. BRCA1 interacts with the receptor-associated protein 80 (RAP80). RAP80 recruitment to DSBs is dependent on γ-H2AX, MDC1 and RNF8 (Kim et al, 2007; Kolas et al, 2007; Mailand

et al, 2007). RAP80 contains two ubiquitin interacting motifs (UIMs) which are capable of specifically recognizing K-63 linked polybiquitin chains (Kim et al, 2007). The interaction of RAP80 and BRCA1 is mediated by another protein named Abraxas (Mailand et al, 2007; Wang et al, 2007). The RAP80-Abraxas-BRCA1 complex is thought to bind DSB sites through the recognition of RNF8- and RNF168-ubiquitylated chromatin by the RAP80 UIM domains (Wang et al, 2007). The way 53BP1 is recruited to the break sites is less well understood. 53BP1 recruitment to DSBs is mediated by the binding of its two TUDOR domains to di-methylated histone H4 at lysine (K) 20. Histone methylation is not increased from its constitutive level following ionizing radiation suggesting that changes in chromatin structure following DNA damage might be responsible for the uncovering of the methylated histones and the binding of 53BP1. It is therefore plausible that ubiquitylation of H2A and H2B by RNF8 and RNF168 triggers conformational changes in the chromatin that lead to a better accessibility of 53BP1 to the methylated histones (Mailand et al, 2007). However, this hypothesis still remains to be tested. The ubiquitylation of chromatin components leads to the rapid amplification of the DNA damage response. However, once the DNA is repaired, a rapid deubiquitination of histone H2A, H2B and H2AX should occur to return cells to their steady-state levels. This is accomplished by ubiquitin isopeptidases known as deubiquitinating enzymes or DUBs. Several DUBs have been described to negatively regulate DSB signaling. Ubiquitin-specific protease 3 (USP3) was shown to deubiquitylate H2A and H2B (Nicassio et al, 2007) and to negatively regulate the activity of RNF8 (Doil et al, 2009). BRCC36 binds to RAP80 and is in the BRCA1 complex that also includes Abraxas. BRCC36 along with RAP80 can antagonize the activity of RNF8-UBC13 by acting as a deubiquitinating enzyme for γ-H2AX. It also leads to decreased ubiquitylation signal at DSB sites (Shao et al, 2009). Recently, OTUB1 (OTU domain, ubiquitin aldehyde binding 1) was identified as an RNF168 DUB. OTUB1 does not use its catalytic activity to deubiquitylate RNF168 but rather acts by binding to and inhibiting UBC13, the RNF168 E2 conjugating enzyme (Nakada et al, 2010).

2.3 Role of SUMOylation in DNA double strand break signaling

SUMOylation is a posttranslational modification that involves the covalent linkage of a small ubiquitin-like modifier (SUMO) polypeptide to a target protein (Al-Hakim et al, 2010; Ciccia & Elledge, 2010). The process of SUMOylation is similar to that of ubiquitylation in that it also requires a SUMO-specific E1 (SAE1/SAE2), an E2 conjugating enzyme (Ubc9) and substrate-specific E3 ligases. Three types of SUMO molecules have been identified, SUMO1, SUMO2 and SUMO3. SUMO2 and SUMO3 have strong homology and share the same function and are therefore usually referred to as SUMO2/3. Both SUMO1 and SUMO2/3 are recruited to DSBs and this recruitment is dependent on the presence of RNF8 and RNF168. The E3 ligases PIAS1 and PIAS4 are needed for the accumulation of SUMO molecules to the break sites. PIAS1 is involved in the accumulation of SUMO2/3 but not SUMO1 at DSBs whereas PIAS4 is involved in the accumulation of all three SUMO moieties. PIAS1 and PIAS4 were both found to be important for accumulation of RNF168 and ubiquitylated H2A at DSB sites. Furthermore, PIAS1 and PIAS4 SUMOylate BRCA1 which is thought to increase its ubiquitin E3 ligase activity and the ubiquitylation of H2A by BRCA1 which would further amplify the DNA damage signal (Morris et al, 2009). SUMOylation of 53BP1 by PIAS1 and PIAS4 was also demonstrated and shown to be required for the efficient recruitment of 53BP1 to DSBs (Galanty et al, 2009). In summary, complex posttranslation modifications such as ubiquitylation, SUMOylation, phosphorylation and methylation, at the sites of DSBs lead to recruitment of proteins that are involved in DNA repair and the regulation of cell cycle checkpoints following DNA damage as will be discussed in the next section.

2.4 Cellular responses following DNA double strand breaks

Following DNA damage, cells are faced with different options. Either to undergo cell cycle arrest and repair the damaged DNA, to undergo senescence or to die by apoptosis. There are three checkpoints put in place to arrest the cell cycle following DNA damage. The G1/S checkpoint, the intra-S checkpoint and the G2/M checkpoint (Warmerdam & Kanaar, 2010). These checkpoints are carefully regulated by ATM and its downstream effectors. ATM phosphorylates and activates the protein kinase Chk2 and the tumor suppressor p53 which then act to enforce cell cycle arrest or apoptosis. Chk2 activation requires phosphorylation by ATM at Thr68 and autophosphorylation at multiple other residues. Chk2 phosphorylation of the cdc25 phosphatases which are needed for cell cycle progression lead to either their degradation (in the case of cdc25A) or their export from the nucleus (for cdc25B and cdc25C) thereby preventing interaction with their respective cdk/cyclin substrates (Donzelli & Draetta, 2003). Chk2 also phosphorylates p53 at Ser20 whereas ATM phosphorylates it at Ser15. This results in the accumulation of p53 and its activation as a transcription factor which transactivates many genes whose products are involved in cell cycle arrest such as p21, GADD45 and 14-3-3σ. p53 also transactivates several proapoptotic genes such as Noxa, PUMA and Bax, thus triggering apoptotic cell death of the damaged cells. The mechanisms that lead to p53-dependent cell cycle arrest versus p53-dependent apoptosis remain poorly understood but are likely to depend on the multiple posttranslational modifications of p53 (Vousden, 2006) .

3. DNA repair

Cells have evolved different pathways to repair DSBs. Currently, homologous recombination (HR) and non-homologous end joining (NHEJ) are recognized as the two major pathways for DSB repair (Kass & Jasin, 2010). The presence of undamaged sister chromatid is required for the error-free HR-mediated DSB repair, whereas NHEJ repair can occur in the absence of a homologous template sequence and is therefore considered to be more error-prone. Alternative NHEJ is another form of DNA repair that does not necessitate the presence of classical NHEJ DNA repair proteins and is characterized by sequence deletion and the introduction of microhomologies within the repaired DNA (Kotnis et al, 2009).

3.1 Non–homologous end joining

NHEJ is the most commonly used pathway for the repair of DSBs. Since it does not require the presence of a homologous sequence on a sister chromatid, it can occur throughout the cell cycle but particularly during G0, G1 and early S-phase (Kass & Jasin, 2010).

The first step of NHEJ is the recognition of the DSBs by the Ku70/Ku80 heterodimer which consists of the Ku70 and Ku80 subunit (Figure 2). The Ku70/Ku80 complex then slides inwards, away from the edge of the DSBs to allow binding of two molecules of the catalytic subunit of DNA-PK, DNA-PKcs. When DNA-PKcs binds to DNA and Ku70/Ku80 it is known as DNA-PK. The two DNA-PKcs molecules bind to each other, thereby bringing

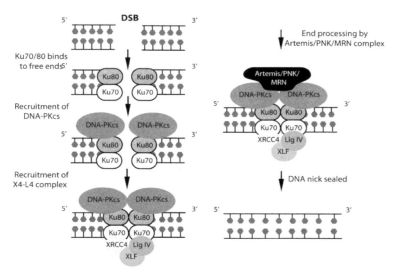

Fig. 2. Repair of DNA double strand breaks by non-homologous end joining

together the DNA ends in a process called synapsis. Binding of Ku70/Ku80 and DNA-PKcs to the DNA ends in this manner protects them against nuclease degradation in the cell. DNA-PKcs is a serine-threonine kinase whose activity is stimulated by binding to double stranded DNA and the Ku heterodimer. Phosphorylation of DNA-PKcs is needed to bring the proteins involved in DNA end processing such as Artemis, the DNA polymerase family members polymerase μ and polymerase λ, and the Polynucleotide kinase (PNK) to the break sites. End processing of the DNA at DSBs allows the removal of DNA lesions that interfere in the ligation process (Mahaney et al, 2009). Artemis is thought to be recruited to DSBs by binding to autophosphorylated DNA-PKcs. While Artemis has inherent 5′→3′ exonuclease activity, in the presence of DNA-PK and ATP it also acquires endonuclease activity. DNA-PK promotes the endonucleolytic activity of Artemis versus its exonucleolytic activity and decreases the speed of nucleotide removal. This is important to limit the amount of trimming done at the DNA ends to the minimum. DNA polymerases μ and λ are brought to the DSB sites via their interactions with either Ku70/Ku80 or the XRCC4/DNA ligase complex. Their role at the DSBs involves filling in gaps to allow ligation. DNA polymerase μ is less dependent than DNA polymerase λ on the presence of a template. PNK was also shown to play a role in NHEJ. It associates with XRCC4 and is dependent on its presence for its activity. It can phosphorylate 5′-OH terminal groups and dephosphorylate 3′-ends to restore normal DNA ends that can be ligated by the XRCC4/DNA ligase complex (Chappell et al, 2002). Aprataxin and PNK–like factor (APLF) is an endo-exonuclease that was shown to be required for full NHEJ activity. It can interact with other NHEJ factors such as Ku and XRCC4 and is phosphorylated by ATM in a DNA damage–dependent manner (Macrae et al, 2008). XRCC4 is thought to act as a scaffolding protein that brings many factors involved in NHEJ to the break sites. XRCC4 and DNA ligase IV, along with XLF (also known as Cernunnos) form a complex known as X4-L4. DNA ligase activity is thought to be stimulated by its binding to XRCC4 and to XLF. XRCC4 and XLF can bind to Ku proteins and to DNA. The X4-L4 complex is capable of ligating one strand of DNA at a time which would allow for concomitant processing and ligation of the ends (Hartlerode & Scully, 2009).

3.2 Alternative non-homologous end joining

When one or more classical NHEJ factors (Ku, DNA-PKcs, XRCC4, DNA ligase IV) are missing, DSBs can be repaired through the alternative NHEJ (Alt-NHEJ) pathway. This type of DNA repair relies on the presence of microhomologies at the terminal ends of the DNA breaks. It was found that Alt-NHEJ can occur in the absence of DNA ligase IV suggesting that one of the two remaining ligases (LigI or LigIII in eukaryotes) can function in DSB end ligation. End joining in the absence of LigIV requires 2-3 nucleotides of homology to stabilize the DNA at broken ends whereas no microhomology is needed in normal cells for NHEJ to occur. Furthermore it was found that a 4 nucleotide long microhomology at the break ends greatly decreases the requirement for Ku70, probably because of the increased stabilization of the DNA ends. Alt-NHEJ is stimulated by the presence of CtIP (CtBP-interacting protein) and suppressed by the classical NHEJ factors Ku and XRCC4-LigIV (Bennardo et al, 2008; Simsek & Jasin, 2010). It was found that Alt-NHEJ promotes chromosomal translocations which might explain the increase of hematological cancer incidence in the absence of one or more classical NHEJ factors (Simsek & Jasin, 2010).

3.3 Homologous recombination

Homologous recombination requires the presence of homologous sequences for the accurate repair of DSBs. It usually occurs in the late S phase or G2 phase when a sister chromatid is available to be used as a template for repair (Ciccia & Elledge, 2010; Kass & Jasin, 2010). The first step of HR is the generation of 3'- ssDNA (single stranded DNA) overhangs with 3'-hydroxyl ends which subsequently invade a homologous duplex DNA sequence (Figure 3). Initial processing of the DNA ends requires the MRN complex along with CtIP. Further processing is done by Exo1 in association with the helicase Bloom syndrome protein BLM (Nimonkar et al, 2008). The 3'-ssDNA overhangs generated by this process are then be bound by RPA (replication protein A) which is needed to melt the secondary structures of the DNA and protect the DNA ends before the binding of other HR proteins can occur. RPA is required for the recruitment of HR factors such as the DNA-dependent ATPase Rad51 to the break sites (Sleeth et al, 2007).

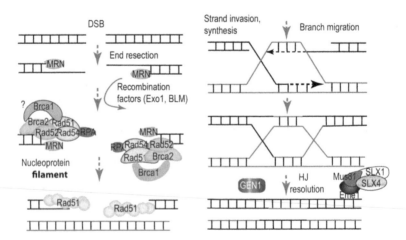

Fig. 3. Double strand break repair by homologous recombination

Rad51, a key HR player, belongs to the Rad52 epistasis group in yeast which is involved in recombinational DNA repair. Rad51 competes with RPA for binding to the DNA. Since it has lower affinity to DNA than RPA, other factors are needed to displace RPA and lead to the formation of Rad51-DNA nucleofilaments. This step requires the presence of the breast cancer susceptibility protein 2 (BRCA2). BRCA2 binds to Rad51 through its BRC repeats and its carboxy-terminus. BRCA2 facilitates the binding of Rad51 to the DNA by promoting RPA displacement and decreasing its ability to bind double stranded DNA. In addition, it inhibits the ATPase activity of Rad51, thereby stabilizing the Rad51-ssDNA complexes (Jensen et al, 2010). Once it binds to the ssDNA, Rad51 catalyzes invasion of a homologous duplex DNA sequence, thereby forming a displacement loop (D-loop). This process is known as synapsis and requires the presence of the Rad54 motor protein. Rad54, a member of the Rad52 epistasis group, binds to the Rad51-DNA nucleofilament, stabilizes it and therefore enhances D-loop formation. However, following synapsis, Rad54 promotes dissociation of Rad51 from double stranded DNA (dsDNA) which allows synthesis of the DNA strand. Rad54-mediated dissociation of Rad51 from dsDNA also allows for rapid Rad51 turnover (Heyer et al, 2010). After the D-loop is formed, DNA repair can occur in three distinct pathways: break-induced replication (BIR), synthesis-dependent strand annealing (SDSA) and double Holliday junctions (dHJ) (Heyer et al, 2010). BIR occurs when only one DNA strand is available to invade duplex DNA. This could occur during replication fork collapse or the uncapping of telomeres. This leads to the formation of a *bona fide* replication fork at this site. DNA synthesis at this site occurs using the regular DNA polymerases (Llorente et al, 2008). During SDSA the invading strand is elongated by DNA synthesis. The D-loop is then reversed, allowing the newly synthesized end to anneal to the resected opposite end of the break. The remaining gaps in the DNA are then filled by DNA synthesis and ligation. SDSA results in non-crossover recombination and is the main pathway used in somatic cells (Sung & Klein, 2006). Finally dHJ mediated recombination involves invasion of the second DNA break into the D loop, DNA synthesis and ligation to join the two invading DNA ends and then dHJ resolution in either a crossover or a non-crossover manner (Sung & Klein, 2006). BLM helicase in conjunction with topoisomerase IIIa leads to the dissolution of HJs to form non-crossover products. The Mus81-Eme1 endonuclease complex, SLX1-SLX4 complex or the human 5'-flap endonuclease GEN1 are capable of resolving dHJ to form both crossover and non-crossover products (Ciccia & Elledge, 2010; Hartlerode & Scully, 2009; Rass et al, 2010).

3.4 Choosing between homologous recombination and non-homologous end joining

The choice of the DNA repair pathway following DSB formation is dependent on many factors. One of the important determinants that allow the cells to choose whether the damaged DNA should be repaired by HR or NHEJ is the cell cycle phase in which it is in. NHEJ can occur throughout the whole cell cycle and is the pathway of choice during the G1 phase whereas DSBs in cells in late S and G2 phases are most likely to be repaired by HR. DNA resection to form 3'ssDNA overhangs is a tightly regulated step because if it occurs it actually commits the cells to repair their DNA using HR versus NHEJ. Binding of CtIP to DSBs promotes resection of the break ends. CtIP levels are regulated in a cell cycle-dependent manner and are elevated during the S, G2 and M phases of the cell cycle but are low during the G1 phase. In addition, CtIP activity is regulated through posttranslational modifications. CtIP is phosphorylated by CDK2 (cyclin dependent kinase 2) during the S and G2 phases of the cell cycle at two different sites S327 and T847. Phosphorylation of CtIP at S327 allows it to interact with the BRCT domain of BRCA1 and with the MRN complex. This then results in the ubiquitylation of CtIP by BRCA1 (Yu et al, 2006). Posttranslational modification of CtIP by phosphorylation and ubiquitination as well as its interaction with BRCA1 were found to be necessary for it binding to DNA and its role in DNA resection. CtIP is also predicted to be a target of ATM phosphorylation and ATM is required for end resection.

There are many lines of evidence showing competition between the NHEJ and HR pathways for DSB repair. In the absence of the NHEJ factors Ku and XRCC4-LigIV there is an increase in end resection and HR. Conversely, mutations in resection factors such as CtIP result in increased NHEJ (Kass & Jasin, 2010). Recently, 53BP1, a protein involved in cell cycle checkpoint and DNA repair has been implicated in the regulation of the switch between NHEJ and HR repair pathways. Some studies have shown that 53BP1 is important for NHEJ. In addition, 53BP1 is thought to bind to the DSB sites and inhibit DNA resection. Loss of 53BP1 in Brca1-null cells results in increased HR activity in these cells suggesting a model whereby 53BP1 inhibition of end resection is overcome by BRCA1, thereby leading to HR-mediated DNA repair (Bouwman et al, 2010; Bunting et al, 2010) . The mechanisms by which BRCA1 can counteract 53BP1 function and promote HR are still unknown but promise to be the focus of intense research in the future.

4. Double strand break repair in normal physiological processes

4.1 Meotic recombination

Meosis is a specialized type of cell division occurring during gametogenesis. It allows the production of haploid cells, containing one copy of the genetic material, from diploid cells containing two copies of the genetic material (Kumar et al, 2010). Meotic recombination is a crucial process during gametogenesis. It occurs during the prophase of the first meiotic division (prophase I) and allows the formation of physical links called chiasmata between two homologous chromosomes. This ensures proper alignment and segregation of the homologous chromosomes during the later phases of meiosis I. DNA recombination during meiosis also allows the exchange of genetic material between homologous chromosomes. This is required to ensure genetic diversity of the organisms and for introduction of mutations needed for the evolution of species. Meiotic recombination requires a highly regulated generation of DSBs followed by their repair through HR. The first step of meiotic recombination is the generation of DSBs during the leptotene stage of prophase I. This stage occurs directly following S phase when DNA replication has occurred. Spo11, a highly conserved type II-like topoisomerase, generates the DSBs needed to initiate meiotic recombination through a transesterification reaction (Keeney et al, 1997). Spo11 binds to both strands of the DNA as a homodimer. Once the DSB is generated, the DNA on which Spo11 is attached is cleaved, thereby releasing a Spo11-oligonucleotide complex. In addition to Spo11, several other proteins were identified as been involved in DSB formation although their mechanism of action is still poorly understood. One of them, Mei4 (MEIosis-specific 4), is needed for DSB formation in both yeast and mammals (Kumar et al., 2010). Mei4 binds to another protein, Rec114 (RECombination 114) which is also essential for DSB formation in yeast. Although the role of Rec114 in mammals is still unknown, its interaction with Mei4 makes it plausible that they function together in DSB generation in mammals (Kumar et al, 2010).

DSBs do not occur evenly throughout the genome but arise more frequently in specific areas called "hotspots". In yeast and mouse it was found that these hotspots are marked by the trimethylation of histone 3 at Lys4 (H3K4Me3) (Borde et al, 2009). Recently, a histone methyltransferase, PRDM9 (PR domain containing 9), was identified as a protein that can bind to and activate hotspots in mammalian genomes (Baudat et al, 2010). After end processing to form 3'-ssDNA, the resected DNA is bound by Rad51 and Dmc1 (Disrupted meiotic cDNA1), a meiosis-specific recombinase. In the yeast *Saccharomyces cerevisiae*, recruitment of Dmc1 to resected DNA ends is dependent upon the two proteins Mei5 and Sae3. Mei5 and Sae3 (Sporulation in the Absence of Spo Eleven 3) form a complex that allows Dmc1 binding to the single stranded DNA and enhances its recombinase activity (Ferrari et al, 2009). The resected ends can then invade double stranded DNA and form a D-loop. Two proteins, Hop2 and Mnd1 which exist in cells as a heterodimeric complex help in the stabilization of the Rad51 and Dmc1 nucleofilaments and increase their ability to invade homologous duplex DNA. Hop2 and Mnd1 function both in yeast and higher eukaryotes, including mammals (Petukhova et al, 2005; Tsubouchi & Roeder, 2002). In contrast to HR occurring in somatic cells which use sister chromatids as a template, the use of a non-sister homologous chromatid is favored during meiotic recombination (Shinohara et al, 1992). The Holliday junctions that form following strand invasion are then resolved to form crossover and non-crossover products. In contrast to what happens during HR in somatic cells, meiotic recombination generates a much higher proportion of crossover products as compared to non-crossover products (Andersen & Sekelsky, 2010). In both *S. cerevisiae* and higher eukaryotes the Msh4-Msh5 (MutS homolog 4-5) complex plays an important role in the resolution of HJs and in crossover formation. It was also suggested that GEN1 could play a role in HJ resolution during human meiotic recombination (Lorenz et al, 2009), however further investigation is needed to prove this hypothesis.

4.2 V(D)J recombination

V(D)J recombination is a crucial process in lymphocyte development through which diverse B and T cell receptors can be generated (Soulas-Sprauel et al, 2007). It involves the assembly of a variable (V), diversity (D) and joining (J) exons to form a B cell or T cell antigen receptor. The multiple combinations that can be obtained by joining together different V, D and J segments are the underlying mechanism for antigen receptor diversity and the ability of the immune system to respond to different types of pathogens. RAG1 and RAG2 (recombination activating genes 1 and 2) are two lymphocyte-specific recombinases that introduce DSBs at specific recombination signal (RS) sequences that border every V, D and J gene segment (Dudley et al, 2005). RS sequences consist of a conserved heptamer and a conserved nonamer separated by a nonconserved 12 bp or 23 bp spacer sequence. In the heavy chain immunoglobulin gene (IgH) for example, RS sequences that surround D sequences have a 12 bp spacer whereas those surrounding the V and J segments have 23 bp. Since recombination can occur only between RS sequences containing a 12 bp spacer and one containing a 23 bp spacer this ensures productive joining of V, D and J sequences (Dudley et al, 2005). RAG mediated cutting of the DNA generates hairpin loops at the joining DNA ends. These hairpin loops are cleaved by the endonuclease Artemis which is recruited and activated by the DNA-PKcs and Ku70/80 complex. The XRCC4/DNAligase IV/XLF complex then religates the joining ends (Soulas-Sprauel et al, 2007).

4.3 Class switch recombination

Class switch recombination (CSR) is a specialized mechanism occurring in B cells that allows the cells to switch from expressing immunoglobulin (Ig) M (IgM) to IgG, IgA or IgE (Stavnezer et al, 2008). This involves replacement of the IgH constant region Cμ encoded in IgM with more downstream constant regions such as Cγ, Cε and Cα which code for IgG, IgE and IgA heavy chain constant regions respectively. This replacement of IgH constant regions is mediated through deletion of parts of the chromosome and subsequent recombination. CSR occurs within or nearby specific sequences called the switch regions that precede every constant region. CSR is initiated upon antigenic stimulation of mature B cells and requires at least two rounds of cell division and the presence of a B cell-specific enzyme activation induced cytidine deaminase (AID) that converts deoxycytosine (dC) to deoxyuracil (dU) in the donor and receiver S regions (Muramatsu et al, 2000). The dU is then removed through the base excision repair pathway. The enzyme that cleaves dU in S regions is the uracil DNA glycosylase UNG. The phosphate backbone of the resulting abasic site is then cleaved by the apurinic/apyrimidinic endonucleases APE1 and APE2, two proteins which were found to be essential for CSR, to form a single strand DNA break (Guikema et al, 2007). In order for CSR to occur, DSBs must be created in the donor and acceptor S regions and the single stranded breaks generated by APE1 and 2 are not enough. When single stranded breaks are generated close enough to each other they might lead to the formation of DSBs. Otherwise, DSBs must be generated by mismatch repair (MMR) proteins. It is hypothesized that the MMR heterodimer Msh2-Msh6 (MutS homolog 2-6) recognizes the mismatched U:G pair and binds to it. Mlh1-Pms2 (MutL homolog 1-PostMeiotic Segregation 2) then binds to Msh2-Msh6 to form a heterotetramer capable of recruiting the exonuclease Exo1. Exo1 cuts the DNA between two single stranded breaks thereby resulting in a DSB (Stavnezer et al, 2008).

DSBs in the S regions are religated using the NHEJ repair machinery. However NHEJ factors are not the only proteins involved in CSR. Studies of mouse knockout models have implicated Atm, Mdc-1, γ-H2ax and 53bp1 in the CSR process (Kotnis et al, 2009). More recently, the E3 ligases Rnf8 and Rnf168 have also been implicated in the process of CSR (Bohgaki et al, 2011; Li et al, 2010; Santos et al, 2010; Stewart et al, 2007). Interestingly, in B cells of mice that are deficient in classical NHEJ repair proteins, sequencing of switch junctions have shown a pattern of increased microhomology suggesting that CSR could be occurring through alternative NHEJ pathways in these cells (Kotnis et al, 2009). Of all of the DSB repair proteins, loss of 53bp1 seems to have the most severe effect on CSR with a 90% decrease in CSR in 53bp1-null B cells (Kotnis et al, 2009). There have been several roles proposed for 53BP1 in CSR. One of them is that that 53BP1 inhibits intraswitch religation of DSBs and promotes synapsis between DSBs occurring in distal switch sequences. In addition, 53BP1 inhibits DSB resection which is needed for alternative NHEJ, thereby leading to increased DSB repair through the classical NHEJ pathway and to increased CSR (Bothmer et al, 2010). Despite many advances in the field of CSR and in the function of factors required for this process, further investigation is still required to determine the precise role of each DSB repair protein in CSR.

5. DSB signaling and repair defects: Human diseases and mouse models

The study of rare hereditary diseases and knockout mouse models in which DSB signaling and repair genes are mutated has greatly increased our understanding of the DNA damage signaling and repair pathways and the underlying mechanisms regulating them (Bohgaki et al, 2010; Hakem, 2008). In this section, a summary of the human syndromes and mouse phenotypes associated with the loss of the major DSB signaling and repair proteins is provided.

5.1 ATM

Mutations in the *ATM* gene result in the devastating disease ataxia-telangiectasia (A-T). A-T is an autosomal recessive disorder. Clinical symptoms of A-T include cerebellar ataxia, oculocutaneous telangiectasias, immunodeficiency, growth retardation, lack of gonadal development, insulin resistance and increased susceptibility to lymphoid cancers (Lavin, 2008). The ataxia manifests itself at an early age when the child starts to walk and worsens with time as the patients usually becomes wheel-chair bound by the end of the first decade of their life. Ataxia in A-T patients is caused by degeneration of Purkinje and granular cells in the cerebellum. A-T patients are immunodeficient, have reduced thymus size and lower serum levels of IgG, IgA and IgE. One of the striking features of A-T is a severe sensitivity to ionizing radiation. This has been observed in both A-T patients who were undergoing radiotherapy and in A-T cells grown in culture. Some patients with A-T develop insulin resistance and diabetes. Although this particular symptom was initially hard to explain through the DNA damage signaling functions of ATM, it has recently become clear that ATM is also a key player in insulin signaling and that it can protect against metabolic disorders (Halaby et al, 2008; Matsuoka et al, 2007). About one third of A-T patients develop lymphoid malignancies.

The phenotype of Atm-deficient mice closely resembles what has been observed in A-T patients. The mice are growth-deficient, sterile, immunodeficient and display increased radiosensitivity. In addition, most mice succumb to thymic lymphoma by 6 months of age (Barlow et al, 1996). Furthermore, it has been reported that $Atm^{-/-}$ mice have CSR defects (Kotnis et al, 2009). Interestingly, $Atm^{-/-}$ mice do not recapitulate entirely the severe neurodegeneration observed in A-T patients. Mild ataxia has been reported in $Atm^{-/-}$ mice, however there were no signs of degeneration in the cerebellum such as those observed in A-T patients (Barlow et al, 1996). This suggests that although ATM functions are mostly conserved from mice to humans, it might not be the case in neuronal cells of these organisms.

5.2 The MRN complex
5.2.1 MRE11

Hypomorphic mutations in the human *MRE11* gene lead to A-T like disorder (ATLD). ATLD is a very rare disorder that shares many similarities with A-T disease (Stewart et al, 1999). ATLD patients display progressive cerebellar ataxia and their cells are radiosensitive. However, in contrast with A-T patients, ATLD patients display normal Ig levels, lack of telangiectasia occurrence and they do not have increased susceptibility for cancer development (Taylor et al, 2004).

Straight knockout mice for *Mre11* are embryonic lethal, suggesting that Mre11 is necessary for embryonic development (Xiao & Weaver, 1997). An ATLD mouse model was developed in which a hypomorphic Mre11 is expressed ($Mre11^{ATLD1/ATLD1}$ mice). These mice appear to have normal growth; however mouse embryonic fibroblasts derived from these mice have increased radiosensitivity, blunted intra-S and G2/M checkpoints and higher levels of genomic instability (Theunissen et al, 2003). However, $Mre11^{ATLD1/ATLD1}$ mice did not develop lymphomas. Interestingly, female $Mre11^{ATLD1/ATLD1}$ mice have a severely reduced fertility due to an inability of developing embryos to proliferate properly.

5.2.2 NBS1

NBS1 hypomorphic mutations are the underlying cause for the Nijmegen Breakage syndrome (NBS) (Carney et al, 1998). NBS patients display stunted growth, microencephaly, immunodeficiency, increased radiosensitivity and increased cancer incidence (Digweed & Sperling, 2004). NBS patients have decreased IgA and IgG level which shows that NBS1 plays an important in CSR (van Engelen et al, 2001). Some female patients also showed ovarian failure and amenorrhea. Lymphomas are the most common malignancies observed in NBS patients although other cancers such as medulloblastomas were also diagnosed in these patients (Digweed & Sperling, 2004).

As with *Mre11*, straight knockout mice of *Nbs1* are not viable (Zhu et al, 2001). Mice with conditional deletion of Nbs1 in B cells had increased genomic instability in B cells and CSR defects (Reina-San-Martin et al, 2005). However and interestingly so, mice with hypomorphic mutation of *Nbs1* that mimics a mutation observed in NBS1 patients display a generally milder phenotype than what is observed in NBS patients (Williams et al, 2002). Mouse embryonic fibroblasts derived from these mice show increased sensitivity to DNA damaging compounds, defects in cell cycle checkpoints and increased chromosomal instability. However, these mice with homozygous *Nbs1* hypomorph mutation do not show immunodeficiency, increased susceptibility to tumor development or female sterility.

5.2.3 RAD50

Recently, a human disorder caused by mutations in the *RAD50* gene was characterized (Waltes et al, 2009). This disorder was described as being NBS-like since the only known patient with this disorder shares similar features with NBS patients. Clinical features of the RAD50 (NBS-like) disorder patient include microencephaly, growth retardation and slight ataxia. The patient has a normal immune system and did not develop any tumors by the age of 23. Cells derived from the patient displayed radiosensitivity, G1/S and G2/M checkpoint defects, radioresistant DNA synthesis and increased genomic instability.

Rad50-null mutant mice are not viable and die early during embryonic development. Viable *Rad50* hypomorphic mice were generated (Bender et al, 2002). These mice have strong growth defects and most die from anemia caused by hematopoietic stem cell failure. Mutant mice that survive develop lymphomas and leukemia and males exhibit degeneration in the testes. Mouse embryonic fibroblasts with the *Rad50* hypomorphic mutation are not sensitive to radiation or DNA damaging agents and do not perform radioresistant DNA synthesis.

5.3 RNF168

RNF168 was recently identified as the gene mutated in the RIDDLE (radiosensitivity, immunodeficiency, dysmorphic features and learning difficulties) syndrome (Stewart et al, 2009; Stewart et al, 2007). The RIDDLE syndrome was identified in only one patient to date and is characterized by immunodeficiency with decreased IgG levels but slightly increased IgA and IgM levels. The RIDDLE patient also displayed a mild decrease in motor and learning abilities, shorter stature and facial dysmorphism. Fibroblasts derived from the RIDDLE patient showed increased radiosensitivity. Interestingly, another patient with

RNF168 gene mutation was recently identified (Devgan et al, 2011). This patient also displayed short stature, cellular radiosensitivity and low serum IgA. In addition, this patient was reported to also display A-T like symptoms including ataxia, ocular telangiectasias, microencephaly, and immunodeficiency with very low IgA levels. Both patients with RNF168 deficiency did not develop tumors.

Rnf168 null mice were recently generated (Bohgaki et al, 2011). These mice display normal growth and development and do not develop malignancies. They do however exhibit immunodeficiency mainly characterized by defects in CSR. Cells deficient for Rnf168 display increased radiosensitivity and genomic instability and elevated cancer risk was observed in mice lacking both Rnf168 and p53.

5.4 RNF8

Human syndromes caused by mutations of the *RNF8* gene have yet to be identified. However, Rnf8 mouse knockout models have been generated and have produced interesting phenotypes that are worth discussing here. *Rnf8-/-* mice are viable and are born in normal mendelian ratio (Li et al, 2010; Santos et al, 2010). They have growth defects, male sterility, increased radiosensitivity and immunodeficiency. *Rnf8-/-* mice display reduced CSR and increased genomic instability. A broad spectrum of tumors including lymphomas, sarcomas and breast tumors developed in *Rnf8-/-* mice (Li et al, 2010). It would be interesting to determine whether mutations of *RNF8* gene lead to human genetic disorders or if RNF8 loss correlates with cancer development in humans.

5.5 BRCA1 and BRCA2

BRCA1 and *BRCA2* are two breast and ovarian cancer susceptibility genes (O'Donovan & Livingston, 2010). Germline mutation of one *BRCA1* allele results in an up to 80% cumulative risk of breast cancer and a 30-40% risk of ovarian cancer by 70 years of age. Carriers of a *BRCA2* mutation have a 50% cumulative risk of breast cancer and a 10-15% risk of developing ovarian cancer by age 70. In addition, germline *BRCA2* mutations have been implicated in familial prostate cancer (McKinnon & Caldecott, 2007). Tumors in *BRCA1* or *BRCA2* mutation carriers most often lose the second *BRCA1* or *BRCA2* allele through loss of heterozygocity. Recently, it has been discovered that BRCA1 and BRCA2-negative tumors are very sensitive to a class of compounds known as PARP inhibitors. PARP inhibitors leave unrepaired single strand breaks in the DNA. If these unrepaired breaks meet a replication fork either fork collapse or DSBs. In the absence of BRCA1 and BRCA2 DSBs are left unrepaired, thereby leading to cell death. In this way PARP inhibitors are able to specifically target and kill *BRCA1* and *BRCA2*-null cells, making these inhibitors powerful therapeutic candidates for BRCA1 and BRCA2 negative breast and ovarian tumors. This treatment strategy might also work for tumors with somatic inactivation of BRCA1 and BRCA2 (Carden et al, 2010).

Brca1 and *Brca2* knockout mice are embryonic lethal, reflecting the essential requirement for these two proteins (Hakem et al, 1996; Suzuki et al, 1997). Brca1-deficient cells displayed radiosensitivity and increased chromosomal abnormalities (Mak et al, 2000; McPherson et al, 2004). Females carrying *Brca1* targeted mutations in mammary tissue exhibit a long latency time before development of mammary tumors, however this latency time is reduced considerably in the absence of tumor suppressor proteins such as p53 and Chk2 (McPherson et al, 2004; Xu et al, 1999). Interestingly, it was recently shown that loss of 53bp1 in Brca1-null mammary epithelium prevented mammary tumor development (Bunting et al, 2010), suggesting that 53bp1 could eventually be targeted to treated Brca1-deficient breast cancer.

Similar to what was observed with *Brca1* conditional mutant mice, loss of Brca2 expression in mouse mammary epithelium leads to increased incidence of mammary tumors, the latency of which is shortened in the absence of a *p53* allele (Jonkers et al, 2001). Recently, study of a conditional knockout of Brca2 in mouse prostate epithelium showed that loss of Brca2 leads to increased prostate cancer incidence which is accelerated in the absence of p53 (Francis et al, 2010).

5.6 DNA ligase IV

Hypomorphic mutations in the *DNA ligase IV* gene in humans give rise to the ligase IV (Lig4) syndrome. Lig4 syndrome is an autosomal recessive disorder characterized by microencephaly, growth retardation, mental retardation, decreased red and white blood cell count, immunodeficiency and increased cancer susceptibility (O'Driscoll et al, 2001). Cells from Lig4 patients display increased radiosensitivity and are defective in NHEJ DSB repair, but they have normal cell cycle checkpoints (O'Driscoll et al, 2001).

Knocking out *DNA ligase IV* in mice results in late embryonic lethality with massive neuronal apoptosis and lymphocyte development arrest due to lack of V(D)J recombination (Frank et al, 1998). Mice with hypomorphic mutation of *DNA ligase IV* were obtained through a mutagenesis screen. These mice have growth defects, are immunodeficient and have hematopoietic stem cell exhaustion with age (Nijnik et al, 2007).

5.7 Artemis

Artemis is the gene mutated in radiosensitive-severe combined immunodeficiency (RS-SCID) (Moshous et al, 2001). RS-SCID is characterized by normal development but increased radiosensitivity and a complete absence of mature B and T cells that can be attributable to defects in V(D)J recombination. While null mutations of *Artemis* give rise to RD-SCID, hypomorphic mutations lead to a plethora of less severe immunodeficiency syndromes that are characterized by increased incidence of Esptein-Barr virus-induced lymphomas (Moshous et al, 2003).

Artemis knockout mice are viable and display normal growth. B cell development in these mice is arrested at early progenitor stages. In contrast to what is observed in humans some T cells are able to undergo V(D)J recombination and mature normally leading to a "leaky" SCID phenotype (Rooney et al, 2002). Artemis-deficient cells display increased radiosensitivity and genomic instability. Recently, Artemis-null mice were generated in a different genetic background (Xiao et al, 2009). These mice exhibit complete arrest of B and T lymphocyte development and do not present a leaky phenotype and thus recapitulate more closely RS-SCID symptoms.

5.8 DNA-PKcs

The first *DNA-PKcs* human gene mutation was recently identified in a patient presenting classical symptoms of RS-SCID (van der Burg et al, 2009). This patient did not have mature B or T cells but had normal natural killer cell numbers. Cells from the patient were unable to properly repair DNA double strand breaks and were deficient in NHEJ.

DNA-PKcs was initially identified as the gene inactivated in the classical scid mice. Later on, knockout mice for *DNA-PKcs* recapitulated the phenotypes of the scid mice (Gao et al, 1998). *DNA-PKcs*-/- mice exhibited no growth defects but they displayed arrested B and T cell development at early progenitor stages, impaired V(D)J recombination and increased cellular radiosensitivity.

5.9 NHEJ1

NHEJ1 (*Cernunnos-XLF*) gene mutations were identified in patients with immunodeficiency and microencephaly (Buck et al, 2006). These patients are characterized by bird-like features, microencephaly, progressive loss of B and T cells and growth retardation. They have low levels of circulating IgA and IgG. Cells derived from these patients are radiosensitive but display normal cell cycle checkpoint.

A mouse model in which *Nhej1* is deleted has been generated (Li et al, 2008). These mice display a much milder phenotype than what is seen in humans. *Nhej1*-null mice are viable, born at the mendelian ratio and have normal growth and development. Although B and T cell numbers are reduced in *Nhej1*-deficient mice, a normal development of immune cells is observed and V(D)J recombination was not impaired in Nhej1-null lymphocytes. On the other hand, B cells from Nhej1-deficient mice had defective CSR. Concomitant loss of Nhej1 and p53 resulted in the rapid occurrence of thymic lymphomas and medulloblastomas.

5.10 Ku70 and Ku80

Mutations in *Ku70* or *Ku80* genes have not yet been described in humans. However knockout mice have been generated for these two proteins. Similar to what has been observed for knockout mice of other NHEJ factors described above, Ku70 and Ku80 deficient mice display immunodeficiency with arrested B and T cell development and defective V(D)J recombination (Gu et al, 1997; Nussenzweig et al, 1996). Interestingly though, *Ku70*[-/-] and *Ku80*[-/-] mice displayed significant growth defects and reduced size compared to wild-type mice.

6. Conclusion

DNA double strand breaks are constantly generated in our cells either through external stressors such as radiation or through internal programmed events that are needed for normal physiological processes such as gametogenesis, V(D)J recombination and class switch recombination. The importance of quickly detecting and repairing these breaks is underscored by the plethora of human syndromes caused by mutation of genes coding for DSB signaling and repair proteins. These syndromes share many similarities which include neurological defects, growth defects, immunodeficiency, radiosensitivity, sterility and increased cancer incidence. Although many of these symptoms have been recapitulated in knockout mouse models of DSB response proteins, some discrepancies between human syndromes and mouse models are sometimes observed which highlight differential role or redundancy between DSB response proteins in humans and mice. Nevertheless, study of these models have provided great insight into the physiological functions of DSB response proteins and have led to rapid discoveries in this field. Finally, these studies resulted in a better understanding of the etiology of certain diseases such as cancer and provided potential new ways of treating these diseases.

7. Acknowledgements

We would like to acknowledge S el-Ghamarasni and Drs. M Bohgaki, T Bohgaki and N Chan for the critical reading of this manuscript. RH was supported by the Cancer Research Society, the Association for International Cancer research, the Canadian Breast Cancer Foundation, and the Canadian Institutes of Health Research.

8. References

Al-Hakim A., Escribano-Diaz, C., LandryM.C, O' Donnel, L., Panier S., Szilard R.K. & Durocher D. (2010) The ubiquitous role of ubiquitin in the DNA damage response. DNA repair, Vol. 9, No. 12, pp. 1229-1240, ISSN 1568-7856

Andersen, S.L. & Sekelsky, J. (2010) Meiotic Versus Mitotic Recombination: Two Different Routes for Double-Strand Break Repair: The Different Functions of Meiotic Versus Mitotic Dsb Repair Are Reflected in Different Pathway Usage and Different Outcomes. *Bioessays,* Vol.32, No.12, pp.1058-1066, ISSN 1521-1878

Bakkenist, C.J. & Kastan, M.B. (2003) DNA Damage Activates Atm through Intermolecular Autophosphorylation and Dimer Dissociation. *Nature,* Vol.421, No.6922, pp.499-506, ISSN 0028-0836

Barlow, C., Hirotsune, S., Paylor, R., Liyanage, M., Eckhaus, M., Collins, F., Shiloh, Y., Crawley, J.N., Ried, T., Tagle, D. & Wynshaw-Boris, A. (1996) Atm-Deficient Mice: A Paradigm of Ataxia Telangiectasia. *Cell,* Vol.86, No.1, pp.159-171, ISSN 0092-8674

Baudat, F., Buard, J., Grey, C., Fledel-Alon, A., Ober, C., Przeworski, M., Coop, G. & de Massy, B. (2010) Prdm9 Is a Major Determinant of Meiotic Recombination Hotspots in Humans and Mice. *Science,* Vol.327, No.5967, pp.836-840, ISSN 1095-9203

Bekker-Jensen, S., Rendtlew Danielsen, J., Fugger, K., Gromova, I., Nerstedt, A., Lukas, C., Bartek, J., Lukas, J. & Mailand, N. (2010) Herc2 Coordinates Ubiquitin-Dependent Assembly of DNA Repair Factors on Damaged Chromosomes. *Nat Cell Biol,* Vol.12, No.1, pp.80-86; sup pp 81-12, ISSN 1476-4679

Bender, C.F., Sikes, M.L., Sullivan, R., Huye, L.E., Le Beau, M.M., Roth, D.B., Mirzoeva, O.K., Oltz, E.M. & Petrini, J.H. (2002) Cancer Predisposition and Hematopoietic Failure in Rad50(S/S) Mice. *Genes Dev,* Vol.16, No.17, pp.2237-2251, ISSN 0890-9369

Bennardo, N., Cheng, A., Huang, N. & Stark, J.M. (2008) Alternative-Nhej Is a Mechanistically Distinct Pathway of Mammalian Chromosome Break Repair. *PLoS Genet,* Vol.4, No.6, pp.e1000110, ISSN 1553-7404

Bohgaki, T., Bohgaki, M., Cardoso, R., Panier, S., Stewart, G.S., Sanchez, O., Durocher, D., Hakem, A. & Hakem, R. (2011) Genomic Instability, Defective Spermatogenesis, Immunodeficiency and Cancer in a Mouse Model of the Riddle Syndrome. *Plos Genetics,* In press.

Bohgaki, T., Bohgaki, M. & Hakem, R. (2010) DNA Double-Strand Break Signaling and Human Disorders. *Genome Integr,* Vol.1, No.1, pp.15, ISSN 2041-9414

Borde, V., Robine, N., Lin, W., Bonfils, S., Geli, V. & Nicolas, A. (2009) Histone H3 Lysine 4 Trimethylation Marks Meiotic Recombination Initiation Sites. *EMBO J,* Vol.28, No.2, pp.99-111, ISSN 1460-2075

Bothmer, A., Robbiani, D.F., Feldhahn, N., Gazumyan, A., Nussenzweig, A. & Nussenzweig, M.C. (2010) 53bp1 Regulates DNA Resection and the Choice between Classical and Alternative End Joining During Class Switch Recombination. *J Exp Med,* Vol.207, No.4, pp.855-865, ISSN 1540-9538

Bouwman, P., Aly, A., Escandell, J.M., Pieterse, M., Bartkova, J., van der Gulden, H., Hiddingh, S., Thanasoula, M., Kulkarni, A., Yang, Q., Haffty, B.G., Tommiska, J., Blomqvist, C., Drapkin, R., Adams, D.J., Nevanlinna, H., Bartek, J., Tarsounas, M., Ganesan, S. & Jonkers, J. (2010) 53bp1 Loss Rescues Brca1 Deficiency and Is

Associated with Triple-Negative and Brca-Mutated Breast Cancers. *Nat Struct Mol Biol,* Vol.17, No.6, pp.688-695, ISSN 1545-9985

Buck, D., Malivert, L., de Chasseval, R., Barraud, A., Fondaneche, M.C., Sanal, O., Plebani, A., Stephan, J.L., Hufnagel, M., le Deist, F., Fischer, A., Durandy, A., de Villartay, J.P. & Revy, P. (2006) Cernunnos, a Novel Nonhomologous End-Joining Factor, Is Mutated in Human Immunodeficiency with Microcephaly. *Cell,* Vol.124, No.2, pp.287-299, ISSN 0092-8674

Bunting, S.F., Callen, E., Wong, N., Chen, H.T., Polato, F., Gunn, A., Bothmer, A., Feldhahn, N., Fernandez-Capetillo, O., Cao, L., Xu, X., Deng, C.X., Finkel, T., Nussenzweig, M., Stark, J.M. & Nussenzweig, A. (2010) 53bp1 Inhibits Homologous Recombination in Brca1-Deficient Cells by Blocking Resection of DNA Breaks. *Cell,* Vol.141, No.2, pp.243-254, ISSN 1097-4172

Carden, C.P., Yap, T.A. & Kaye, S.B. (2010) Parp Inhibition: Targeting the Achilles' Heel of DNA Repair to Treat Germline and Sporadic Ovarian Cancers. *Curr Opin Oncol,* Vol.22, No.5, pp.473-480, ISSN 1531-703X

Carney, J.P., Maser, R.S., Olivares, H., Davis, E.M., Le Beau, M., Yates, J.R., 3rd, Hays, L., Morgan, W.F. & Petrini, J.H. (1998) The Hmre11/Hrad50 Protein Complex and Nijmegen Breakage Syndrome: Linkage of Double-Strand Break Repair to the Cellular DNA Damage Response. *Cell,* Vol.93, No.3, pp.477-486, ISSN 0092-8674

Chappell, C., Hanakahi, L.A., Karimi-Busheri, F., Weinfeld, M. & West, S.C. (2002) Involvement of Human Polynucleotide Kinase in Double-Strand Break Repair by Non-Homologous End Joining. *EMBO J,* Vol.21, No.11, pp.2827-2832, ISSN 0261-4189

Ciccia, A. & Elledge, S.J. (2010) The DNA Damage Response: Making It Safe to Play with Knives. *Molecular Cell* Vol.40, No.2, pp.179-204

Cook, P.J., Ju, B.G., Telese, F., Wang, X., Glass, C.K. & Rosenfeld, M.G. (2009) Tyrosine Dephosphorylation of H2ax Modulates Apoptosis and Survival Decisions. *Nature,* Vol.458, No.7238, pp.591-596, ISSN 1476-4687

D'Amours, D. & Jackson, S.P. (2002) The Mre11 Complex: At the Crossroads of Dna Repair and Checkpoint Signalling. *Nat Rev Mol Cell Biol,* Vol.3, No.5, pp.317-327, ISSN 1471-0072

Devgan, S.S., Sanal, O., Doil, C., Nakamura, K., Nahas, S.A., Pettijohn, K., Bartek, J., Lukas, C., Lukas, J. & Gatti, R.A. (2011) Homozygous Deficiency of Ubiquitin-Ligase Ring-Finger Protein Rnf168 Mimics the Radiosensitivity Syndrome of Ataxia-Telangiectasia. *Cell Death Differ,* ISSN 1476-5403

Digweed, M. & Sperling, K. (2004) Nijmegen Breakage Syndrome: Clinical Manifestation of Defective Response to DNA Double-Strand Breaks. *DNA Repair (Amst),* Vol.3, No.8-9, pp.1207-1217, ISSN 1568-7864

Doil, C., Mailand, N., Bekker-Jensen, S., Menard, P., Larsen, D.H., Pepperkok, R., Ellenberg, J., Panier, S., Durocher, D., Bartek, J., Lukas, J. & Lukas, C. (2009) Rnf168 Binds and Amplifies Ubiquitin Conjugates on Damaged Chromosomes to Allow Accumulation of Repair Proteins. *Cell,* Vol.136, No.3, pp.435-446, ISSN 1097-4172

Donzelli, M. & Draetta, G.F. (2003) Regulating Mammalian Checkpoints through Cdc25 Inactivation. *EMBO Rep,* Vol.4, No.7, pp.671-677, ISSN 1469-221X

Dudley, D.D., Chaudhuri, J., Bassing, C.H. & Alt, F.W. (2005) Mechanism and Control of V(D)J Recombination Versus Class Switch Recombination: Similarities and Differences. *Adv Immunol*, Vol.86, pp.43-112, ISSN 0065-2776

Ferrari, S.R., Grubb, J. & Bishop, D.K. (2009) The Mei5-Sae3 Protein Complex Mediates Dmc1 Activity in Saccharomyces Cerevisiae. *J Biol Chem*, Vol.284, No.18, pp.11766-11770, ISSN 0021-9258

Francis, J.C., McCarthy, A., Thomsen, M.K., Ashworth, A. & Swain, A. (2010) Brca2 and Trp53 Deficiency Cooperate in the Progression of Mouse Prostate Tumourigenesis. *PLoS Genet*, Vol.6, No.6, pp.e1000995, ISSN 1553-7404

Frank, K.M., Sekiguchi, J.M., Seidl, K.J., Swat, W., Rathbun, G.A., Cheng, H.L., Davidson, L., Kangaloo, L. & Alt, F.W. (1998) Late Embryonic Lethality and Impaired V(D)J Recombination in Mice Lacking DNA Ligase Iv. *Nature*, Vol.396, No.6707, pp.173-177, ISSN 0028-0836

Galanty, Y., Belotserkovskaya, R., Coates, J., Polo, S., Miller, K.M. & Jackson, S.P. (2009) Mammalian Sumo E3-Ligases Pias1 and Pias4 Promote Responses to DNA Double-Strand Breaks. *Nature*, Vol.462, No.7275, pp.935-939, ISSN 1476-4687

Gao, Y., Chaudhuri, J., Zhu, C., Davidson, L., Weaver, D.T. & Alt, F.W. (1998) A Targeted DNA-Pkcs-Null Mutation Reveals DNA-Pk-Independent Functions for Ku in V(D)J Recombination. *Immunity*, Vol.9, No.3, pp.367-376, ISSN 1074-7613

Goldberg, M., Stucki, M., Falck, J., D'Amours, D., Rahman, D., Pappin, D., Bartek, J. & Jackson, S.P. (2003) Mdc1 Is Required for the Intra-S-Phase DNA Damage Checkpoint. *Nature*, Vol.421, No.6926, pp.952-956, ISSN 0028-0836

Gu, Y., Seidl, K.J., Rathbun, G.A., Zhu, C., Manis, J.P., van der Stoep, N., Davidson, L., Cheng, H.L., Sekiguchi, J.M., Frank, K., Stanhope-Baker, P., Schlissel, M.S., Roth, D.B. & Alt, F.W. (1997) Growth Retardation and Leaky Scid Phenotype of Ku70-Deficient Mice. *Immunity*, Vol.7, No.5, pp.653-665, ISSN 1074-7613

Guikema, J.E., Linehan, E.K., Tsuchimoto, D., Nakabeppu, Y., Strauss, P.R., Stavnezer, J. & Schrader, C.E. (2007) Ape1- and Ape2-Dependent DNA Breaks in Immunoglobulin Class Switch Recombination. *J Exp Med*, Vol.204, No.12, pp.3017-3026, ISSN 1540-9538

Hakem, R. (2008) DNA-Damage Repair; the Good, the Bad, and the Ugly. *EMBO J*, Vol.27, No.4, pp.589-605, ISSN 1460-2075

Hakem, R., de la Pompa, J.L., Sirard, C., Mo, R., Woo, M., Hakem, A., Wakeham, A., Potter, J., Reitmair, A., Billia, F., Firpo, E., Hui, C.C., Roberts, J., Rossant, J. & Mak, T.W. (1996) The Tumor Suppressor Gene Brca1 Is Required for Embryonic Cellular Proliferation in the Mouse. *Cell*, Vol.85, No.7, pp.1009-1023, ISSN 0092-8674

Halaby, M.J., Hibma, J.C., He, J. & Yang, D.Q. (2008) Atm Protein Kinase Mediates Full Activation of Akt and Regulates Glucose Transporter 4 Translocation by Insulin in Muscle Cells. *Cell Signal*, Vol.20, No.8, pp.1555-1563, ISSN 0898-6568

Hartlerode, A.J. & Scully, R. (2009) Mechanisms of Double-Strand Break Repair in Somatic Mammalian Cells. *Biochem J*, Vol.423, No.2, pp.157-168, ISSN 1470-8728

Heyer, W.D., Ehmsen, K.T. & Liu, J. (2010) Regulation of Homologous Recombination in Eukaryotes. *Annu Rev Genet*, Vol.44, pp.113-139, ISSN 1545-2948

Huen, M.S., Grant, R., Manke, I., Minn, K., Yu, X., Yaffe, M.B. & Chen, J. (2007) Rnf8 Transduces the DNA-Damage Signal Via Histone Ubiquitylation and Checkpoint Protein Assembly. *Cell*, Vol.131, No.5, pp.901-914, 0092-8674

Jensen, R.B., Carreira, A. & Kowalczykowski, S.C. (2010) Purified Human Brca2 Stimulates Rad51-Mediated Recombination. *Nature,* Vol.467, No.7316, pp.678-683, ISSN 1476-4687

Jonkers, J., Meuwissen, R., van der Gulden, H., Peterse, H., van der Valk, M. & Berns, A. (2001) Synergistic Tumor Suppressor Activity of Brca2 and P53 in a Conditional Mouse Model for Breast Cancer. *Nat Genet,* Vol.29, No.4, pp.418-425, ISSN 1061-4036

Kass, E.M. & Jasin, M. (2010) Collaboration and Competition between DNA Double-Strand Break Repair Pathways. *FEBS Lett,* Vol.584, No.17, pp.3703-3708, ISSN 1873-3468

Keeney, S., Giroux, C.N. & Kleckner, N. (1997) Meiosis-Specific DNA Double-Strand Breaks Are Catalyzed by Spo11, a Member of a Widely Conserved Protein Family. *Cell,* Vol.88, No.3, pp.375-384, ISSN 0092-8674

Kim, H., Chen, J. & Yu, X. (2007) Ubiquitin-Binding Protein Rap80 Mediates Brca1-Dependent DNA Damage Response. *Science,* Vol.316, No.5828, pp.1202-1205, ISSN 1095-9203

Kolas, N.K., Chapman, J.R., Nakada, S., Ylanko, J., Chahwan, R., Sweeney, F.D., Panier, S., Mendez, M., Wildenhain, J., Thomson, T.M., Pelletier, L., Jackson, S.P. & Durocher, D. (2007) Orchestration of the DNA-Damage Response by the Rnf8 Ubiquitin Ligase. *Science,* Vol.318, No.5856, pp.1637-1640, ISSN 1095-9203

Kotnis, A., Du, L., Liu, C., Popov, S.W. & Pan-Hammarstrom, Q. (2009) Non-Homologous End Joining in Class Switch Recombination: The Beginning of the End. *Philos Trans R Soc Lond B Biol Sci,* Vol.364, No.1517, pp.653-665, ISSN 1471-2970

Kumar, R., Bourbon, H.M. & de Massy, B. (2010) Functional Conservation of Mei4 for Meiotic DNA Double-Strand Break Formation from Yeasts to Mice. *Genes Dev,* Vol.24, No.12, pp.1266-1280, ISSN 1549-5477

Lamarche, B.J., Orazio, N.I. & Weitzman, M.D. (2010) The Mrn Complex in Double-Strand Break Repair and Telomere Maintenance. *FEBS Lett,* Vol.584, No.17, pp.3682-3695, ISSN 1873-3468

Lavin, M.F. (2008) Ataxia-Telangiectasia: From a Rare Disorder to a Paradigm for Cell Signalling and Cancer. *Nat Rev Mol Cell Biol,* Vol.9, No.10, pp.759-769, ISSN 1471-0080

Li, G., Alt, F.W., Cheng, H.L., Brush, J.W., Goff, P.H., Murphy, M.M., Franco, S., Zhang, Y. & Zha, S. (2008) Lymphocyte-Specific Compensation for Xlf/Cernunnos End-Joining Functions in V(D)J Recombination. *Mol Cell,* Vol.31, No.5, pp.631-640, ISSN 1097-4164

Li, L., Halaby, M.J., Hakem, A., Cardoso, R., El Ghamrasni, S., Harding, S., Chan, N., Bristow, R., Sanchez, O., Durocher, D. & Hakem, R. (2010) Rnf8 Deficiency Impairs Class Switch Recombination, Spermatogenesis, and Genomic Integrity and Predisposes for Cancer. *J Exp Med,* Vol.207, No.5, pp.983-997, ISSN 1540-9538

Llorente, B., Smith, C.E. & Symington, L.S. (2008) Break-Induced Replication: What Is It and What Is It For? *Cell Cycle,* Vol.7, No.7, pp.859-864, ISSN 1551-4005

Lorenz, A., West, S.C. & Whitby, M.C. (2009) The Human Holliday Junction Resolvase Gen1 Rescues the Meiotic Phenotype of a Schizosaccharomyces Pombe Mus81 Mutant. *Nucleic Acids Res,* Vol.38, No.6, pp.1866-1873, ISSN 1362-4962

Lou, Z., Minter-Dykhouse, K., Franco, S., Gostissa, M., Rivera, M.A., Celeste, A., Manis, J.P., van Deursen, J., Nussenzweig, A., Paull, T.T., Alt, F.W. & Chen, J. (2006) Mdc1

Maintains Genomic Stability by Participating in the Amplification of Atm-Dependent DNA Damage Signals. *Mol Cell,* Vol.21, No.2, pp.187-200, ISSN 1097-2765

Macrae, C.J., McCulloch, R.D., Ylanko, J., Durocher, D. & Koch, C.A. (2008) Aplf (C2orf13) Facilitates Nonhomologous End-Joining and Undergoes Atm-Dependent Hyperphosphorylation Following Ionizing Radiation. *DNA Repair (Amst),* Vol.7, No.2, pp.292-302, ISSN 1568-7864

Mahaney, B.L., Meek, K. & Lees-Miller, S.P. (2009) Repair of Ionizing Radiation-Induced DNA Double-Strand Breaks by Non-Homologous End-Joining. *Biochem J,* Vol.417, No.3, pp.639-650, ISSN 1470-8728

Mailand, N., Bekker-Jensen, S., Faustrup, H., Melander, F., Bartek, J., Lukas, C. & Lukas, J. (2007) Rnf8 Ubiquitylates Histones at DNA Double-Strand Breaks and Promotes Assembly of Repair Proteins. *Cell,* Vol.131, No.5, pp.887-900, ISSN 0092-8674

Mak, T.W., Hakem, A., McPherson, J.P., Shehabeldin, A., Zablocki, E., Migon, E., Duncan, G.S., Bouchard, D., Wakeham, A., Cheung, A., Karaskova, J., Sarosi, I., Squire, J., Marth, J. & Hakem, R. (2000) Brca1 Is Required for T Cell Lineage Development but Not Tcr Loci Rearrangement. *Nat Immunol,* Vol.1, No.1, pp.77-82, ISSN 1529-2908

Matsuoka, S., Ballif, B.A., Smogorzewska, A., McDonald, E.R., 3rd, Hurov, K.E., Luo, J., Bakalarski, C.E., Zhao, Z., Solimini, N., Lerenthal, Y., Shiloh, Y., Gygi, S.P. & Elledge, S.J. (2007) Atm and Atr Substrate Analysis Reveals Extensive Protein Networks Responsive to DNA Damage. *Science,* Vol.316, No.5828, pp.1160-1166, ISSN 1095-9203

McKinnon, P.J. & Caldecott, K.W. (2007) DNA Strand Break Repair and Human Genetic Disease. *Annu Rev Genomics Hum Genet,* Vol.8, pp.37-55, ISSN 1527-8204

McPherson, J.P., Lemmers, B., Hirao, A., Hakem, A., Abraham, J., Migon, E., Matysiak-Zablocki, E., Tamblyn, L., Sanchez-Sweatman, O., Khokha, R., Squire, J., Hande, M.P., Mak, T.W. & Hakem, R. (2004) Collaboration of Brca1 and Chk2 in Tumorigenesis. *Genes Dev,* Vol.18, No.10, pp.1144-1153, ISSN 0890-9369

Modesti, M. & Kanaar, R. (2001) DNA Repair: Spot(Light)S on Chromatin. *Curr Biol,* Vol.11, No.6, pp.R229-232, ISSN 0960-9822

Morris, J.R., Boutell, C., Keppler, M., Densham, R., Weekes, D., Alamshah, A., Butler, L., Galanty, Y., Pangon, L., Kiuchi, T., Ng, T. & Solomon, E. (2009) The Sumo Modification Pathway Is Involved in the Brca1 Response to Genotoxic Stress. *Nature,* Vol.462, No.7275, pp.886-890, ISSN 1476-4687

Moshous, D., Pannetier, C., Chasseval Rd, R., Deist Fl, F., Cavazzana-Calvo, M., Romana, S., Macintyre, E., Canioni, D., Brousse, N., Fischer, A., Casanova, J.L. & Villartay, J.P. (2003) Partial T and B Lymphocyte Immunodeficiency and Predisposition to Lymphoma in Patients with Hypomorphic Mutations in Artemis. *J Clin Invest,* Vol.111, No.3, pp.381-387, ISSN 0021-9738

Muramatsu, M., Kinoshita, K., Fagarasan, S., Yamada, S., Shinkai, Y. & Honjo, T. (2000) Class Switch Recombination and Hypermutation Require Activation-Induced Cytidine Deaminase (Aid), a Potential Rna Editing Enzyme. *Cell,* Vol.102, No.5, pp.553-563, ISSN 0092-8674

Nakada, S., Tai, I., Panier, S., Al-Hakim, A., Iemura, S., Juang, Y.C., O'Donnell, L., Kumakubo, A., Munro, M., Sicheri, F., Gingras, A.C., Natsume, T., Suda, T. &

Durocher, D. (2010) Non-Canonical Inhibition of DNA Damage-Dependent Ubiquitination by Otub1. *Nature,* Vol.466, No.7309, pp.941-946, ISSN 1476-4687

Nicassio, F., Corrado, N., Vissers, J.H., Areces, L.B., Bergink, S., Marteijn, J.A., Geverts, B., Houtsmuller, A.B., Vermeulen, W., Di Fiore, P.P. & Citterio, E. (2007) Human Usp3 Is a Chromatin Modifier Required for S Phase Progression and Genome Stability. *Curr Biol,* Vol.17, No.22, pp.1972-1977, ISSN 0960-9822

Nijnik, A., Woodbine, L., Marchetti, C., Dawson, S., Lambe, T., Liu, C., Rodrigues, N.P., Crockford, T.L., Cabuy, E., Vindigni, A., Enver, T., Bell, J.I., Slijepcevic, P., Goodnow, C.C., Jeggo, P.A. & Cornall, R.J. (2007) DNA Repair Is Limiting for Haematopoietic Stem Cells During Ageing. *Nature,* Vol.447, No.7145, pp.686-690, ISSN 1476-4687

Nimonkar, A.V., Ozsoy, A.Z., Genschel, J., Modrich, P. & Kowalczykowski, S.C. (2008) Human Exonuclease 1 and Blm Helicase Interact to Resect DNA and Initiate DNA Repair. *Proc Natl Acad Sci U S A,* Vol.105, No.44, pp.16906-16911, ISSN 1091-6490

Nussenzweig, A., Chen, C., da Costa Soares, V., Sanchez, M., Sokol, K., Nussenzweig, M.C. & Li, G.C. (1996) Requirement for Ku80 in Growth and Immunoglobulin V(D)J Recombination. *Nature,* Vol.382, No.6591, pp.551-555, ISSN 0028-0836

O'Donovan, P.J. & Livingston, D.M. (2010) Brca1 and Brca2: Breast/Ovarian Cancer Susceptibility Gene Products and Participants in DNA Double-Strand Break Repair. *Carcinogenesis,* Vol.31, No.6, pp.961-967, ISSN 1460-2180

O'Driscoll, M., Cerosaletti, K.M., Girard, P.M., Dai, Y., Stumm, M., Kysela, B., Hirsch, B., Gennery, A., Palmer, S.E., Seidel, J., Gatti, R.A., Varon, R., Oettinger, M.A., Neitzel, H., Jeggo, P.A. & Concannon, P. (2001) DNA Ligase Iv Mutations Identified in Patients Exhibiting Developmental Delay and Immunodeficiency. *Mol Cell,* Vol.8, No.6, pp.1175-1185, ISSN 1097-2765

Panier, S. & Durocher, D. (2009) Regulatory Ubiquitylation in Response to DNA Double-Strand Breaks. *DNA Repair (Amst),* Vol.8, No.4, pp.436-443, ISSN 1568-7864

Petukhova, G.V., Pezza, R.J., Vanevski, F., Ploquin, M., Masson, J.Y. & Camerini-Otero, R.D. (2005) The Hop2 and Mnd1 Proteins Act in Concert with Rad51 and Dmc1 in Meiotic Recombination. *Nat Struct Mol Biol,* Vol.12, No.5, pp.449-453, ISSN 1545-9993

Rass, U., Compton, s.A., Matos, J., Singleton, M.R., Ip, S.C.Y., Blanco, M.G., Griffith, J.D. & West, S.C. (2010) Mechanism of Holliday Junction Resolution by the Human Gen1 Protein. *Genes and Development,* Vol.24, pp.1559-1569

Reina-San-Martin, B., Nussenzweig, M.C., Nussenzweig, A. & Difilippantonio, S. (2005) Genomic Instability, Endoreduplication, and Diminished Ig Class-Switch Recombination in B Cells Lacking Nbs1. *Proc Natl Acad Sci U S A,* Vol.102, No.5, pp.1590-1595, ISSN 0027-8424

Rooney, S., Sekiguchi, J., Zhu, C., Cheng, H.L., Manis, J., Whitlow, S., DeVido, J., Foy, D., Chaudhuri, J., Lombard, D. & Alt, F.W. (2002) Leaky Scid Phenotype Associated with Defective V(D)J Coding End Processing in Artemis-Deficient Mice. *Mol Cell,* Vol.10, No.6, pp.1379-1390, ISSN 1097-2765

Santos, M.A., Huen, M.S., Jankovic, M., Chen, H.T., Lopez-Contreras, A.J., Klein, I.A., Wong, N., Barbancho, J.L., Fernandez-Capetillo, O., Nussenzweig, M.C., Chen, J. & Nussenzweig, A. (2010) Class Switching and Meiotic Defects in Mice Lacking the E3 Ubiquitin Ligase Rnf8. *J Exp Med,* Vol.207, No.5, pp.973-981, ISSN 1540-9538

Shao, G., Lilli, D.R., Patterson-Fortin, J., Coleman, K.A., Morrissey, D.E. & Greenberg, R.A. (2009) The Rap80-Brcc36 De-Ubiquitinating Enzyme Complex Antagonizes Rnf8-Ubc13-Dependent Ubiquitination Events at DNA Double Strand Breaks. *Proc Natl Acad Sci U S A*, Vol.106, No.9, pp.3166-3171, ISSN 1091-6490

Shinohara, A., Ogawa, H. & Ogawa, T. (1992) Rad51 Protein Involved in Repair and Recombination in S. Cerevisiae Is a Reca-Like Protein. *Cell,* Vol.69, No.3, pp.457-470, ISSN 0092-8674

Simsek, D. & Jasin, M. (2010) Alternative End-Joining Is Suppressed by the Canonical Nhej Component Xrcc4-Ligase Iv During Chromosomal Translocation Formation. *Nat Struct Mol Biol,* Vol.17, No.4, pp.410-416, ISSN 1545-9985

Sleeth, K.M., Sorensen, C.S., Issaeva, N., Dziegielewski, J., Bartek, J. & Helleday, T. (2007) Rpa Mediates Recombination Repair During Replication Stress and Is Displaced from DNA by Checkpoint Signalling in Human Cells. *J Mol Biol,* Vol.373, No.1, pp.38-47, ISSN 0022-2836

Soulas-Sprauel, P., Rivera-Munoz, P., Malivert, L., Le Guyader, G., Abramowski, V., Revy, P. & de Villartay, J.P. (2007) V(D)J and Immunoglobulin Class Switch Recombinations: A Paradigm to Study the Regulation of DNA End-Joining. *Oncogene,* Vol.26, No.56, pp.7780-7791, ISSN 1476-5594

Stavnezer, J., Guikema, J.E. & Schrader, C.E. (2008) Mechanism and Regulation of Class Switch Recombination. *Annu Rev Immunol,* Vol.26, pp.261-292, ISSN 0732-0582

Stewart, G.S., Maser, R.S., Stankovic, T., Bressan, D.A., Kaplan, M.I., Jaspers, N.G., Raams, A., Byrd, P.J., Petrini, J.H. & Taylor, A.M. (1999) The DNA Double-Strand Break Repair Gene Hmre11 Is Mutated in Individuals with an Ataxia-Telangiectasia-Like Disorder. *Cell,* Vol.99, No.6, pp.577-587, ISSN 0092-8674

Stewart, G.S., Panier, S., Townsend, K., Al-Hakim, A.K., Kolas, N.K., Miller, E.S., Nakada, S., Ylanko, J., Olivarius, S., Mendez, M., Oldreive, C., Wildenhain, J., Tagliaferro, A., Pelletier, L., Taubenheim, N., Durandy, A., Byrd, P.J., Stankovic, T., Taylor, A.M. & Durocher, D. (2009) The Riddle Syndrome Protein Mediates a Ubiquitin-Dependent Signaling Cascade at Sites of DNA Damage. *Cell,* Vol.136, No.3, pp.420-434, ISSN 1097-4172

Stewart, G.S., Stankovic, T., Byrd, P.J., Wechsler, T., Miller, E.S., Huissoon, A., Drayson, M.T., West, S.C., Elledge, S.J. & Taylor, A.M. (2007) Riddle Immunodeficiency Syndrome Is Linked to Defects in 53bp1-Mediated DNA Damage Signaling. *Proc Natl Acad Sci U S A*, Vol.104, No.43, pp.16910-16915, ISSN 0027-8424

Stewart, G.S., Wang, B., Bignell, C.R., Taylor, A.M. & Elledge, S.J. (2003) Mdc1 Is a Mediator of the Mammalian DNA Damage Checkpoint. *Nature,* Vol.421, No.6926, pp.961-966, ISSN 0028-0836

Sung, P. & Klein, H. (2006) Mechanism of Homologous Recombination: Mediators and Helicases Take on Regulatory Functions. *Nat Rev Mol Cell Biol,* Vol.7, No.10, pp.739-750, ISSN 1471-0072

Suzuki, A., de la Pompa, J.L., Hakem, R., Elia, A., Yoshida, R., Mo, R., Nishina, H., Chuang, T., Wakeham, A., Itie, A., Koo, W., Billia, P., Ho, A., Fukumoto, M., Hui, C.C. & Mak, T.W. (1997) Brca2 Is Required for Embryonic Cellular Proliferation in the Mouse. *Genes Dev,* Vol.11, No.10, pp.1242-1252, ISSN 0890-9369

Taylor, A.M., Groom, A. & Byrd, P.J. (2004) Ataxia-Telangiectasia-Like Disorder (Atld)-Its Clinical Presentation and Molecular Basis. *DNA Repair (Amst)*, Vol.3, No.8-9, pp.1219-1225, ISSN 1568-7864

Theunissen, J.W., Kaplan, M.I., Hunt, P.A., Williams, B.R., Ferguson, D.O., Alt, F.W. & Petrini, J.H. (2003) Checkpoint Failure and Chromosomal Instability without Lymphomagenesis in Mre11(Atld1/Atld1) Mice. *Molecular Cell*, Vol.12, No.6, pp.1511-1523

Tsubouchi, H. & Roeder, G.S. (2002) The Mnd1 Protein Forms a Complex with Hop2 to Promote Homologous Chromosome Pairing and Meiotic Double-Strand Break Repair. *Mol Cell Biol*, Vol.22, No.9, pp.3078-3088, ISSN 0270-7306

van der Burg, M., Ijspeert, H., Verkaik, N.S., Turul, T., Wiegant, W.W., Morotomi-Yano, K., Mari, P.O., Tezcan, I., Chen, D.J., Zdzienicka, M.Z., van Dongen, J.J. & van Gent, D.C. (2009) A DNA-Pkcs Mutation in a Radiosensitive T-B- Scid Patient Inhibits Artemis Activation and Nonhomologous End-Joining. *J Clin Invest*, Vol.119, No.1, pp.91-98, ISSN 0021-9738

van Engelen, B.G., Hiel, J.A., Gabreels, F.J., van den Heuvel, L.P., van Gent, D.C. & Weemaes, C.M. (2001) Decreased Immunoglobulin Class Switching in Nijmegen Breakage Syndrome Due to the DNA Repair Defect. *Hum Immunol*, Vol.62, No.12, pp.1324-1327, ISSN 0198-8859

Vousden, K.H. (2006) Outcomes of P53 Activation--Spoilt for Choice. *J Cell Sci*, Vol.119, No.Pt 24, pp.5015-5020, ISSN 0021-9533

Waltes, R., Kalb, R., Gatei, M., Kijas, A.W., Stumm, M., Sobeck, A., Wieland, B., Varon, R., Lerenthal, Y., Lavin, M.F., Schindler, D. & Dork, T. (2009) Human Rad50 Deficiency in a Nijmegen Breakage Syndrome-Like Disorder. *Am J Hum Genet*, Vol.84, No.5, pp.605-616, ISSN 1537-6605

Wang, B., Matsuoka, S., Ballif, B.A., Zhang, D., Smogorzewska, A., Gygi, S.P. & Elledge, S.J. (2007) Abraxas and Rap80 Form a Brca1 Protein Complex Required for the DNA Damage Response. *Science*, Vol.316, No.5828, pp.1194-1198, ISSN 1095-9203

Warmerdam, D.O. & Kanaar, R. (2010) Dealing with DNA Damage: Relationships between Checkpoint and Repair Pathways. *Mutat Res*, Vol.704, No.1-3, pp.2-11, ISSN 0027-5107

Williams, B.R., Mirzoeva, O.K., Morgan, W.F., Lin, J., Dunnick, W. & Petrini, J.H. (2002) A Murine Model of Nijmegen Breakage Syndrome. *Curr Biol*, Vol.12, No.8, pp.648-653, ISSN 0960-9822

Xiao, Y. & Weaver, D.T. (1997) Conditional Gene Targeted Deletion by Cre Recombinase Demonstrates the Requirement for the Double-Strand Break Repair Mre11 Protein in Murine Embryonic Stem Cells. *Nucleic Acids Res*, Vol.25, No.15, pp.2985-2991, ISSN 0305-1048

Xiao, Z., Yannone, S.M., Dunn, E. & Cowan, M.J. (2009) A Novel Missense Rag-1 Mutation Results in T-B-Nk+ Scid in Athabascan-Speaking Dine Indians from the Canadian Northwest Territories. *Eur J Hum Genet*, Vol.17, No.2, pp.205-212, ISSN 1476-5438

Xu, X., Wagner, K.U., Larson, D., Weaver, Z., Li, C., Ried, T., Hennighausen, L., Wynshaw-Boris, A. & Deng, C.X. (1999) Conditional Mutation of Brca1 in Mammary Epithelial Cells Results in Blunted Ductal Morphogenesis and Tumour Formation. *Nat Genet*, Vol.22, No.1, pp.37-43, ISSN 1061-4036

Yu, X., Fu, S., Lai, M., Baer, R. & Chen, J. (2006) Brca1 Ubiquitinates Its Phosphorylation-Dependent Binding Partner Ctip. *Genes and Development,* Vol.20, pp.1721-1726

Zhu, J., Petersen, S., Tessarollo, L. & Nussenzweig, A. (2001) Targeted Disruption of the Nijmegen Breakage Syndrome Gene Nbs1 Leads to Early Embryonic Lethality in Mice. *Curr Biol,* Vol.11, No.2, pp.105-109, ISSN 0960-9822

4

The Role of Error-Prone Alternative Non-Homologous End-Joining in Genomic Instability in Cancer

Li Li[1], Carine Robert[2] and Feyruz V. Rassool[2]
[1]Department of Oncology, Johns Hopkins University School of Medicine
[2]Department of Radiation Oncology and Greenebaum Cancer Center
University of Maryland School of Medicine, Baltimore, MD
USA

1. Introduction

To maintain the integrity of the genome, cells have evolved a complex set of pathways that function in response to DNA damage. Components of this response include *(i)* cell cycle checkpoints that prevent damaged DNA from being replicated, *(ii)* induction of programmed cell death to prevent the transmission of potentially mutagenic genetic changes and *(iii)* DNA repair pathways that remove various types of DNA lesions such as single base lesions, single strand breaks (SSB)s or double strand breaks (DSB)s.

DSBs are considered the most lethal form of DNA damage because, unlike almost any other types of DNA damage that have an intact undamaged template strand to guide the repair, the integrity of both strands of the duplex is lost (Khanna and Jackson, 2001). DSBs can be induced by environmental factors such as ionizing radiation, ultraviolet light, therapeutic treatment but also occur as a consequence of specific physiological processes such as DNA replication, the V(D)J recombination in B and T-lymphocytes or the immunoglobulin class switch recombination (CSR) within immunoglobulin variable domains in B-lymphocytes occurring during the development and maturation of the immune system (Ferguson and Alt, 2001, Revy et al., 2005). In order to maintain the integrity of the DNA information, cells recruit stringent DSB repair machinery to ensure the efficient repair of various types of DNA damage. Thus, failure to properly repair the DSBs may cause chromosomal abnormalities, which in turn, may lead to genomic instability and predispose the cells to malignant transformation. Moreover, the importance of DNA repair in protecting against DSB-induced genomic instability is suggested by the increased incidence of cancer in autosomal recessive DNA repair deficient human syndromes, such as BRCA1/2 deficient breast cancers (Futreal et al., 1994). Thus, since genomic instability is a common characteristic of both inherited and sporadic forms of cancer cells, it is likely that abnormalities in DNA repair contribute to the development and progression of sporadic cancers (Khanna and Jackson, 2001).

DSBs can be repaired by two major pathways, homology–directed repair (HR) and non-homologous end-joining (NHEJ) (Helleday et al., 2007). HR is active during the late S and G2 phases of the cell cycle and uses the intact sister chromatid as the template for repair

(Khanna and Jackson, 2001, Hartlerode and Scully, 2009). This pathway is a highly efficacious and error-free form of repair and is mainly responsible for the repair of DSBs caused by stalled/or collapsed replication forks induced for example by chemotherapeutic agents that abrogate DNA replication (Keller et al., 2001). HR mechanisms and their implication in genomic stability are reviewed in detail in Khanna and Jackson, 2001, Helleday et al., 2007, Hartlerode and Scully, 2009.

NHEJ repairs DSBs quite differently from HR by joining DNA ends directly. This form of repair is independent of extensive DNA sequence homology, and therefore errors can be introduced during the processing and joining of non-compatible DNA ends (Khanna and Jackson, 2001, Lieber, 2008, Hartlerode and Scully, 2009). NHEJ occurs throughout the cell cycle and is the major DSB repair pathway in G0, G1 and early S phase. NHEJ is the preferential pathway for repair of DSBs in mammalian cells (Lieber et al., 2003, Lieber, 2008).

Here, we describe the mechanism(s) and the role(s) of the error-prone NHEJ pathway in the maintenance of genomic instability in cancer and discuss how targeting NHEJ is a promising therapeutic strategy in cancer.

2. Error-prone NHEJ pathway: Mechanisms and properties in normal and cancer cells

Classical or C-NHEJ contributes to the repair of DSBs caused by endogenous and exogenous DNA damaging agents and also plays an important role in the repair of programmed DSBs in normal mammalian cells, made during V(D)J or CSR (Lieber et al., 2006). In addition, evidence now exists for an alternative version of NHEJ (ALT-NHEJ) (Nussenzweig and Nussenzweig, 2007) that exists at low levels in normal cells (Sallmyr et al., 2008b) and is enhanced in the absence of C-NHEJ. Here, we discuss the mechanisms and properties of C-NHEJ and ALT-NHEJ in normal and cancer cells.

2.1 The C-NHEJ pathway

There appears to be two phases of C-NHEJ: a rapid phase and a slower phase (Riballo et al., 2004). The rapid phase will repair most of the simple lesions which do not require any type of processing. In contrast, the slower phase of NHEJ reflects both the repair of (i) DSBs that occur in condensed chromatin and (ii) more complex DSBs that require processing before ligation (Riballo et al., 2004, Goodarzi et al., 2008).

The C-NHEJ pathway is initiated by the Ku70/Ku86 heterodimer also called Ku, a ring shaped complex that binds DSBs (Walker et al., 2001). This leads to the recruitment of the catalytic subunit of DNA dependent protein kinase (DNA PKcs) (Mimori and Hardin, 1986, Falzon et al., 1993, Gottlieb and Jackson, 1993) to form the activated DNA PK (Calsou et al., 1999, Singleton et al., 1999). The kinase activity of DNA PK is critical for C-NHEJ (Lees-Miller et al., 1990). DNA PK also phosphorylates other proteins, such as Artemis, which binds to DNA PKcs (Ma et al., 2002), activating its endonuclease activity at both 3' and 5' overhangs. The physical juxtaposition of DNA ends involves interactions between DNA-bound DNA PKcs molecules (Yaneva et al., 1997, DeFazio et al., 2002). If DNA ends can be directly ligated then the repair only requires ligation by XLF/DNA ligase IV/XRCC4, after interaction with DNA PK (Ahnesorg et al., 2006, Buck et al., 2006). However, a large fraction of DSBs generated by agents such as, ionizing radiation, are not directly ligatable, and require additional processing (Chen et al., 2000, Lobrich and Jeggo, 2005). Many proteins are involved in processing these DNA ends, including polynucleotide kinase (PNK) which interacts with XRCC4 (Chappell et al., 2002), the nucleases Flap endonuclease-1 (FEN-1) (Wu et al., 1999) and Artemis (Chen et al., 2000), and the Polymerase X family members, Pol μ and λ (Ma et al., 2004). As a consequence of these processing reactions, the joining of DSBs by C-NHEJ often results in the loss or addition of a few nucleotides and the presence of short complementary sequences, microhomologies, at the break site that presumably contribute to the alignment of the DNA ends (Roth et al., 1985, Roth and Wilson, 1986). A schematic of the C-NHEJ is presented in **Figure 1**.

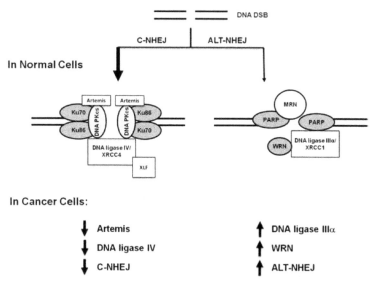

Fig. 1. In normal cells (upper panel), ALT-NHEJ pathway is a minor DSB repair pathway compared with C-NHEJ. In cancer cells (lower panel), the steady state levels of key C-NHEJ proteins are reduced whereas the steady state levels of key ALT-NHEJ are increased. This results in increased activity of the ALT-NHEJ pathway and reduced activity of the C-NHEJ pathway. Figure modified from Rassool and Tomkinson, 2010.

2.2 The ALT-NHEJ pathway

There are several lines of evidence for an alternative or back-up version of NHEJ that is enhanced in the absence of C-NHEJ (Riballo et al., 2004, Wang et al., 2006, Nussenzweig and Nussenzweig, 2007) **(Figure 1)**. While these studies have begun to define more precisely the characteristics, mechanisms, regulation and roles of ALT-NHEJ in the development and maintenance of cancer, much of this pathway(s) remains to be elucidated. In the next section, the current state of our knowledge of ALT-NHEJ will be discussed.

2.2.1 Key signatures of ALT-NHEJ

The key features of the ALT-NHEJ pathway are that the repair junctions are characterized by larger deletions, insertions, and longer tracts of microhomology compared with those generated by C-NHEJ, and a much higher frequency of chromosomal translocations (Nussenzweig and Nussenzweig, 2007).

2.2.1.1 Microhomologies

Mechanistically, 3′ single stranded overhangs containing longer tracts of microhomology are used to mediate ALT-NHEJ (Corneo et al., 2007, Yan et al., 2007, Bennardo et al., 2008, Deriano et al., 2009, Dinkelmann et al., 2009, Rass et al., 2009, Xie et al., 2009). This generally involves the loss of the intervening DNA sequences between the microhomology containing regions, resulting in larger DNA deletions. The regions of microhomology always reside at the precise site of repair and can be used as a marker to define these repair events. Moreover, while, ALT-NHEJ is associated with the generation of 3′ single stranded overhang at the sites of DSBs, the presence of the DNA end-processing factor CtIP, appears to be required for microhomology-mediated joins upon depletion of the C-NHEJ component Ku70 (Lee-Theilen et al., 2011). Notably, microhomology sequences suggestive of ALT-NHEJ have been found at the recombination junctions of radiation-induced genomic rearrangements (Morris and Thacker, 1993, Nohmi et al., 1999) implying that radiation-induced DSBs can be repaired by ALT-NHEJ. Moreover, microhomologies are frequently detected at the breakpoints of chromosomal deletions and translocations in human cancer cells (Canning and Dryja, 1989, Dryja et al., 1989, Smanik et al., 1995, Wiemels and Greaves, 1999).

2.2.1.2 Translocation frequency

Several groups have observed that in the absence of C-NHEJ proteins, chromosomal translocations occur with increased frequency (Boboila et al., 2010b, Simsek and Jasin, 2010). These authors thus suggested that C-NHEJ suppresses chromosomal translocations. An alternative explanation for the increase in translocation frequency when C-NHEJ is absent, is that end-joining may be inefficient due to missing or mutant NHEJ components, and this may lead to the accumulation of multiple unrepaired DSBs. There is evidence that the repair kinetics of ALT-NHEJ is slower than that of C-NHEJ, in that end-joining assays performed in cells lacking DNA ligase IV are about 10 times slower than in cells proficient for C-NHEJ (Yan et al., 2007, Han and Yu, 2008). Thus, slowed NHEJ would be expected to increase the time of overlap during which two breaks would remain unrepaired, thereby increasing the chance of translocation events (Lieber, 2010).

Recent studies have suggested that oncogenes critical in the pathogenesis of leukemias directly or indirectly down regulate steady state levels of key C-NHEJ proteins, and in concert, upregulate key ALT-NHEJ proteins, leading to an increase in the frequency of deletions and translocations, which likely drive genomic instability, disease progression or resistance to treatment (Chen et al., 2008, Sallmyr et al., 2008b, Fan et al., 2010, Li et al., 2011).

2.2.2 Components involved in ALT-NHEJ

The presence or absence of Ku at the DSB dictate whether repair occurs *via* C-NHEJ or ALT-NHEJ, respectively (Fattah et al., 2010, Cheng et al., 2011). Several DNA repair proteins have been implicated in ALT-NHEJ repair. These include, DNA ligase IIIα/XRCC1, poly(ADP) ribose polymerase-1 (PARP-1), the MRN complex (Mre11/Rad50/Nbs1), WRN and CtIP (Audebert et al., 2004, Wang et al., 2005, Wang et al., 2006, Rass et al., 2009, Robert et al., 2009, Xie et al., 2009, Lee-Theilen et al., 2011, Cheng et al., 2011, Zhang and Jasin, 2011).

Given that ALT-NHEJ is initiated by resected DNA ends, the question arises, which factors can bind resected DSBs to start this repair process? Recent work identified PARP-1 as an additional potential contributor to ALT-NHEJ (Audebert et al., 2004). PARP-1 recognizes DNA strand interruptions *in vivo* and triggers its own modification as well as that of other proteins by the sequential addition of ADP-ribose to form polymers. PARP-1 intervenes in base excision and single strand annealing (SSA) and now also operates in ALT-NHEJ (Audebert et al., 2004, Wang et al., 2006). While its role in ALT-NHEJ remains to be clearly elucidated, Wang et al. showed that PARP-1 binds to DNA ends in direct competition with Ku (Wang et al., 2006). When essential components of C-NHEJ are absent, PARP-1 is recruited for DSB repair, particularly in the absence of Ku proteins (Wang et al., 2006, Cheng et al., 2011).

The next question that arises is, which factor(s) is involved in the final joining reaction of ALT-NHEJ? Several studies implicate DNA ligase IIIα in ALT-NHEJ (Audebert et al., 2004, Wang et al., 2005, Haber, 2008). For example, using extract fractionation studies, Wang et al., showed that the majority of DNA end joining activity in extracts of HeLa cells could be attributed to DNA ligase IIIα (Wang et al., 2005). In addition, immunodepletion of DNA ligase IIIα from cell extracts caused loss of activity that could be recovered by the addition of the joining activity contributed by the purified enzyme. These experiments also ruled out a significant contribution to the end joining activity by DNA ligase I and DNA ligase IV. Furthermore, Wang et al., also addressed this question using RNA interference to investigate the requirements for DNA ligase IIIα and DNA ligase IV in the repair of DSBs (Wang et al., 2005). *In vivo* plasmid assays showed that DNA ligase IV-deficient mouse embryonic fibroblasts (MEFs) retained significant DNA end joining activity that could be reduced by up to 80% in cells knocked down for DNA ligase IIIα using RNAi (Wang et al., 2005). These *in vivo* observations are in line with DNA ligase IIIα being a candidate component for ALT-NHEJ. Other studies have implicated additional factors in ALT-NHEJ, such as PNK, FEN-1 (Gottlich et al., 1998, Wang et al., 2003, Audebert et al., 2004, Wang et al., 2006), and it is expected that additional factors will also be identified in the future **(Figure 1)**.

2.2.3 Where ALT-NHEJ fits into the hierarchy of DSB repair?

While there is strong evidence that ALT-NHEJ is enhanced in cells that are defective for C-NHEJ, the question of where ALT-NHEJ fits into the hierarchy of DSB repair with respect to the cell cycle, and what would be the consequences of this repair at the genomic level, are still relatively unclear **(Figure 2)**.

2.2.3.1 ALT-NHEJ and cell cycle

While it is well documented that HR is efficiently carried out only in the late S and G2 phases of the cell cycle using the newly synthesized sister chromatid, whereas C-NHEJ is the major DSB repair pathway in G0, G1 and early S phase (Lieber et al., 2003, Lieber et al., 2006), recent studies suggest that ALT-NHEJ may also be cell cycle dependent. During DNA replication, the newly replicated chromatids are held together by cohesin and this sister chromatid cohesion is maintained until mitosis. When a DSB occurs, the intact sister chromatid is preferentially used to repair the DSB by HR. If HR is defective, as it is demonstrated in BRCA 1/2 deficient cells, DSB is likely to be repaired by the following error-prone pathways (Tutt et al., 2001, Venkitaraman, 2001): *(i)* SSA that generates intrachromosomal deletions between repeated sequences, *(ii)* C-NHEJ pathway that generates small intrachromosomal deletions and insertions, and *(iii)* ALT-NHEJ pathway that generates larger deletions and chromosomal translocations. One of the roles of the DNA PK complex assembled on the DNA end is to protect the DNA end from resection (Huertas, 2010). If C-NHEJ is defective, it is likely that end resection will occur (**Figure 2**). While the above hypothetical scenarios for error-prone repair of DSBs are envisioned, recent studies suggest that ALT-NHEJ may occur more frequently in G2. Mladenov and Iliakis enquired whether ALT-NHEJ was cell cycle dependent. In this study, MEFs with defects in C-NHEJ and/or HR were irradiated, G1 and G2 cells were isolated by cell sorting, and repair was examined by using pulse field gel electrophoresis (Mladenov and Iliakis, 2011). They found that wild-type and HR defective (*Rad54$^{-/-}$*) MEFs repaired DSBs with similar efficiency in G1 and G2 phases. In contrast, C-NHEJ defective (*DNA ligase IV$^{-/-}$*, *DNA PKcs$^{-/-}$*, and *Ku70$^{-/-}$*) MEFs showed a more pronounced repair defect in G1 phase than in G2 phase. Importantly, *DNA ligase IV$^{-/-}$/Rad54$^{-/-}$* MEFs repaired DSBs as efficiently as *DNA ligase IV$^{-/-}$* MEFs in G2 suggesting that the increased repair efficiency in G2 phase relies on the enhanced function of ALT-NHEJ rather than on HR. Furthermore, *in vivo* and *in vitro* plasmid end joining assays confirmed an enhanced function of ALT-NHEJ in G2 phase (Mladenov and Iliakis, 2011). Additional studies along the same lines using mutant Chinese hamster cells with defects in the DNA PKcs, Ku86 or XRCC4 components of C-NHEJ, or in the XRCC2 and XRCC3 components of HR confirmed these observations (Wu et al., 2008). Wild-type cells and mutants of HR repaired DSBs with similar efficiency in G1 and G2 phases. Mutants of C-NHEJ, showed more pronounced repair in G2 phase than in G1. These results in aggregate demonstrate a new and potentially important cell cycle regulation of ALT-NHEJ and generate a framework to investigate the mechanistic basis of HR contribution to DSB repair and its possible interactions with ALT-NHEJ.

Yet another study by Shibata et al., also examined the regulation of repair pathway usage at DSBs in G2 (Shibata et al., 2011). They identified the speed of DSB repair as a major component influencing repair pathway usage showing that DNA damage and chromatin complexity are factors influencing DSB repair rate and pathway choice. They found that loss of C-NHEJ proteins slowed DSB repair allowing increased resection. In contrast, loss of HR does not impair repair by C-NHEJ although CtIP-dependent end-resection precludes C-NHEJ usage. These data suggest that C-NHEJ initially attempts the repair of DSBs and, if rapid rejoining does not ensue, then resection occurs promoting repair by HR using the homologous chromosome as template, but this may result in loss of heterozygosity (LOH). It is likely that if repair does not occur by HR, DNA ends will be repaired by error-prone pathways, such as SSA and ALT-NHEJ, pathways that require end-resected DSBs (Shibata et al., 2011) (**Figure 2**).

2.2.3.2 Factors regulating ALT-NHEJ

Unlike C-NHEJ, the mechanism(s) for regulation of ALT-NHEJ and the factors involved in this repair pathway(s) are not clearly understood. The presence of Ku proteins appear to determine whether DSBs are repaired by C-NHEJ *vs.* ALT-NHEJ (Bennardo et al., 2008, Fattah et al., 2010, Cheng et al., 2011). Fattah et al., utilized an end-joining assay in isogenic human colon carcinoma cell lines and human somatic HCT116 with targeted deletions of the key C-NHEJ factors (Ku, DNA PKcs, XLF, and DNA ligase IV). The end-joining assay was a plasmid based repair assay of a DSB made within reporter plasmid pEGFP-Pem1-Ad2 and reconstitution of green fluorescent protein (GFP). They found that absence of key C-NHEJ factors resulted in cell lines that were profoundly impaired in DSB repair activity. Unexpectedly, Ku86-deleted cells showed wild-type levels of DNA DSB repair activity but the events were mainly repaired by microhomology joining. Using siRNA technology, ALT-

NHEJ repair activity could also be efficiently activated in *DNA ligase IV$^{-/-}$* and *DNA PKcs$^{-/-}$* cells by subsequently reducing the level of Ku70. Recently, Cheng et al., demonstrated that Ku is the main factor preventing PARP-1 and MRN mobilization to the site of DSBs (Cheng et al., 2011). These studies demonstrate that Ku proteins are the critical C-NHEJ factors that regulate DSB repair pathway choice. Similarly, studies of Bennardo et al., compared the genetic requirements for ALT-NHEJ, using a series of chromosome integrated reporters to monitor repair of DSBs by the I-SceI endonuclease in mouse embryonic stem (ES) cells and the HEK293 cell line (Bennardo et al., 2008). Each individual reporter was designed such that repair of I-SceI-induced DSBs by a specific pathway restored a GFP expression cassette. Such repair was then scored in individual cells as green fluorescence using flow cytometric analysis. They found that the *Ku70$^{-/-}$* cells exhibited a 4-fold increase in the restoration of the GFP$^+$ gene over wild-type cells, and that this increase was reversed by co-transfection of a Ku70 expression vector (Bennardo et al., 2008). Thus, the ALT-NHEJ repair events appeared not only to be Ku-independent, but also appear to be inhibited by Ku proteins (Bennardo et al., 2008, Cheng et al., 2011). Bennardo and Stark have also highlighted the importance of the presence of ataxia telangiectasia-mutated (ATM) in matching correct DNA ends during end-joining and preventing the joining of multiple chromosome ends that can lead to chromosomal translocation and genomic instability (Bennardo and Stark, 2010). They found that genetic or chemical disruption of ATM caused a substantial increase in incorrect end joining (Distal-EJ), but not correct end joining (Proximal-EJ). Moreover, the increase in Distal-EJ caused by ATM disruption was dependent on the presence of C-NHEJ factors, specifically DNA PKcs, XRCC4, and XLF. Thus, these authors concluded that ATM is important to limit incorrect end utilization during C-NHEJ. In yet another study, Zha et al. showed that ATM and XLF have fundamental roles in processing and joining DNA ends during V(D)J recombination, but that these roles were masked by functional redundancies. They found that combined deficiency of ATM and XLF nearly blocked mouse lymphocyte development due to an inability to process and join chromosomal V(D)J recombination DSB intermediates. Combined XLF and ATM deficiency also severely impaired C-NHEJ, but not ALT-NHEJ, during CSR. Redundant ATM and XLF functions in C-NHEJ appeared to be mediated by ATM kinase activity and are not required for extra-chromosomal V(D)J recombination, indicating a role for chromatin-associated ATM substrates. These authors also found a role for H2AX, protein involved in the recruitment of DNA repair factors to nuclear foci after DSBs (Rogakou et al., 1998). Conditional H2AX inactivation in XLF-deficient pro-B lines leads to V(D)J recombination defects associated with marked degradation of unjoined V(D)J ends, revealing that H2AX also has a role in the repair process (Zha et al., 2011).

Mechanistically, it is believed that during ALT-NHEJ both broken ends are resected to generate 3'-single-stranded overhangs (Huertas, 2010). Given that Ku-deficiency can lead to elevated DSB end-processing, these results raise the possibility that ALT-NHEJ, SSA and HR share end-processing as a common intermediate. Thus, Bennardo et al., determined also whether end-resecting factor CtIP is important for ALT-NHEJ, by performing siRNA knock-down of CtIP in HEK293 cell lines with integrated GFP reporter plasmids and stable expression of the inducible I-SceI protein and examined ALT-NHEJ repair in CtIP-depleted cells *vs.* control cells. They observed that ALT-NHEJ was significantly reduced in CtIP-depleted cells suggesting that CtIP-mediated DSB end-processing promotes ALT-NHEJ but also SSA and HR (Bennardo et al., 2008). Interestingly, disrupting RAD51 and RAD52 expression decrease HR and SSA activity respectively without perturbing ALT-NHEJ repair

(Bennardo et al., 2008). In recent studies, Zhang and Jasin, showed that depletion of CtIP, resulted in a substantial decrease in the chromosomal translocation frequency in mouse cells and a significantly lower usage of microhomology at the translocation breakpoint junctions. This suggests that CtIP-mediated ALT-NHEJ has a primary role in translocation formation (Zhang and Jasin, 2011).

Several studies have also implicated the MRN complex in ALT-NHEJ repair (Rass et al., 2009, Xie et al., 2009). Recent studies examined the role of the nuclease MRE11 in CSR. They showed that loss of the nuclease MRE11 resulted in milder defects, compared with loss of the whole MRN complex. This suggested that the MRN complex performed activities in end-joining, in addition to the nuclease activity of MRE11. Studies employing atomic force microscopy have visualized the MRN complex bridging DNA at distances of 1200 angstroms (Moreno-Herrero et al., 2005). Thus, MRN may perform bridging functions that may be particularly suited for CSR. In addition, since chromosomal translocations are frequently observed in ALT-NHEJ, the MRN complex may also play a role in end-bridging of distant DSBs, resulting in chromosomal rearrangements (**Figure 2**).

A schematic representation of the regulation and the hierarchy of the DSB repair pathways is presented in **Figure 2**.

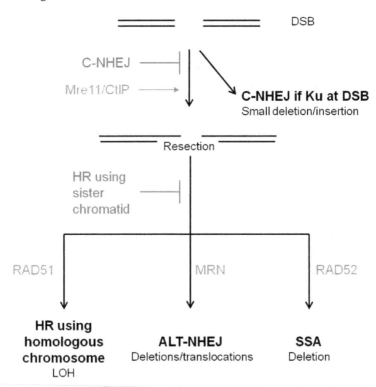

Fig. 2. The majority of the DSBs are repaired by C-NHEJ. If this pathway is inactive, DSBs can be repaired by HR using the homologous chromosome as template or by SSA or ALT-NHEJ. Positive regulators of specific stage as described in text are represented in blue while defective pathways are represented in red.

2.2.4 ALT-NHEJ at dysfunctional telomeres

Mammalian telomeres are regions of repetitive DNA sequences at the ends of chromosomes, which protect them from e or from fusion with neighbouring chromosomes. Critically shortened telomeres are recognized as DSBs and are highly susceptible to be repaired by HR or NHEJ pathways (Palm et al., 2009, Rai et al., 2010). However, unequal exchange of telomeric sequences by HR or misrepair by C- and/or ALT-NHEJ, can lead to loss of cell viability or can result in genomic instability and cancer. In mammals, telomeres form single-stranded G-rich overhangs that associate with and are protected by shelterin, a core complex of telomere-binding proteins that includes the double-stranded DNA-binding proteins TRF1 and TRF2 and protection of telomeres 1 (POT1a/b) that interacts with its binding partner TPP1 to protect them from resection, recombination and alteration (Palm et al., 2009). Telomeres are maintained by the enzyme telomerase, which is limited in human somatic cells, resulting in progressive telomere shortening. Celli et al., showed that Ku and TRF2 repress HR and represent an important aspect of telomere protection (Celli et al., 2006). Recent evidence suggests that dysfunctional telomeres that can no longer exert end-protective functions are recognized as DSBs by the DNA damage repair pathway. Thus, removal of TRF2 with retrovirus-mediated shTrf2, resulted in end-to-end chromosome fusions mediated by the C-NHEJ pathway (Rai et al., 2010). In addition, the data of Deng et al., indicated a critical role for the MRN complex in sensing these dysfunctional telomeres. They showed that in the absence of TRF2, MRE11 nuclease activity removes the 3' telomeric overhang to promote chromosome fusions. MRE11 can also protect newly replicated leading strand telomeres from NHEJ by promoting 5' strand resection to generate POT1a-TPP1-bound 3' overhangs (Deng et al., 2009). Rai et al. used also MEFs in which specific components of the C-NHEJ had been deleted to determine how dysfunctional telomeres are joined together (Rai et al., 2010). They showed that DSB marker 53BP1 (Schultz et al., 2000, Anderson et al., 2001) was necessary for end to end fusion in TRF2 deficient MEFs. Surprisingly, they showed that removal of *Tpp1-Pot1a/b* from *53BP1⁻/⁻* MEFs or *DNA ligase IV⁻/⁻* MEFs resulted in robust end to end fusions. They also examined chromosome fusion in MEFs from telomerase knock-out cells that generate naturally shortened telomeres, and which had also been knocked out for *53BP1⁻/⁻*. Lymphomas derived from these mice demonstrated an increase in the number of fused chromosomes. These data suggested that fusion of naturally shortened telomeres do not require 53BP1 and occur through mechanisms independent of C-NHEJ. They concluded that telomeres engage distinct DNA repair pathways depending on how they are rendered dysfunctional, and that ALT-NHEJ is a major pathway for processing of dysfunctional telomeres (Rai et al., 2010).

2.2.5 NHEJ-defective mouse models of cancers and leukemias

2.2.5.1 NHEJ in V(D)J recombination and CSR

In addition to DSBs generated by exogenous and endogenous DNA damaging agents, DSBs also occur as a consequence of specific physiological processes such as the V(D)J recombination in B and T-lymphocytes and the immunoglobulin CSR within immunoglobulin variable domains in B-lymphocytes during the development and maturation of the immune system (Ferguson and Alt, 2001, Revy et al., 2005). The organism recruits stringent DNA repair machinery to ensure the efficient repair of the damage or the elimination of the damaged cells. Failure to properly repair the DNA damage may cause chromosomal abnormalities, which in turn may lead to genomic instability and predispose the cells to malignant transformation.

The immune system provides a unique platform for understanding the NHEJ pathway because of its requirement for V(D)J recombination and CSR for development and maturation. In these systems, DNA damage is initiated by recombination activating gene 1 and 2 (RAG1/RAG2) in the case of V(D)J recombination, activation-induced cytidine deaminase (AID) in the case of CSR (Oettinger et al., 1990, McBlane et al., 1995, Petersen et al., 2001, Manis et al., 2002), that is uniquely expressed in specialized B- or T-lymphocytes. The rejoining of the broken DNA ends is then completed by C- and/or ALT-NHEJ pathway (Bassing et al., 2002). Notably, V(D)J recombination specifically recruits the C-NHEJ pathway components (Corneo et al., 2007). In contrast, approximately 50% of CSR events are completed by the ALT-NHEJ pathways (Soulas-Sprauel et al., 2007b, Yan et al., 2007, Han and Yu, 2008). Animal models and human conditions have demonstrated that defects in any of the C-NHEJ pathway components may cause immunodeficiency. The resultant erroneous DNA repair may predispose the cells to genomic instability and the development of cancer.

2.2.5.2 Defective C-NHEJ in immunodeficiency

Spontaneous mutant and genetically engineered animal models deficient for the various C-NHEJ components have in common impaired V(D)J recombination and consequent immunodeficiency, together with increased sensitivity to ionizing radiation.

Severe combined immune deficiency (SCID) mouse is a naturally occurring mutant mouse strain (Bosma and Carroll, 1991) which harbors a non-sense mutation in their highly conserved C-terminal part of DNA PKcs gene (Blunt et al., 1996, Araki et al., 1997). These mice lack mature B and T lymphocytes (Bosma and Carroll, 1991), accompanied by an increased cellular radiosensitivity (RS-SCIDs), indicative of a defect in DNA repair. Similarly, DNA PKcs knockout mice do not show overt cellular growth defects but exhibit immunodeficiency and ionizing radiation hypersensitivity (Gao et al., 1998, Taccioli et al., 1998, Kurimasa et al., 1999). Artemis-deficient mice resemble DNA PKcs-deficient mice, including a leaky SCID and increased cellular ionizing radiation sensitivity, supporting the idea that Artemis cooperates with DNA PKcs in a subset of C-NHEJ functions (Rooney et al., 2002).

Like the DNA-PKcs mutant SCID mice, Ku70 and Ku86 knockout mice demonstrate "leaky" immunodeficiency and are hypersensitive to irradiation (Nussenzweig et al., 1996, Zhu et al., 1996, Gu et al., 1997, Ouyang et al., 1997). In addition, they also show signs of growth retardation and extensive apoptosis of the newly generated neurons. Mice lacking either XRCC4 or DNA ligase IV die *in utero* with massive neuronal apoptosis and a complete block in lymphocyte development, suggesting the requirement for Ku, XRCC4 and DNA ligase IV in growth control and neuron development (Barnes et al., 1998, Frank et al., 1998, Gao et al., 1998). Mice lacking XLF are also immunodeficient and hypersensitive to ionizing radiation. However, they have modestly reduced lymphocyte numbers, nearly normal V(D)J recombination and moderately defective immunoglobulin heavy chain CSR (Li et al., 2008). Combined deficiency of ATM and XLF severely impairs V(D)J recombination and nearly blocks mouse lymphocyte development, indicative of the compensatory roles of ATM and XLF in C-NHEJ pathway (Zha et al., 2011), as discussed earlier in this chapter.

2.2.5.3 Involvement of ALT-NHEJ pathways in leukemia/lymphoma in mouse models

In the absence of C-NHEJ, the microhomology-based ALT-NHEJ is thought to be employed to ligate the broken DNA ends generated during V(D)J recombination and CSR.

Mice defective for one or more C-NHEJ components show various degrees of genomic instability. The absence of Ku, XRCC4, DNA ligase IV, XLF, Artemis, or DNA PKcs leads to the accumulation of DNA breaks and translocations in ES cells, fibroblasts or stimulated B cells (Guidos et al., 1996, Nacht et al., 1996, Karanjawala et al., 1999, Difilippantonio et al., 2000, Ferguson and Alt, 2001, Zhu et al., 2002, Rooney et al., 2003, Yan et al., 2007, Franco et al., 2008, Li et al., 2008, Boboila et al., 2010a). In the presence of the p53-null background, deletion of any one of the key components of the C-NHEJ pathway invariably leads to the early onset of very aggressive tumors, mostly pro-B-cell lymphomas, which generally harbor chromosomal translocations. Mice defective for *P53* and *Ku86* develop pro-B-cell lymphoma at an early age (Difilippantonio et al., 2000). These tumors display a specific set of chromosomal translocations and gene amplifications involving the immunoglobulin heavy chain IgH/Myc locus, reminiscent of Burkitt lymphoma. Combined deficiency in p53/XRCC4 or p53/DNA ligase IV results in live births. However, the offspring are immunodeficient and develop pro-B cell lymphomas (Frank et al., 2000, Gao et al., 2000). Mice lacking both Artemis and p53 develop pro–B cell lymphomas harboring N-myc-IgH, but not the Myc-Igh translocations observed in tumors in other C-NHEJ/p53 deficient mice (Rooney et al., 2004). XLF/p53-double-deficient mice are not markedly prone to pro-B lymphomas. However, like other C-NHEJ/p53-deficient mice, they still develop medulloblastomas (Li et al., 2008).

Recent studies based on C-NHEJ deficient mutant models also revealed that Ku or DNA ligase IV/XRCC4 are not required for, but rather suppress chromosomal translocations (Corneo et al., 2007, Soulas-Sprauel et al., 2007a, Yan et al., 2007, Boboila et al., 2010a). It has recently been reported that translocation breakpoint junctions are similar in wild-type and Ku or XRCC4 deficient mutants, including an unchanged bias toward microhomology. Complex insertions at some breakpoint junctions show that joining can be iterative, encompassing successive processing steps before joining, implying that ALT-NHEJ contributes to the translocation formation in mammalian cells (Simsek and Jasin, 2010).

Altogether, the development of leukemia/lymphoma in C-NHEJ deficient mouse models suggests that ALT-NHEJ pathways play important roles in the DSB repair in V(D)J recombination and CSR. Its low fidelity predisposes the cells to genomic instability and the development of malignancy. Further investigations of the molecular mechanisms underlying these pathways will provide insights into the roles of ALT-NHEJ in the occurrence of genomic instability and the development of cancer.

2.2.6 ALT-NHEJ in human cancer and leukemia

Many of the studies characterizing ALT-NHEJ have been conducted in a background of experimentally induced deficiency of components of the C-NHEJ pathway. This has drawn criticism that the results demonstrating ALT-NHEJ are biased by artificial experimental conditions that do not exist in reality. Many human cancers are characterized by recurrent chromosome abnormalities and microhomologous sequences have been identified at the breakpoint junctions of these abnormalities. Therefore, human cancers may represent model systems in which to study ALT-NHEJ.

2.2.6.1 Leukemia and lymphoma cells as models for the study of ALT-NHEJ

Like the SCID phenotype observed in mice, defective V(D)J recombination in humans causes arrest of B and T lymphocyte maturation, conferring severe combined immune deficiency (T-B-SCID). 70% of T-B-SCID patients have mutations in RAG1 or RAG2, which disables the initiation steps in V(D)J recombination. The remaining 30% patients also show hypersensitivity to ionizing radiation, and therefore referred to as RS-SCID. They are caused by defects in the C-NHEJ pathway (de Villartay et al., 2003). So far, most genetic defects reported are found in the Artemis gene. In other cases, mutations in DNA ligase IV, XLF and DNA PKcs are reported. EBV-associated B-cell lymphomas and leukemia have been reported in patients with Artemis and DNA ligase IV mutations, respectively, indicative of the genomic instability associated with the impaired C-NHEJ (Riballo et al., 1999, Moshous et al., 2003). Patients with mutations in the gene encoding XLF also have greater chromosomal instability (Dai et al., 2003, Buck et al., 2006). These findings suggest that RS-SCID patients defective for C-NHEJ have elevated genomic instability which may predispose the cells to cancer. It is also likely that ALT-NHEJ among other error-prone pathways may drive genomic instability in these cases.

2.2.6.2 Microhomologies at breakpoints junction of recurrent alterations in cancer and leukemia

In vivo and *in vitro* assays in cancer and leukemia cells demonstrate increased errors following repair, with the majority of errors resulting from large DNA deletions occurring at the repair sites characterized by sequence microhomologies. Using *in vitro* end-joining assays based on repair of pUC18 plasmids containing a DSB in cell lines derived from myeloid leukemias, Gaymes et al. demonstrated a significant increase in errors characterized by increased size of deletions and microhomologies at the repair junctions further suggestive of the importance of ALT-NHEJ repair in these malignancies (Gaymes et al., 2002). Analyzing actual genomic deletions in tumors, Canning and Dryja found genomic deletions involving the retinoblastoma gene in 12 of 49 tumors from patients with retinoblastoma or osteosarcoma. They mapped the deletion breakpoints and sequenced 200 base pairs surrounding each deletion breakpoint in DNA from 4 tumor samples. Three deletions had termini characterized by direct repeats ranging in size from 4 to 7 base pairs (Canning and Dryja, 1989).

Recurrent chromosome translocations characterize leukemia and lymphoma and are specifically associated with their classification and prognosis. They occur frequently in both *de novo* and therapy-related in acute myeloid leukemia (AML) and myelodysplastic syndromes (MDS). Cloning of the genomic breakpoints in the common chromosome translocations in leukemia reveal that most of the genomic breakpoints tend to cluster in a restricted intronic region (Zhang and Rowley, 2006). In addition, sequencing of the translocation junctions identified regions of microhomology, strongly indicative of the involvement of ALT-NHEJ in the repair of DSBs and the generation of these chromosomal abnormalities (Reichel et al., 1998, Gillert et al., 1999, Strissel et al., 2000, Rassool, 2003, Zhang and Rowley, 2006; Wiemels and Greaves, 1999, Xiao et al., 2001, Reiter et al., 2003, Zhang and Rowley, 2006). An important example of such a study is sequencing of the TEL AML1 gene fusions found in pediatric leukemias and approximately 25% of adult acute B cell lymphomas. Analysis of the DNA sequence and structure surrounding the breakpoints revealed clues to their possible formation (Wiemels and Greaves, 1999). A long-distance inverse PCR strategy was used to amplify *TEL-AML1* genomic fusion sequences from diagnostic DNA from nine patients. Breakpoints were scattered within the 14 kb of intronic DNA between exons 5 and 6 of *TEL* and in two putative cluster regions within intron 1 of *AML1*. DNA sequences containing the breakpoint junctions exhibited characteristic signs of C- and ALT-NHEJ, including microhomologies at the breakpoints, small deletions and duplications. Wiemels and Greaves concluded that the data was compatible with the possibility that *TEL-AML1* translocations occur by nonhomologous recombination involving imprecise, constitutive repair processes following DSBs (Wiemels and Greaves, 1999, Zelent et al., 2004).

2.2.6.3 Origins of DNA damage?

Genes such as *AML1, TEL* or *mixed lineage leukemia (MLL)* have been found rearranged with different partner genes in lymphoid and myeloid leukemias (Zelent et al., 2004). These translocations have been shown to correlate with sites of double-strand DNA cleavage by agents to which the cells or patients have been exposed, including exogenous rare-cutting endonucleases, radiomimetic compounds, and topoisomerase inhibitors (Greaves and Wiemels, 2003). The nature of the DNA damage leading to *MLL* translocations in leukemia in infants have been examined by several investigators (Greaves and Wiemels, 2003). The finding of identical *MLL* rearrangements in the leukemias from pairs of monozygotic twins where both twins were affected, but not in their constitutional DNA, established that *MLL* translocations in infant leukemias are non-hereditary, non-constitutional, *in utero* events. Furthermore, the most likely explanation was that cells with the translocation were transferred from one twin to the other *via* the placenta (Felix et al., 2000). The retrospective finding of leukemia-associated *MLL* genomic breakpoint junction sequences by PCR analysis of genomic DNAs contained in bloodspots on neonatal Guthrie cards of infants who were diagnosed later with leukemia showed that *MLL* translocations also occur *in utero* in the non-twin cases (Gale et al., 1997). Molecular cloning and analysis of *MLL* genomic breakpoint junctions sequences in infant leukemias suggested staggered and/or multiple sites of breakage as elements of damage and DNA repair by C- and/or ALT-NHEJ. This provided further evidence that DNA damage and repair underlie the formation of the translocations (Greaves and Wiemels, 2003, Gilliland et al., 2004). Because *MLL* translocations are much less frequent in *de novo* leukemias of older patients but frequent in leukemias following chemotherapeutic DNA topoisomerase II poisons, e.g., etoposide, it has been proposed that leukemia in infants may have an etiology resembling treatment-related cases (Gilliland et al., 2004). The chemotherapy-leukemia association in the treatment-related cases suggests that chromosomal breakage resulting from DNA topoisomerase II cleavage and attempted repair of DSBs may play a role in the formation of these translocations. The precision of the breakpoint junction sequences and the results of DNA topoisomerase II *in vitro* cleavage assays in treatment-related leukemias are consistent with the processing of 4-base, staggered DSB (Gilliland et al., 2004). In the infant leukemias, the breakpoint junction sequences and *in vitro* cleavage assays suggest a mechanism in which DNA topoisomerase II introduce separate single-stranded nicks in duplex DNA that are staggered by up to several hundred bases. This leads to a DNA damage-repair model in which various naturally occurring DNA topoisomerase II poisons induce DNA topoisomerase II-mediated damage in leukemia *in utero* (Gilliland et al., 2004). The large deleted regions observed in other infant cases are consistent with multiple sites of breakage or, alternatively, more extensive processing (Raffini et al., 2002).

2.2.6.4 Increased ALT-NHEJ activity in leukemia

In addition to increased DNA damage providing a substrate for error-prone repair and genomic instability, increased repair activity may also drive the acquisition of genomic alterations. Recently, Sallmyr at al. demonstrated increased activity of the ALT-NHEJ pathway in chronic myeloid leukemia (CML) cells characterized by the oncogenic fusion tyrosine kinase, BCR-ABL (Gaymes et al., 2002, Sallmyr et al., 2008b). They showed that key proteins in the major C-NHEJ pathway, Artemis and DNA ligase IV, were down-regulated, whereas DNA ligase IIIα, and the protein deleted in Werner syndrome, WRN, are up-regulated in CML cells. Furthermore, they showed that DNA ligase IIIα and WRN form a complex that is recruited to DSBs, and that "knockdown" of either DNA ligase IIIα or WRN leads to increased accumulation of unrepaired DSBs, demonstrating that these DNA repair proteins contribute to their repair. To determine whether knockdown of either DNA ligase IIIα or WRN leads to differences in repair using DNA sequence microhomologies, Sallmyr et al. sequenced the breakpoint junctions of 15 repaired plasmids from each of the LacZα reactivation experiments. The majority (80%) of plasmids in CML cell line, K562 were repaired using DNA microhomologies of 1 to 6 bp. In contrast, plasmids from cells with reduced levels of either DNA ligase IIIα or WRN had a reduction in the overall percentage of microhomologies and these constituted 1 to 3 bp in length (DNA ligase IIIα, 25%; WRN, 40%) at the breakpoint junctions in repaired plasmids. Notably, in cell lines established from normal lymphocytes, end-joining assays reveal that the DSBs are repaired mainly using the C-NHEJ pathway. Furthermore, sequencing of the rare DSBs that were misrepaired (1 in approximately 10,000) revealed deletions of only a few base pairs. These results indicate that while ALT-NHEJ is possibly operative at very low levels in normal cells, altered DSB repair in CML cells may be caused at least in part by the increased activity of ALT-NHEJ repair pathway, involving DNA ligase IIIα and WRN. In AML characterized by expression of the constitutively activated receptor tyrosine kinase Fms Like tyrosine 3/Internal tandem duplication (FLT3/ITD), Sallmyr et al. reported that this constitutively activated tyrosine kinase initiates a cycle of genomic instability that is likely to promote both aggressive disease and resistance to therapy (Sallmyr et al., 2008a). Specifically, Sallmyr et al. showed that expression of FLT3/ITD induces increased reactive oxygen species production and that cells transformed by FLT3/ITD, including primary AML cells and cell lines established from FLT3/ITD-positive AML patients, have increased endogenous DSBs (Sallmyr et al., 2008a). Furthermore, repair of DSBs by NHEJ is less efficient and more error-prone in FLT3/ITD-expressing cells (Sallmyr et al., 2008a). More recently, Fan et al. reported that the steady state levels of Ku86 and to a lesser extent, Ku70, are significantly reduced in FLT3/ITD-expressing cells (Fan et al., 2010). In turn, there is a concomitant increase in the steady state levels of ALT-NHEJ components, PARP-1 and DNA ligase IIIα (Fan et al., 2010). Similar alterations in Ku86 and PARP-1 are also observed in FLT3/ITD knock-in mice, but increased levels of DNA ligase IIIα are only seen in the homozygote mice (Fan et al, 2010). Similar changes in C-NHEJ and ALT-NHEJ components are observed at the transcript level (Li et al., 2011) (**Figure 3**). In the FLT3/ITD mouse model, the impairment of C-NHEJ decreases the ability of cells to complete post-cleavage DSB ligation, resulting in failure to complete V(D)J recombination inhibiting B-lymphocyte maturation (Li et al, 2011). As a consequence of these changes in NHEJ proteins, the frequency of DNA sequence microhomologies and the size of deletions at repair sites are increased, reflecting the increased contribution of ALT-NHEJ to DSB repair. This suggests that FLT3/ITD signaling is involved in regulating both C- and ALT-NHEJ, directly or indirectly (**Figure 3**). Importantly, they reported that reducing the levels of DNA ligase IIIα in AML cells not only reduces the frequency of DNA sequence microhomologies and the size of deletions at repair sites but also increases the steady state levels of unrepaired DSBs, indicating that the ALT-NHEJ pathway is particularly important for the survival of FLT3/ITD expressing AML cells (Li et al., 2011).

2.2.7 ALT-NHEJ as therapeutic targets

Several lines of evidence suggest that both hereditary and sporadic cancers have abnormal level of DNA damage and repair responses that lead to the generation of structural chromosomal abnormalities and genomic instability, which are critical for survival, disease progression and resistance. The identification of defects in the DNA damage response between normal and cancer cells at the molecular level will guide the development of more targeted therapies by identifying biomarkers that are indicative of the abnormal DNA repair in cancer cells. To exploit the differences in the DNA damage response between normal and cancer cells, it will be necessary to characterize the DNA repair abnormalities and develop agents that target the abnormal DNA repair pathways that are specific for cancer cells, thereby reducing survival of cancer but not normal cells. In addition to participating in base excision and SSB repair, PARP-1 and DNA ligase IIIα also appear to be involved in ALT-NHEJ. In recent studies, we and others have shown that PARP-1 and DNA ligase IIIα are upregulated in certain cancers and leukemias (Chen et al., 2008, Sallmyr et al., 2008b, Fan et al., 2010, Li et al., 2011) (**Figure 4**).

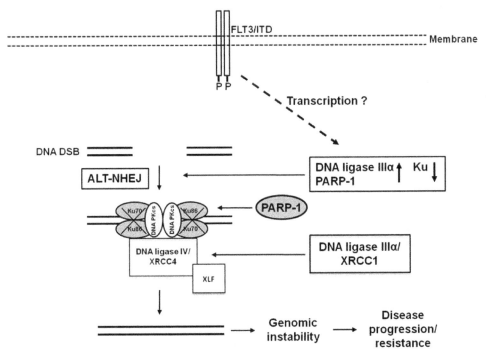

Fig. 3. Schematic for the mechanism of regulation of C- and ALT-NHEJ by FLT3/ITD. FLT3/ITD signalling leads to upregulation of DNA ligase IIIα and PARP-1 and downregulation of Ku70/86. The consequent increase in ALT-NHEJ activity promotes the acquisition of genomic changes that lead to disease progression or resistance to treatment.

2.2.7.1 PARP inhibitors

The abundant nuclear protein PARP-1 binds avidly to SSBs, an event that activates PARP-1 polymerase (Ame et al., 2004). Activated PARP-1 utilizes nicotinamide to synthesize poly(ADP-ribose) polymers on itself and other nuclear proteins. Poly(ADP-ribosylated) PARP-1 serves as a recruitment factor for DNA ligase IIIα/XRCC1 and other factors involved in the repair of SSBs (Okano et al., 2003). Although there are other PARP family members, PARP-1 is the predominant enzyme that synthesizes poly(ADP-ribose) in response to DNA damage (Menissier de Murcia et al., 2003). The replication of DNA containing SSBs cause DSBs and so preventing the repair of SSBs by inhibiting PARP-1 results in an increase in DSBs. Since these replication-associated DSBs would normally be repaired by HR, cells that are defective in HR are hypersensitive to PARP inhibitors. Based on this rationale, potent and specific inhibitors of PARP were developed as therapeutic agents for inherited forms of breast and ovarian cancer as the PARP inhibitors should be cytotoxic for *BRCA* mutant tumors but not normal tissues with a functional *BRCA* allele (Bryant et al., 2005, Farmer et al., 2005). As expected, PARP inhibitors increased the cytotoxicity of a range of anti-cancer agents including temozolomide and ionizing radiation that cause SSBs (Tentori et al., 2002, Liu et al., 2008) and both *BRCA1*- and *BRCA2*-mutant cell lines were hypersensitive to PARP inhibitors in cell culture and mouse xenograft assays (Lord and Ashworth, 2008). These results formed the basis for a phase I clinical trial, which demonstrated that the PARP inhibitor AZD2281 exhibited antitumor activity in patients with ovarian and breast tumors resulting from either *BRCA1* or *BRCA2* mutations (Evers et al., 2008). The promising results from this clinical trial have prompted the evaluation of PARP inhibitors in combination with other cancer therapeutics in the treatment of different types of cancer.

Unfortunately, resistance to PARP-1 inhibitors has led to the failure of phase III clinical trials in triple negative breast cancers, and thus there is an urgency for elucidating the mechanisms by which resistance occurs in cells with defects in HR (Guha, 2011). One potential mechanism for resistance to PARP inhibitors in BRCA-deficient cells is that spontaneous or induced DSBs are rerouted for repair by error-prone mechanisms, including NHEJ, because the preferred mode of error-free repair by HR is unavailable (Venkitaraman, 2001). Patel et al. recently showed that in *BRCA2* deficient ovarian cancer cell lines PARP inhibitor treatment induces phosphorylation of DNA PK substrates and stimulates C-NHEJ selectively. Previous studies provided evidence for interplay between key C-NHEJ proteins and PARP-1: *(i)* PARP-1 can interact *in vitro* and *in vivo* with Ku (Galande and Kohwi-Shigematsu, 1999) and has been shown to compete with Ku80 for DNA ends *in vitro* (Wang et al., 2006), *(ii)* Ablation of C-NHEJ restores the survival of PARP-1-deficient cells treated with agents inducing DSBs (Hochegger et al., 2006). All together those results suggest that C-NHEJ and perhaps ALT-NHEJ could be involved in the genomic instability observed in HR-deficient cells treated with PARP inhibitors (Patel et al., 2011). Patel et al. showed that inhibiting DNA PK activity reverses the genomic instability induced by PARP inhibition in *BRCA2* deficient cells. Moreover, disabling C-NHEJ by using genetic or pharmacologic approaches diminished the toxicity of PARP inhibition in HR-deficient cells. These results not only implicate PARP-1 catalytic activity in the regulation of C-NHEJ and perhaps ALT-NHEJ in HR-deficient cells, but also indicate that deregulated C-NHEJ and perhaps ALT-NHEJ plays a major role in generating cytotoxicity and genomic instability in HR-deficient cells treated with PARP inhibitors (Patel et al., 2011). Recently Chen et al. showed that C-NHEJ protein DNA ligase IV was down regulated in cell lines derived from sporadic breast cancer (Chen et al., 2008). Thus, it would be important to evaluate C-NHEJ and ALT-NHEJ activity in *BRCA* deficient tumors in assessment of clinical response and resistance to PARP inhibitors.

2.2.7.2 DNA ligase inhibitors

DNA joining events are required for the completion of almost all DNA repair pathways. Thus, inhibitors of DNA ligase are predicted to sensitize cells to a variety of DNA damaging agents depending upon the inhibitor specificity for the three mammalian DNA ligases. Using computer-aided drug design based on the structure of human DNA ligase I in complex with nicked DNA, a series of small molecule inhibitors of human DNA ligases have been identified (Chen et al., 2008, Zhong et al., 2008). Briefly, an in silico data base of about 1.5 million commercially available small molecules was screened for candidates that were predicted to bind to a DNA binding pocket within the DNA binding domain (DBD) of human DNA ligase I. This binding pocket makes key contacts with nicked DNA (Chen et al., 2008). Out of 233 candidate molecules, 192 were assayed for their ability to inhibit human DNA ligase I but not T4 DNA ligase and for their ability to inhibit cell proliferation because human DNA ligase I is the major replicative DNA ligase. The *in vitro* DNA joining assays identified 10 small molecules that specifically inhibit human DNA ligase I by more than 50% at 100 mM, with 5 of these molecules also inhibiting the proliferation of cultured human cells. Since the amino acid sequences of the DBDs of human DNA ligases III and IV are closely related to that of the human DNA ligase I DBD, Chen et al. enquired whether the inhibitors of human DNA ligase I are also active against the other human DNA ligases. Molecules that inhibit DNA ligase I alone (L82), DNA ligase I and III (L67), and all three human DNA ligases (L189) *in vitro*, that were also active in cell culture assays, were further characterized. In accord with the screening strategy, all the ligase inhibitors with the exception of L82 act as competitive inhibitors with respect to nicked DNA. The structure of L67 and the other inhibitors consists of heterocyclic rings separated by a flexible linker. Interestingly, L67 and L189 are cytotoxic, whereas L82 is cytostatic. It is possible that this reflects the different mechanisms of inhibition. Alternatively, while inhibition of DNA ligase I alone is not toxic, inhibition of either DNA ligase III or DNA ligase IV alone or in combination with human DNA ligase I may be cytotoxic. Another interesting feature of the ligase inhibitors is that sub-toxic concentrations specifically potentiate the cytotoxicity of DNA-damaging agents in cancer cells (**Figure 4**). As in cell lines expressing BCR-ABL and FLT3/ITD (Sallmyr et al., 2008b, Fan et al., 2010), DNA ligase IIIα is also overexpressed in cancer cell lines, whereas the levels of DNA ligase IV are reduced compared to a non-cancerous breast epithelial cell line (Chen et al., 2008). Together these results suggests that ligase inhibitors will not only provide a novel approach to delineating the cellular functions of these enzyme, but may also serve as lead compounds for the development of therapeutic agents that target DNA replication and/or repair (Chen et al., 2008).

Notably, these compounds exhibit different specificities for the three human DNA ligases *in vitro* and a subset of these molecules preferentially sensitize cancer cells to DNA alkylating agents and ionizing radiation, suggesting that they may have utility as lead compounds for the development of novel therapeutic agents. Notably, the ligase inhibitors would constitute an extremely versatile group of agents in that, depending on their specificity, they can be used to target a variety of DNA repair pathways that would be chosen based on the DNA damaging agent. For example, a DNA ligase IV specific inhibitor would sensitize cells with a functional C-NHEJ pathway to ionizing radiation whereas a DNA ligase III specific inhibitor would sensitize cancer cells that are dependent upon ALT-NHEJ to ionizing radiation and other agents that cause DSBs, such as PARP inhibitors (**Figure 4**).

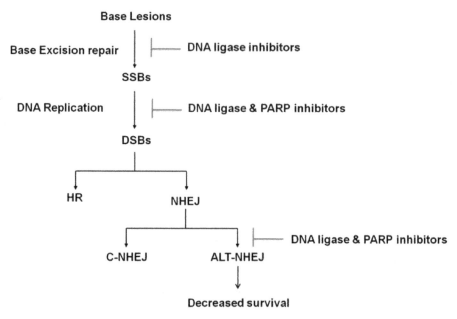

Fig. 4. Schematic of the effect of DNA ligase and PARP inhibitors on base excision repair, DNA replication and ALT-NHEJ in cancer and leukemia cells.

3. Conclusion

ALT-NHEJ is involved in the development of a variety of cancers, including leukemias, and is likely to play a key role in the generation of chromosomal abnormalities, including translocations, that drive cancer progression. It appears that cancer cells are more dependent on ALT-NHEJ for the repair of DSBs and survival, compared with normal cells. Thus targeting this pathway may be an attractive therapeutic strategy. Elucidation of the pathways components, and how they are regulated, will further guide the design of these therapies. Finally, investigation of the molecular mechanisms underlying abnormal DNA damage and repair in cancers and leukemias, together with the development of new animal models, will better our understanding of the complex relations between DNA repair and neoplastic transformation, which will provide new targets for the treatment of cancer.

4. References

Ahnesorg, P., Smith, P. & Jackson, S.P. (2006). XLF interacts with the XRCC4-DNA ligase IV complex to promote DNA nonhomologous end-joining. *Cell*, 124, 2, 301-13.

Ame, J.C., Spenlehauer, C. & de Murcia, G. (2004). The PARP superfamily. *Bioessays*, 26, 8, 882-93.

Anderson, L., Henderson, C. & Adachi, Y. (2001). Phosphorylation and rapid relocalization of 53BP1 to nuclear foci upon DNA damage. *Molecular and cellular biology*, 21, 5, 1719-29.

Araki, R., Fujimori, A., Hamatani, K., Mita, K., Saito, T., Mori, M., Fukumura, R., Morimyo, M., Muto, M., Itoh, M., Tatsumi, K. & Abe, M. (1997). Nonsense mutation at Tyr-4046 in the DNA-dependent protein kinase catalytic subunit of severe combined immune deficiency mice. *Proc Natl Acad Sci U S A*, 94, 6, 2438-43.

Audebert, M., Salles, B. & Calsou, P. (2004). Involvement of poly(ADP-ribose) polymerase-1 and XRCC1/DNA ligase III in an alternative route for DNA double-strand breaks rejoining. *J Biol Chem*, 279, 53, 55117-26.

Barnes, D.E., Stamp, G., Rosewell, I., Denzel, A. & Lindahl, T. (1998). Targeted disruption of the gene encoding DNA ligase IV leads to lethality in embryonic mice. *Curr Biol*, 8, 25, 1395-8.

Bassing, C.H., Swat, W. & Alt, F.W. (2002). The mechanism and regulation of chromosomal V(D)J recombination. *Cell*, 109 Suppl, S45-55.

Bennardo, N., Cheng, A., Huang, N. & Stark, J.M. (2008). Alternative-NHEJ is a mechanistically distinct pathway of mammalian chromosome break repair. *PLoS Genet*, 4, 6, e1000110.

Bennardo, N. & Stark, J.M. (2010). ATM limits incorrect end utilization during non-homologous end joining of multiple chromosome breaks. *PLoS genetics*, 6, 11, e1001194.

Blunt, T., Gell, D., Fox, M., Taccioli, G.E., Lehmann, A.R., Jackson, S.P. & Jeggo, P.A. (1996). Identification of a nonsense mutation in the carboxyl-terminal region of DNA-dependent protein kinase catalytic subunit in the scid mouse. *Proc Natl Acad Sci U S A*, 93, 19, 10285-90.

Boboila, C., Jankovic, M., Yan, C.T., Wang, J.H., Wesemann, D.R., Zhang, T., Fazeli, A., Feldman, L., Nussenzweig, A., Nussenzweig, M. & Alt, F.W. (2010a). Alternative end-joining catalyzes robust IgH locus deletions and translocations in the combined absence of ligase 4 and Ku70. *Proc Natl Acad Sci U S A*, 107, 7, 3034-9.

Boboila, C., Yan, C., Wesemann, D.R., Jankovic, M., Wang, J.H., Manis, J., Nussenzweig, A., Nussenzweig, M. & Alt, F.W. (2010b). Alternative end-joining catalyzes class switch recombination in the absence of both Ku70 and DNA ligase 4. *The Journal of experimental medicine*, 207, 2, 417-27.

Bosma, M.J. & Carroll, A.M. (1991). The SCID mouse mutant: definition, characterization, and potential uses. *Annu Rev Immunol*, 9, 323-50.

Bryant, H.E., Schultz, N., Thomas, H.D., Parker, K.M., Flower, D., Lopez, E., Kyle, S., Meuth, M., Curtin, N.J. & Helleday, T. (2005). Specific killing of BRCA2-deficient tumours with inhibitors of poly(ADP-ribose) polymerase. *Nature*, 434, 7035, 913-7.

Buck, D., Malivert, L., de Chasseval, R., Barraud, A., Fondaneche, M.C., Sanal, O., Plebani, A., Stephan, J.L., Hufnagel, M., le Deist, F., Fischer, A., Durandy, A., de Villartay, J.P. & Revy, P. (2006). Cernunnos, a novel nonhomologous end-joining factor, is mutated in human immunodeficiency with microcephaly. *Cell*, 124, 2, 287-99.

Calsou, P., Frit, P., Humbert, O., Muller, C., Chen, D.J. & Salles, B. (1999). The DNA-dependent protein kinase catalytic activity regulates DNA end processing by means of Ku entry into DNA. *J Biol Chem*, 274, 12, 7848-56.

Canning, S. & Dryja, T.P. (1989). Short, direct repeats at the breakpoints of deletions of the retinoblastoma gene. *Proc Natl Acad Sci U S A*, 86, 13, 5044-8.

Celli, G.B., Denchi, E.L. & de Lange, T. (2006). Ku70 stimulates fusion of dysfunctional telomeres yet protects chromosome ends from homologous recombination. *Nat Cell Biol*, 8, 8, 885-90.

Chappell, C., Hanakahi, L.A., Karimi-Busheri, F., Weinfeld, M. & West, S.C. (2002). Involvement of human polynucleotide kinase in double-strand break repair by non-homologous end joining. *Embo J*, 21, 11, 2827-32.

Chen, L., Trujillo, K., Sung, P. & Tomkinson, A.E. (2000). Interactions of the DNA ligase IV-XRCC4 complex with DNA ends and the DNA-dependent protein kinase. *J Biol Chem*, 275, 34, 26196-205.

Chen, X., Zhong, S., Zhu, X., Dziegielewska, B., Ellenberger, T., Wilson, G.M., MacKerell, A.D., Jr. & Tomkinson, A.E. (2008). Rational design of human DNA ligase inhibitors that target cellular DNA replication and repair. *Cancer Res*, 68, 9, 3169-77.

Cheng, Q., Barboule, N., Frit, P., Gomez, D., Bombarde, O., Couderc, B., Ren, G. S., Salles, B. & Calsou, P. (2011). Ku counteracts mobilization of PARP1 and MRN in chromatin damaged with DNA double-strand breaks. *Nucleic acids research*, Epud ahead of print

Corneo, B., Wendland, R.L., Deriano, L., Cui, X., Klein, I.A., Wong, S.Y., Arnal, S., Holub, A.J., Weller, G.R., Pancake, B.A., Shah, S., Brandt, V.L., Meek, K. & Roth, D.B. (2007). Rag mutations reveal robust alternative end joining. *Nature*, 449, 7161, 483-6.

Dai, Y., Kysela, B., Hanakahi, L.A., Manolis, K., Riballo, E., Stumm, M., Harville, T.O., West, S.C., Oettinger, M.A. & Jeggo, P.A. (2003). Nonhomologous end joining and V(D)J recombination require an additional factor. *Proc Natl Acad Sci U S A*, 100, 5, 2462-7.

de Villartay, J.P., Poinsignon, C., de Chasseval, R., Buck, D., Le Guyader, G. & Villey, I. (2003). Human and animal models of V(D)J recombination deficiency. *Curr Opin Immunol*, 15, 5, 592-8.

DeFazio, L.G., Stansel, R.M., Griffith, J.D. & Chu, G. (2002). Synapsis of DNA ends by DNA-dependent protein kinase. *Embo J*, 21, 12, 3192-200.

Deng, Y., Guo, X., Ferguson, D.O. & Chang, S. (2009). Multiple roles for MRE11 at uncapped telomeres. *Nature*, 460, 7257, 914-8.

Deriano, L., Stracker, T.H., Baker, A., Petrini, J.H. & Roth, D.B. (2009). Roles for NBS1 in alternative nonhomologous end-joining of V(D)J recombination intermediates. *Mol Cell*, 34, 1, 13-25.

Difilippantonio, M.J., Zhu, J., Chen, H.T., Meffre, E., Nussenzweig, M.C., Max, E.E., Ried, T. & Nussenzweig, A. (2000). DNA repair protein Ku80 suppresses chromosomal aberrations and malignant transformation. *Nature*, 404, 6777, 510-4.

Dinkelmann, M., Spehalski, E., Stoneham, T., Buis, J., Wu, Y., Sekiguchi, J.M. & Ferguson, D.O. (2009). Multiple functions of MRN in end-joining pathways during isotype class switching. *Nat Struct Mol Biol*, 16, 8, 808-13.

Dryja, T.P., Mukai, S., Petersen, R., Rapaport, J.M., Walton, D. & Yandell, D.W. (1989). Parental origin of mutations of the retinoblastoma gene. *Nature*, 339, 6225, 556-8.

Evers, B., Drost, R., Schut, E., de Bruin, M., van der Burg, E., Derksen, P.W., Holstege, H., Liu, X., van Drunen, E., Beverloo, H.B., Smith, G.C., Martin, N.M., Lau, A., O'Connor, M.J. & Jonkers, J. (2008). Selective inhibition of BRCA2-deficient mammary tumor cell growth by AZD2281 and cisplatin. *Clin Cancer Res*, 14, 12, 3916-25.

Falzon, M., Fewell, J.W. & Kuff, E.L. (1993). EBP-80, a transcription factor closely resembling the human autoantigen Ku, recognizes single- to double-strand transitions in DNA. *J Biol Chem,* 268, 14, 10546-52.

Fan, J., Li, L., Small, D. & Rassool, F. (2010). Cells expressing FLT3/ITD mutations exhibit elevated repair errors generated through alternative NHEJ pathways: implications for genomic instability and therapy. *Blood,* 116, 24, 5298-305.

Farmer, H., McCabe, N., Lord, C.J., Tutt, A.N., Johnson, D.A., Richardson, T.B., Santarosa, M., Dillon, K.J., Hickson, I., Knights, C., Martin, N.M., Jackson, S.P., Smith, G.C. & Ashworth, A. (2005). Targeting the DNA repair defect in BRCA mutant cells as a therapeutic strategy. *Nature,* 434, 7035, 917-21.

Fattah, F., Lee, E.H., Weisensel, N., Wang, Y., Lichter, N. & Hendrickson, E.A. (2010). Ku regulates the non-homologous end joining pathway choice of DNA double-strand break repair in human somatic cells. *PLoS Genet,* 6, 2, e1000855.

Felix, C.A., Lange, B.J. & Chessells, J.M. (2000). Pediatric Acute Lymphoblastic Leukemia: Challenges and Controversies in 2000. *Hematology / the Education Program of the American Society of Hematology. American Society of Hematology. Education Program,* 285-302.

Ferguson, D.O. & Alt, F.W. (2001). DNA double strand break repair and chromosomal translocation: lessons from animal models. *Oncogene,* 20, 40, 5572-9.

Franco, S., Murphy, M.M., Li, G., Borjeson, T., Boboila, C. & Alt, F.W. (2008). DNA-PKcs and Artemis function in the end-joining phase of immunoglobulin heavy chain class switch recombination. *The Journal of experimental medicine,* 205, 3, 557-64.

Frank, K.M., Sekiguchi, J.M., Seidl, K.J., Swat, W., Rathbun, G.A., Cheng, H.L., Davidson, L., Kangaloo, L. & Alt, F.W. (1998). Late embryonic lethality and impaired V(D)J recombination in mice lacking DNA ligase IV. *Nature,* 396, 6707, 173-7.

Frank, K.M., Sharpless, N.E., Gao, Y., Sekiguchi, J.M., Ferguson, D.O., Zhu, C., Manis, J.P., Horner, J., DePinho, R.A. & Alt, F.W. (2000). DNA ligase IV deficiency in mice leads to defective neurogenesis and embryonic lethality via the p53 pathway. *Mol Cell,* 5, 6, 993-1002.

Futreal, P.A., Liu, Q., Shattuck-Eidens, D., Cochran, C., Harshman, K., Tavtigian, S., Bennett, L.M., Haugen-Strano, A., Swensen, J., Miki, Y. & et al. (1994). BRCA1 mutations in primary breast and ovarian carcinomas. *Science,* 266, 5182, 120-2.

Galande, S. & Kohwi-Shigematsu, T. (1999). Poly(ADP-ribose) polymerase and Ku autoantigen form a complex and synergistically bind to matrix attachment sequences. *The Journal of biological chemistry,* 274, 29, 20521-8.

Gale, K.B., Ford, A.M., Repp, R., Borkhardt, A., Keller, C., Eden, O.B. & Greaves, M.F. (1997). Backtracking leukemia to birth: identification of clonotypic gene fusion sequences in neonatal blood spots. *Proceedings of the National Academy of Sciences of the United States of America,* 94, 25, 13950-4.

Gao, Y., Chaudhuri, J., Zhu, C., Davidson, L., Weaver, D.T. & Alt, F.W. (1998). A targeted DNA-PKcs-null mutation reveals DNA-PK-independent functions for KU in V(D)J recombination. *Immunity,* 9, 3, 367-76.

Gao, Y., Ferguson, D.O., Xie, W., Manis, J.P., Sekiguchi, J., Frank, K.M., Chaudhuri, J., Horner, J., DePinho, R.A. & Alt, F.W. (2000). Interplay of p53 and DNA-repair protein XRCC4 in tumorigenesis, genomic stability and development. *Nature,* 404, 6780, 897-900.

Gaymes, T.J., Mufti, G.J. & Rassool, F.V. (2002). Myeloid leukemias have increased activity of the nonhomologous end-joining pathway and concomitant DNA misrepair that is dependent on the Ku70/86 heterodimer. *Cancer Res,* 62, 10, 2791-7.

Gillert, E., Leis, T., Repp, R., Reichel, M., Hosch, A., Breitenlohner, I., Angermuller, S., Borkhardt, A., Harbott, J., Lampert, F., Griesinger, F., Greil, J., Fey, G.H. & Marschalek, R. (1999). A DNA damage repair mechanism is involved in the origin of chromosomal translocations t(4;11) in primary leukemic cells. *Oncogene,* 18, 33, 4663-71.

Gilliland, D.G., Jordan, C.T. & Felix, C.A. (2004). The molecular basis of leukemia. *Hematology (Am Soc Hematol Educ Program),* 80-97.

Goodarzi, A.A., Noon, A.T., Deckbar, D., Ziv, Y., Shiloh, Y., Lobrich, M. & Jeggo, P.A. (2008). ATM signaling facilitates repair of DNA double-strand breaks associated with heterochromatin. *Mol Cell,* 31, 2, 167-77.

Gottlich, B., Reichenberger, S., Feldmann, E. & Pfeiffer, P. (1998). Rejoining of DNA double-strand breaks in vitro by single-strand annealing. *Eur J Biochem,* 258, 2, 387-95.

Gottlieb, T.M. & Jackson, S.P. (1993). The DNA-dependent protein kinase: requirement for DNA ends and association with Ku antigen. *Cell,* 72, 1, 131-42.

Greaves, M.F. & Wiemels, J. (2003). Origins of chromosome translocations in childhood leukaemia. *Nat Rev Cancer,* 3, 9, 639-49.

Gu, Y., Seidl, K.J., Rathbun, G.A., Zhu, C., Manis, J.P., van der Stoep, N., Davidson, L., Cheng, H.L., Sekiguchi, J.M., Frank, K., Stanhope-Baker, P., Schlissel, M.S., Roth, D.B. & Alt, F.W. (1997). Growth retardation and leaky SCID phenotype of Ku70-deficient mice. *Immunity,* 7, 5, 653-65.

Guha, M. (2011). PARP inhibitors stumble in breast cancer. *Nat Biotechnol,* 29, 5, 373-4.

Guidos, C.J., Williams, C.J., Grandal, I., Knowles, G., Huang, M.T. & Danska, J.S. (1996). V(D)J recombination activates a p53-dependent DNA damage checkpoint in scid lymphocyte precursors. *Genes Dev,* 10, 16, 2038-54.

Haber, J.E. (2008). Alternative endings. *Proc Natl Acad Sci U S A,* 105, 2, 405-6.

Han, L. & Yu, K. (2008). Altered kinetics of nonhomologous end joining and class switch recombination in ligase IV-deficient B cells. *J Exp Med,* 205, 12, 2745-53.

Hartlerode, A.J. & Scully, R. (2009). Mechanisms of double-strand break repair in somatic mammalian cells. *Biochem J,* 423, 2, 157-68.

Helleday, T., Lo, J., van Gent, D.C. & Engelward, B.P. (2007). DNA double-strand break repair: from mechanistic understanding to cancer treatment. *DNA repair,* 6, 7, 923-35.

Hochegger, H., Dejsuphong, D., Fukushima, T., Morrison, C., Sonoda, E., Schreiber, V., Zhao, G.Y., Saberi, A., Masutani, M., Adachi, N., Koyama, H., de Murcia, G. & Takeda, S. (2006). Parp-1 protects homologous recombination from interference by Ku and Ligase IV in vertebrate cells. *EMBO J,* 25, 6, 1305-14.

Huertas, P. (2010). DNA resection in eukaryotes: deciding how to fix the break. *Nat Struct Mol Biol,* 17, 1, 11-6.

Karanjawala, Z.E., Grawunder, U., Hsieh, C.L. & Lieber, M.R. (1999). The nonhomologous DNA end joining pathway is important for chromosome stability in primary fibroblasts. *Curr Biol,* 9, 24, 1501-4.

Keller, K.L., Overbeck-Carrick, T.L. & Beck, D.J. (2001). Survival and induction of SOS in Escherichia coli treated with cisplatin, UV-irradiation, or mitomycin C are dependent on the function of the RecBC and RecFOR pathways of homologous recombination. *Mutat Res,* 486, 1, 21-9.

Khanna, K.K. & Jackson, S.P. (2001). DNA double-strand breaks: signaling, repair and the cancer connection. *Nat Genet,* 27, 3, 247-54.

Kurimasa, A., Ouyang, H., Dong, L.J., Wang, S., Li, X., Cordon-Cardo, C., Chen, D.J. & Li, G.C. (1999). Catalytic subunit of DNA-dependent protein kinase: impact on lymphocyte development and tumorigenesis. *Proc Natl Acad Sci U S A,* 96, 4, 1403-8.

Lee-Theilen, M., Matthews, A.J., Kelly, D., Zheng, S. & Chaudhuri, J. (2011). CtIP promotes microhomology-mediated alternative end joining during class-switch recombination. *Nature structural & molecular biology,* 18, 1, 75-9.

Lees-Miller, S.P., Chen, Y.R. & Anderson, C.W. (1990). Human cells contain a DNA-activated protein kinase that phosphorylates simian virus 40 T antigen, mouse p53, and the human Ku autoantigen. *Mol Cell Biol,* 10, 12, 6472-81.

Li, G., Alt, F.W., Cheng, H.L., Brush, J.W., Goff, P.H., Murphy, M.M., Franco, S., Zhang, Y. & Zha, S. (2008). Lymphocyte-specific compensation for XLF/cernunnos end-joining functions in V(D)J recombination. *Mol Cell,* 31, 5, 631-40.

Li, L., Zhang, L., Fan, J., Greenberg, K., Desiderio, S., Rassool, F.V. & Small, D. (2011). Defective nonhomologous end joining blocks B-cell development in FLT3/ITD mice. *Blood,* 117, 11, 3131-9.

Lieber, M.R. (2008). The mechanism of human nonhomologous DNA end joining. *J Biol Chem,* 283, 1, 1-5.

Lieber, M.R. (2010). NHEJ and its backup pathways in chromosomal translocations. *Nat Struct Mol Biol,* 17, 4, 393-5.

Lieber, M.R., Ma, Y., Pannicke, U. & Schwarz, K. (2003). Mechanism and regulation of human non-homologous DNA end-joining. *Nat Rev Mol Cell Biol,* 4, 9, 712-20.

Lieber, M.R., Yu, K. & Raghavan, S.C. (2006). Roles of nonhomologous DNA end joining, V(D)J recombination, and class switch recombination in chromosomal translocations. *DNA Repair (Amst),* 5, 9-10, 1234-45.

Liu, S.K., Coackley, C., Krause, M., Jalali, F., Chan, N. & Bristow, R.G. (2008). A novel poly(ADP-ribose) polymerase inhibitor, ABT-888, radiosensitizes malignant human cell lines under hypoxia. *Radiother Oncol,* 88, 2, 258-68.

Lobrich, M. & Jeggo, P.A. (2005). The two edges of the ATM sword: co-operation between repair and checkpoint functions. *Radiother Oncol,* 76, 2, 112-8.

Lord, C.J. & Ashworth, A. (2008). Targeted therapy for cancer using PARP inhibitors. *Curr Opin Pharmacol,* 8, 4, 363-9.

Ma, Y., Lu, H., Tippin, B., Goodman, M.F., Shimazaki, N., Koiwai, O., Hsieh, C.L., Schwarz, K. & Lieber, M.R. (2004). A biochemically defined system for mammalian nonhomologous DNA end joining. *Mol Cell,* 16, 5, 701-13.

Ma, Y., Pannicke, U., Schwarz, K. & Lieber, M.R. (2002). Hairpin opening and overhang processing by an Artemis/DNA-dependent protein kinase complex in nonhomologous end joining and V(D)J recombination. *Cell,* 108, 6, 781-94.

Manis, J.P., Tian, M. & Alt, F.W. (2002). Mechanism and control of class-switch recombination. *Trends Immunol,* 23, 1, 31-9.

McBlane, J.F., van Gent, D.C., Ramsden, D.A., Romeo, C., Cuomo, C.A., Gellert, M. & Oettinger, M.A. (1995). Cleavage at a V(D)J recombination signal requires only RAG1 and RAG2 proteins and occurs in two steps. *Cell*, 83, 3, 387-95.

Menissier de Murcia, J., Ricoul, M., Tartier, L., Niedergang, C., Huber, A., Dantzer, F., Schreiber, V., Ame, J.C., Dierich, A., LeMeur, M., Sabatier, L., Chambon, P. & de Murcia, G. (2003). Functional interaction between PARP-1 and PARP-2 in chromosome stability and embryonic development in mouse. *Embo J*, 22, 9, 2255-63.

Mimori, T. & Hardin, J.A. (1986). Mechanism of interaction between Ku protein and DNA. *J Biol Chem*, 261, 22, 10375-9.

Mladenov, E. & Iliakis, G. (2011). Induction and repair of DNA double strand breaks: The increasing spectrum of non-homologous end joining pathways. *Mutation research*, 711, 1-2, 61-72.

Moreno-Herrero, F., Holtzer, L., Koster, D.A., Shuman, S., Dekker, C. & Dekker, N.H. (2005). Atomic force microscopy shows that vaccinia topoisomerase IB generates filaments on DNA in a cooperative fashion. *Nucleic acids research*, 33, 18, 5945-53.

Morris, T. & Thacker, J. (1993). Formation of large deletions by illegitimate recombination in the HPRT gene of primary human fibroblasts. *Proc Natl Acad Sci U S A*, 90, 4, 1392-6.

Moshous, D., Pannetier, C., Chasseval Rd, R., Deist Fl, F., Cavazzana-Calvo, M., Romana, S., Macintyre, E., Canioni, D., Brousse, N., Fischer, A., Casanova, J.L. & Villartay, J.P. (2003). Partial T and B lymphocyte immunodeficiency and predisposition to lymphoma in patients with hypomorphic mutations in Artemis. *J Clin Invest*, 111, 3, 381-7.

Nacht, M., Strasser, A., Chan, Y.R., Harris, A.W., Schlissel, M., Bronson, R.T. & Jacks, T. (1996). Mutations in the p53 and SCID genes cooperate in tumorigenesis. *Genes Dev*, 10, 16, 2055-66.

Nohmi, T., Suzuki, M., Masumura, K., Yamada, M., Matsui, K., Ueda, O., Suzuki, H., Katoh, M., Ikeda, H. & Sofuni, T. (1999). Spi(-) selection: An efficient method to detect gamma-ray-induced deletions in transgenic mice. *Environ Mol Mutagen*, 34, 1, 9-15.

Nussenzweig, A., Chen, C., da Costa Soares, V., Sanchez, M., Sokol, K., Nussenzweig, M.C. & Li, G.C. (1996). Requirement for Ku80 in growth and immunoglobulin V(D)J recombination. *Nature*, 382, 6591, 551-5.

Nussenzweig, A. & Nussenzweig, M.C. (2007). A backup DNA repair pathway moves to the forefront. *Cell*, 131, 2, 223-5.

Oettinger, M.A., Schatz, D.G., Gorka, C. & Baltimore, D. (1990). RAG-1 and RAG-2, adjacent genes that synergistically activate V(D)J recombination. *Science*, 248, 4962, 1517-23.

Okano, S., Lan, L., Caldecott, K.W., Mori, T. & Yasui, A. (2003). Spatial and temporal cellular responses to single-strand breaks in human cells. *Mol Cell Biol*, 23, 11, 3974-81.

Ouyang, H., Nussenzweig, A., Kurimasa, A., Soares, V.C., Li, X., Cordon-Cardo, C., Li, W., Cheong, N., Nussenzweig, M., Iliakis, G., Chen, D.J. & Li, G.C. (1997). Ku70 is required for DNA repair but not for T cell antigen receptor gene recombination In vivo. *J Exp Med*, 186, 6, 921-9.

Palm, W., Hockemeyer, D., Kibe, T. & de Lange, T. (2009). Functional dissection of human and mouse POT1 proteins. *Mol Cell Biol*, 29, 2, 471-82.

Patel, A.G., Sarkaria, J.N. & Kaufmann, S.H. (2011). Nonhomologous end joining drives poly(ADP-ribose) polymerase (PARP) inhibitor lethality in homologous recombination-deficient cells. *Proceedings of the National Academy of Sciences of the United States of America,* 108, 8, 3406-11.

Petersen, S., Casellas, R., Reina-San-Martin, B., Chen, H.T., Difilippantonio, M.J., Wilson, P.C., Hanitsch, L., Celeste, A., Muramatsu, M., Pilch, D.R., Redon, C., Ried, T., Bonner, W.M., Honjo, T., Nussenzweig, M.C. & Nussenzweig, A. (2001). AID is required to initiate Nbs1/gamma-H2AX focus formation and mutations at sites of class switching. *Nature,* 414, 6864, 660-5.

Raffini, L.J., Slater, D.J., Rappaport, E.F., Lo Nigro, L., Cheung, N.K., Biegel, J.A., Nowell, P.C., Lange, B.J. & Felix, C.A. (2002). Panhandle and reverse-panhandle PCR enable cloning of der(11) and der(other) genomic breakpoint junctions of MLL translocations and identify complex translocation of MLL, AF-4, and CDK6. *Proceedings of the National Academy of Sciences of the United States of America,* 99, 7, 4568-73.

Rai, R., Zheng, H., He, H., Luo, Y., Multani, A., Carpenter, P.B. & Chang, S. (2010). The function of classical and alternative non-homologous end-joining pathways in the fusion of dysfunctional telomeres. *EMBO J,* 29, 15, 2598-610.

Rass, E., Grabarz, A., Plo, I., Gautier, J., Bertrand, P. & Lopez, B.S. (2009). Role of Mre11 in chromosomal nonhomologous end joining in mammalian cells. *Nat Struct Mol Biol,* 16, 8, 819-24.

Rassool, F.V. (2003). DNA double strand breaks (DSB) and non-homologous end joining (NHEJ) pathways in human leukemia. *Cancer Lett,* 193, 1, 1-9.

Rassool, F.V. & Tomkinson, A.E. (2010). Targeting abnormal DNA double strand break repair in cancer. *Cell Mol Life Sci,* 67, 21, 3699-710.

Reichel, M., Gillert, E., Nilson, I., Siegler, G., Greil, J., Fey, G.H. & Marschalek, R. (1998). Fine structure of translocation breakpoints in leukemic blasts with chromosomal translocation t(4;11): the DNA damage-repair model of translocation. *Oncogene,* 17, 23, 3035-44.

Reiter, A., Saussele, S., Grimwade, D., Wiemels, J.L., Segal, M.R., Lafage-Pochitaloff, M., Walz, C., Weisser, A., Hochhaus, A., Willer, A., Reichert, A., Buchner, T., Lengfelder, E., Hehlmann, R. & Cross, N.C. (2003). Genomic anatomy of the specific reciprocal translocation t(15;17) in acute promyelocytic leukemia. *Genes Chromosomes Cancer,* 36, 2, 175-88.

Revy, P., Buck, D., le Deist, F. & de Villartay, J.P. (2005). The repair of DNA damages/modifications during the maturation of the immune system: lessons from human primary immunodeficiency disorders and animal models. *Adv Immunol,* 87, 237-95.

Riballo, E., Critchlow, S.E., Teo, S.H., Doherty, A.J., Priestley, A., Broughton, B., Kysela, B., Beamish, H., Plowman, N., Arlett, C.F., Lehmann, A.R., Jackson, S.P. & Jeggo, P.A. (1999). Identification of a defect in DNA ligase IV in a radiosensitive leukaemia patient. *Curr Biol,* 9, 13, 699-702.

Riballo, E., Kuhne, M., Rief, N., Doherty, A., Smith, G.C., Recio, M.J., Reis, C., Dahm, K., Fricke, A., Krempler, A., Parker, A.R., Jackson, S.P., Gennery, A., Jeggo, P.A. & Lobrich, M. (2004). A pathway of double-strand break rejoining dependent upon ATM, Artemis, and proteins locating to gamma-H2AX foci. *Mol Cell,* 16, 5, 715-24.

Robert, I., Dantzer, F. & Reina-San-Martin, B. (2009). Parp1 facilitates alternative NHEJ, whereas Parp2 suppresses IgH/c-myc translocations during immunoglobulin class switch recombination. *J Exp Med*, 206, 5, 1047-56.

Rogakou, E.P., Pilch, D.R., Orr, A.H., Ivanova, V.S. & Bonner, W.M. (1998). DNA double-stranded breaks induce histone H2AX phosphorylation on serine 139. *J Biol Chem*, 273, 10, 5858-68.

Rooney, S., Alt, F.W., Lombard, D., Whitlow, S., Eckersdorff, M., Fleming, J., Fugmann, S., Ferguson, D.O., Schatz, D.G. & Sekiguchi, J. (2003). Defective DNA repair and increased genomic instability in Artemis-deficient murine cells. *J Exp Med*, 197, 5, 553-65.

Rooney, S., Sekiguchi, J., Whitlow, S., Eckersdorff, M., Manis, J.P., Lee, C., Ferguson, D.O. & Alt, F.W. (2004). Artemis and p53 cooperate to suppress oncogenic N-myc amplification in progenitor B cells. *Proc Natl Acad Sci U S A*, 101, 8, 2410-5.

Rooney, S., Sekiguchi, J., Zhu, C., Cheng, H.L., Manis, J., Whitlow, S., DeVido, J., Foy, D., Chaudhuri, J., Lombard, D. & Alt, F.W. (2002). Leaky Scid phenotype associated with defective V(D)J coding end processing in Artemis-deficient mice. *Mol Cell*, 10, 6, 1379-90.

Roth, D.B., Porter, T.N. & Wilson, J.H. (1985). Mechanisms of nonhomologous recombination in mammalian cells. *Mol Cell Biol*, 5, 10, 2599-607.

Roth, D.B. & Wilson, J.H. (1986). Nonhomologous recombination in mammalian cells: role for short sequence homologies in the joining reaction. *Mol Cell Biol*, 6, 12, 4295-304.

Sallmyr, A., Fan, J., Datta, K., Kim, K.T., Grosu, D., Shapiro, P., Small, D. & Rassool, F. (2008a). Internal tandem duplication of FLT3 (FLT3/ITD) induces increased ROS production, DNA damage, and misrepair: implications for poor prognosis in AML. *Blood*, 111, 6, 3173-82.

Sallmyr, A., Tomkinson, A.E. & Rassool, F.V. (2008b). Up-regulation of WRN and DNA ligase IIIalpha in chronic myeloid leukemia: consequences for the repair of DNA double-strand breaks. *Blood*, 112, 4, 1413-23.

Schultz, L.B., Chehab, N.H., Malikzay, A. & Halazonetis, T.D. (2000). p53 binding protein 1 (53BP1) is an early participant in the cellular response to DNA double-strand breaks. *The Journal of cell biology*, 151, 7, 1381-90.

Shibata, A., Conrad, S., Birraux, J., Geuting, V., Barton, O., Ismail, A., Kakarougkas, A., Meek, K., Taucher-Scholz, G., Lobrich, M. & Jeggo, P.A. (2011). Factors determining DNA double-strand break repair pathway choice in G2 phase. *EMBO J*, 30, 6, 1079-92.

Simsek, D. & Jasin, M. (2010). Alternative end-joining is suppressed by the canonical NHEJ component Xrcc4-ligase IV during chromosomal translocation formation. *Nat Struct Mol Biol*, 17, 4, 410-6.

Singleton, B.K., Torres-Arzayus, M.I., Rottinghaus, S.T., Taccioli, G.E. & Jeggo, P.A. (1999). The C terminus of Ku80 activates the DNA-dependent protein kinase catalytic subunit. *Mol Cell Biol*, 19, 5, 3267-77.

Smanik, P.A., Furminger, T.L., Mazzaferri, E.L. & Jhiang, S.M. (1995). Breakpoint characterization of the ret/PTC oncogene in human papillary thyroid carcinoma. *Hum Mol Genet*, 4, 12, 2313-8.

Soulas-Sprauel, P., Le Guyader, G., Rivera-Munoz, P., Abramowski, V., Olivier-Martin, C., Goujet-Zalc, C., Charneau, P. & de Villartay, J.P. (2007a). Role for DNA repair factor XRCC4 in immunoglobulin class switch recombination. *J Exp Med*, 204, 7, 1717-27.

Soulas-Sprauel, P., Rivera-Munoz, P., Malivert, L., Le Guyader, G., Abramowski, V., Revy, P. & de Villartay, J.P. (2007b). V(D)J and immunoglobulin class switch recombinations: a paradigm to study the regulation of DNA end-joining. *Oncogene*, 26, 56, 7780-91.

Strissel, P.L., Strick, R., Tomek, R.J., Roe, B.A., Rowley, J.D. & Zeleznik-Le, N.J. (2000). DNA structural properties of AF9 are similar to MLL and could act as recombination hot spots resulting in MLL/AF9 translocations and leukemogenesis. *Hum Mol Genet*, 9, 11, 1671-9.

Taccioli, G.E., Amatucci, A.G., Beamish, H.J., Gell, D., Xiang, X.H., Torres Arzayus, M.I., Priestley, A., Jackson, S.P., Marshak Rothstein, A., Jeggo, P.A. & Herrera, V.L. (1998). Targeted disruption of the catalytic subunit of the DNA-PK gene in mice confers severe combined immunodeficiency and radiosensitivity. *Immunity*, 9, 3, 355-66.

Tentori, L., Leonetti, C., Scarsella, M., d'Amati, G., Portarena, I., Zupi, G., Bonmassar, E. & Graziani, G. (2002). Combined treatment with temozolomide and poly(ADP-ribose) polymerase inhibitor enhances survival of mice bearing hematologic malignancy at the central nervous system site. *Blood*, 99, 6, 2241-4.

Tutt, A., Bertwistle, D., Valentine, J., Gabriel, A., Swift, S., Ross, G., Griffin, C., Thacker, J. & Ashworth, A. (2001). Mutation in Brca2 stimulates error-prone homology-directed repair of DNA double-strand breaks occurring between repeated sequences. *Embo J*, 20, 17, 4704-16.

Venkitaraman, A.R. (2001). Chromosome stability, DNA recombination and the BRCA2 tumour suppressor. *Curr Opin Cell Biol*, 13, 3, 338-43.

Walker, J.R., Corpina, R.A. & Goldberg, J. (2001). Structure of the Ku heterodimer bound to DNA and its implications for double-strand break repair. *Nature*, 412, 6847, 607-14.

Wang, H., Perrault, A.R., Takeda, Y., Qin, W. & Iliakis, G. (2003). Biochemical evidence for Ku-independent backup pathways of NHEJ. *Nucleic Acids Res*, 31, 18, 5377-88.

Wang, H., Rosidi, B., Perrault, R., Wang, M., Zhang, L., Windhofer, F. & Iliakis, G. (2005). DNA ligase III as a candidate component of backup pathways of nonhomologous end joining. *Cancer research*, 65, 10, 4020-30.

Wang, M., Wu, W., Rosidi, B., Zhang, L., Wang, H. & Iliakis, G. (2006). PARP-1 and Ku compete for repair of DNA double strand breaks by distinct NHEJ pathways. *Nucleic Acids Res*, 34, 21, 6170-82.

Wiemels, J.L. & Greaves, M. (1999). Structure and possible mechanisms of TEL-AML1 gene fusions in childhood acute lymphoblastic leukemia. *Cancer Res*, 59, 16, 4075-82.

Wu, W., Wang, M., Mussfeldt, T. & Iliakis, G. (2008). Enhanced use of backup pathways of NHEJ in G2 in Chinese hamster mutant cells with defects in the classical pathway of NHEJ. *Radiat Res*, 170, 4, 512-20.

Wu, X., Wilson, T.E. & Lieber, M.R. (1999). A role for FEN-1 in nonhomologous DNA end joining: the order of strand annealing and nucleolytic processing events. *Proc Natl Acad Sci U S A*, 96, 4, 1303-8.

Xiao, Z., Greaves, M.F., Buffler, P., Smith, M.T., Segal, M.R., Dicks, B.M., Wiencke, J.K. & Wiemels, J.L. (2001). Molecular characterization of genomic AML1-ETO fusions in childhood leukemia. *Leukemia*, 15, 12, 1906-13.

Xie, A., Kwok, A. & Scully, R. (2009). Role of mammalian Mre11 in classical and alternative nonhomologous end joining. *Nat Struct Mol Biol,* 16, 8, 814-8.

Yan, C.T., Boboila, C., Souza, E.K., Franco, S., Hickernell, T.R., Murphy, M., Gumaste, S., Geyer, M., Zarrin, A.A., Manis, J.P., Rajewsky, K. & Alt, F.W. (2007). IgH class switching and translocations use a robust non-classical end-joining pathway. *Nature,* 449, 7161, 478-82.

Yaneva, M., Kowalewski, T. & Lieber, M.R. (1997). Interaction of DNA-dependent protein kinase with DNA and with Ku: biochemical and atomic-force microscopy studies. *Embo J,* 16, 16, 5098-112.

Zelent, A., Greaves, M. & Enver, T. (2004). Role of the TEL-AML1 fusion gene in the molecular pathogenesis of childhood acute lymphoblastic leukaemia. *Oncogene,* 23, 24, 4275-83.

Zha, S., Guo, C., Boboila, C., Oksenych, V., Cheng, H.L., Zhang, Y., Wesemann, D.R., Yuen, G., Patel, H., Goff, P.H., Dubois, R.L. & Alt, F.W. (2011). ATM damage response and XLF repair factor are functionally redundant in joining DNA breaks. *Nature,* 469, 7329, 250-4.

Zhang, Y. & Jasin, M. (2011). An essential role for CtIP in chromosomal translocation formation through an alternative end-joining pathway. *Nat Struct Mol Biol,* 18, 1, 80-4.

Zhang, Y. & Rowley, J.D. (2006). Chromatin structural elements and chromosomal translocations in leukemia. *DNA Repair (Amst),* 5, 9-10, 1282-97.

Zhong, S., Chen, X., Zhu, X., Dziegielewska, B., Bachman, K.E., Ellenberger, T., Ballin, J.D., Wilson, G.M., Tomkinson, A.E. & Mackerell, A.D., Jr. (2008). Identification and Validation of Human DNA Ligase Inhibitors Using Computer-Aided Drug Design. *J Med Chem.*

Zhu, C., Bogue, M.A., Lim, D.S., Hasty, P. & Roth, D.B. (1996). Ku86-deficient mice exhibit severe combined immunodeficiency and defective processing of V(D)J recombination intermediates. *Cell,* 86, 3, 379-89.

Zhu, C., Mills, K.D., Ferguson, D.O., Lee, C., Manis, J., Fleming, J., Gao, Y., Morton, C.C. & Alt, F.W. (2002). Unrepaired DNA breaks in p53-deficient cells lead to oncogenic gene amplification subsequent to translocations. *Cell,* 109, 7, 811-21.

5

Nucleotide Excision Repair and Cancer

Joost P.M. Melis[1,2], Mirjam Luijten[1],
Leon H.F. Mullenders[2] and Harry van Steeg[1,2]
[1]National Institute of Public Health and the Environment
Laboratory for Health Protection Research
[2]Leiden University Medical Center, Department of Toxicogenetics
The Netherlands

1. Introduction

Cancer ranks as one of the most frequent causes of death worldwide and in Western society it is competing with cardiovascular disease as the number one killer. This high frequency in Western countries can be attributed to lifestyle and environmental factors, only 5-10% of all cancers are directly due to heredity. Common environmental factors leading to cancer include: tobacco (25-30%), diet and obesity (30-35%), infections (15-20%), radiation, lack of physical activity and environmental pollutants or chemicals (Anand et al.,2008). Exposure to these environmental factors cause or enhance abnormalities in the genetic material of cells (Kinzler KW et al.,2002). These changes in the DNA or hereditary predisposition can result in respectively uncontrolled cell growth, invasion and metastasis. Cancer cells can damage tissue and disturb homeostasis leading to dysfunctions in the body that can eventually lead to death. Under normal conditions cell growth is under strict conditions and control. Hereditary dysfunctions or introduced DNA damage in tumor suppressor genes, oncogenes or DNA repair genes can create an imbalance that may lead to cancer development. DNA repair and cell cycle arrest pathways are essential cellular mechanisms to prevent or repair substantial DNA damage which, if left unattended, can cause diseases.

Here, one of the most important and versatile DNA repair pathways, the Nucleotide Excision Repair (NER) pathway, will be discussed in relation to DNA damage accumulation and carcinogenesis together with its mechanistic mode of action.

2. DNA damage

One of the initial steps in cancer development is the accumulation of DNA damage. These genomic assaults are abundant due to environmental factors and continuously ongoing metabolic processes inside the cell (Lodish et al.,2004). Endogenous DNA damage occurs at an estimated frequency of approximately 20,000 – 50,000 lesions per cell per day in humans (Lindahl,1993; Friedberg,1995), which roughly adds up to 10 - 40 trillion lesions per second in the human body. Endogenously generated lesions can occur through metabolic cellular processes and result in hydrolysis (e.g. depurination, depyrimidination and deamination), oxidation (8-oxoG, thymine glycol, cytosine hydrates and lipid peroxidation products) and non-enzymatic methylation of the DNA components (Cadet et al.,2003; Friedberg et al.,2006b). Besides these endogenous insults to the DNA, exogenous factors can play a significant role in damaging the DNA. Examples of exogenous insults are ionizing radiation, ultraviolet (UV) radiation and exposure to chemical agents. One hour of sunbathing in Europe for example generates around 80,000 lesions per cell in the human skin (Mullaart et al.,1990). The endogenous and exogenous primary lesions can result in persistent DNA damage if left unattended. Therefore, repair pathways and cellular responses are of vital importance in the prevention of cancer and age-related diseases. DNA repair pathways come in many varieties, Figure 1 shows a schematic overview of biological responses to several types of DNA damage. Reversal of DNA damage and excision repair pathways are responsible for the fundamental repair of damaged nucleotides, resulting into the correct nucleotide sequence and DNA structure. Besides damaged nucleotides, cells often sustain fracture of the sugar-phosphate backbone, resulting in single- or double-strand breaks (SSB or DSB) (Friedberg et al.,2006b). Repairing the DNA damage can occur in an error-free (e.g. Nucleotide Excision Repair (NER), Base Excision Repair (BER), Homologous Recombination (HR)) or by an error-prone pathway like Non-Homologous End-Joining (NHEJ). Besides DNA repair pathways, DNA damage tolerance mechanisms are active to bypass lesion that normally block replication like Translesion Synthesis (TLS) or template switching. Template switching occurs in an error-free way, while TLS acts in an often error-prone manner (although a few polymerases of this pathway are able to handle the lesions in an error-free way). Even though error-prone mechanisms do not result in the original coding information they do enhance the chances of cell survival, which is preferred over correct genomic maintenance in these cases. In light of this, cell cycle checkpoint activation and scheduled cell death (apoptosis) also enhance chances of genomic stability and in some cases cell survival. The responses, in which tumor suppressor factor p53 plays a major role, greatly facilitate the efficiency of repair and damage tolerance. Arrested cell cycle progression will result in an increased time window for DNA repair or damage tolerance to occur. In addition, apoptosis will attenuate the risk of genomic instability by programming the cells with extensive DNA damage for cell death, thereby, annulling the possible negative effect of the DNA damage in those cells and hence maintaining homeostasis.

3. Nucleotide excision repair

The abundant targeting of bases and nucleotides in the genome makes the Nucleotide Excision Repair one of the most essential repair pathways. NER can restore the correct genomic information, but also replication and transcription after these types of damage. The pathway can deal with a broad spectrum of (mostly) structurally unrelated bulky DNA lesions, arisen from either endogenous or exogenous agents. NER for example removes DNA lesions from the genome such as photolesions, crosslinks, bulky aromatic hydrocarbon and alkylation adducts (Figure 1).

Nucleotide excision repair is a multistep pathway using over 30 proteins that eliminate the helix-distorting lesions. As mentioned, lesions of this matter can originate upon exposures to several damaging agents. For instance, UV radiation (sunshine) is a physical DNA damaging agent that mainly produces cyclobutane pyrimidine dimers (CPDs) and pyrimidine-(6,4)-pyrimidone products (6-4PP) but is also believed to induce oxidative DNA damage (Lo et al.,2005). Exposure to numerous chemicals can result in helix-distorting bulky adducts, for example polycyclic aromatic hydrocarbons (present in cigarette smoke or charcoaled meat) (de Boer et al.,2000). Interstrand crosslinks, alkylation adducts and oxygen free-radical induced minor base damage can trigger NER (Friedberg et al.,2006b).

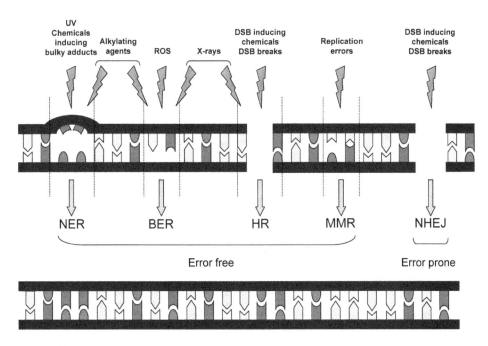

Schematic overview of DNA repair pathways. Several types of induced DNA damage can trigger different repair pathways, which can repair the DNA in an error-free or an error-prone manner. NER (Nucleotide Excision Repair), BER (Base Excision Repair), HR (Homologous Recombination), MMR (Mismatch Repair), NHEJ (Non-Homologous End-Joining).

Fig. 1. DNA Repair pathways.

3.1 Global genome-NER and transcription coupled-NER

NER is divided into two subpathways which mechanistically initiate in a divergent manner, but after damage recognition both pathways proceed along the same molecular route (see Figure 2). The subpathways are designated Global Genome NER (GG-NER) and Transcription Coupled NER (TC-NER). GG-NER recognizes and removes lesions throughout the entire genome, and is considered to be a relatively slow and somewhat more inefficient process, since it scans the whole genome for DNA damage (Guarente et al.,2008). However, UV induced helix-distorting lesions like 6-4PPs, are rapidly cleared by GG-NER (Garinis et al.,2006). TC-NER is responsible for eliminating lesions in the transcribed strand of active genes. This repair process takes care of lesions blocking the transcription machinery and otherwise possible resulting dysfunctions. Since TC-NER is directly coupled to the transcription machinery it is considered to be faster acting and more efficient than GG-NER, but is only initiated when transcription of a gene is blocked.

3.2 DNA damage recognition

The difference between the two sub pathways is the initial damage recognition step (Figure 2). As mentioned previously, a helical distortion and alteration of DNA chemistry appears to be the first structural element that is recognized. For GG-NER, the XPC/hHR23B complex (including centrin2), together with the UV-Damaged DNA Binding (UV-DDB) protein (assembled by the DDB1 (p127) and DDB2/XPE (p48) subunits), are involved in lesion recognition (Dip et al.,2004). The XPC/hHR23B complex is additionally essential for recruitment of the consecutive components of the NER machinery to the damaged site, also known as the preincision complex (Yokoi et al.,2000; Araujo et al.,2001).

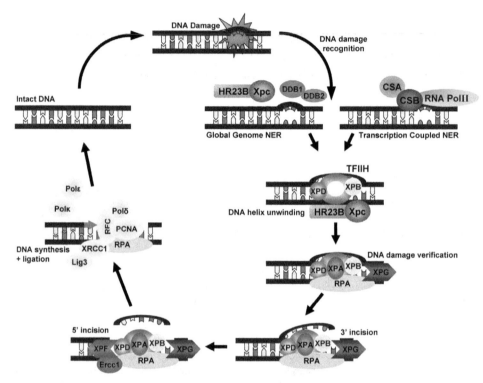

Fig. 2. Nucleotide Excision Repair.

Schematic overview of the Nucleotide Excision Repair (NER) pathway. Damaged DNA is recognized by either initial factors of the Global Genome Repair (e.g. Xpc) or Transcription Coupled Repair (CSA and CSB), which constitute the two different repair pathways in NER. After DNA damage recognition the repair route progresses along the same way. After helix unwinding and verification of the damage incisions are made to remove the faulty stretch of DNA. Finally, DNA synthesis and subsequent ligation reproduce the correct DNA sequence. It has been shown that XPC itself has affinity for DNA and can initiate GG-NER *in vitro*, but its functionality is enhanced when hHR23b and centrin2 are added (Nishi et al.,2005; Araki et al.,2001). The latter two are not able to bind to DNA themselves. Centrin2 as well as hHR23B stabilize the heterotrimer complex, putatively by inhibiting polyubiquitination of XPC and hence preventing subsequent degradation by the 26S proteasome (Nishi et al.,2005). XPC recognizes various helix-distorting base lesions that do not share a common chemical structure. Biochemical studies have revealed that XPC recognizes a specific secondary DNA structure rather than the lesions themselves and the presence of single-stranded DNA seems a crucial factor (Sugasawa et al.,2001; Sugasawa et al.,2002; Min et al.,2007). XPC appears to scan the DNA for distortions by migrating over the DNA, repeatedly binding and dissociating from the helix. When XPC encounters a lesion the protein changes its conformation and aromatic amino acid residues stack with unpaired nucleotides opposite the lesion, thereby increasing its affinity and creating a conformation which makes it possible to interact with other NER factors (Hoogstraten et al.,2008).

Binding affinity of XPC to the DNA seems to correlate with the extent of helical distortion. 6-4PP products substantially distort the DNA structure and are therefore more easily recognized than CPDs, which only induce a minimal helical distortion (Sugasawa et al.,2005). More recent studies have indicated that UV-DDB facilitates recognition of lesions that are less well-recognized by the XPC-hHR23B complex, like CPDs, via ubiquitylation of XPC (Fitch et al.,2003).

The UV-DDB is able to recognize UV-induced photoproducts in the DNA and is now believed to precede the binding of XPC-hHR23B to the UV-damaged site. CPD repair is UV-DDB dependent (Fitch et al.,2003; Tang et al.,2000). Since affinity of the XPC-hHR23B to CPD sites is low, DDB2 is needed for efficient binding (Tang et al.,2000). Affinity of DDB2 for 6-4PP is also extremely high and the protein is furthermore able to bind to DNA lesions such as apurinic/apyrimidinic (AP) sites and mismatches (Nichols et al.,2000; Wittschieben et al.,2005). DDB2 is also part of the E3 ubiquitin ligase complex which is further comprised of CUL4A, ROC1/RBX1, COP9 signalosome (CSN) and DDB1 (Groisman et al.,2003). Live cell imaging studies show prompt recruitment of DDB1, DDB2 and Cul4a to UV induced lesions (Alekseev et al.,2008). CUL4A displays ubiquitin ligase activity and was shown to ubiquitylate DDB2 (Chen et al.,2001; Nag et al.,2001; Matsuda et al.,2005). The CSN subunit contains deubiquitylation capacities. This interactive mechanism is thought to be responsible for (poly)ubiquitylation of XPC and DDB2, but not in a similar fashion and result. Upon ubiquitylation DDB2 is degraded by the 26S proteasome (Fitch et al.,2003; Rapic-Otrin et al.,2002). XPC is not degraded after UV DNA damage, hereby increasing its binding affinity to the DNA as well as stimulating the interaction with hHR23B (Araki et al.,2001; Ortolan et al.,2004; Ng et al.,2003). Degradation of UV-DDB enhances the binding of XPC-hHR23B to the DNA *in vitro* (Sugasawa et al.,2005). Timing of the programmed degradation of DDB2 determines the recruitment of XPC-hHR23B to the UV-damaged site (El Mahdy et al.,2006).

The XPC protein contains several binding domains, a DNA binding domain, a hHR23B binding domain, centrin2 binding domain and a TFIIH binding domain (Sugasawa,2008). TFIIH is a multifunctional transcription factor and NER complex and amongst others contains the helicases XPB and XPD (Figure 2). This complex is essential for the continuation of the NER pathway and is responsible for unwinding the DNA helix after damage recognition by XPC/hHR23B. XPC has been shown to physically interact with TFIIH and *in vivo* and *in vitro* studies have shown the recruitment of the NER complex to unwind the DNA is executed in a XPC-dependent manner (Sugasawa,2008; Friedberg et al.,2006b).

The XPC protein is redundant in TC-NER. Here a stalled RNA polymerase II (RNA polII) is the onset of the NER machinery. The proteins CSA and CSB play a crucial role in setting the transcription coupled repair in motion, but are also implicated in RNA polII transcription functions. The CSB protein interacts with RNA polII (Tantin et al.,1997), while CSA does not (Tantin,1998). CSA mainly interacts with CSB, XAB2 (XPA binding protein 2) and the p44 subunit of the TFIIH complex (Henning et al.,1995; Nakatsu et al.,2000). The function of CSA remains to be elucidated but is implicated to be required for TC-NER during elongation of the transcription process (Groisman et al.,2003; Kamiuchi et al.,2002). CSA is also part of an E3 ubiquitin ligase complex in which CUL4A, CSN and DDB1 are involved. Both CSA and CSB are part of RNA PolII associated complexes, but for CSB additional functions are assigned outside NER (Sunesen et al.,2002).

In TC-NER, CSB is thought to be responsible for displacement of the stalled RNA polymerase. Additionally, as with XPC in GG-NER, the preincision complex of NER is recruited in a CSB-dependent manner (Fousteri et al.,2008; Fousteri et al.,2006). But first, as in GG-NER, the TFIIH complex is recruited after damage recognition.

3.3 DNA helix unwinding

From DNA damage recognition and subsequent recruitment of TFIIH on, GG-NER and TC-NER converge into the same pathway. The TFIIH complex consists of 10 proteins: XPB, XPD, p62, pP52, p44, p34, p8 and the CDK-activating kinase (CAK) complex: MAT1, CDK7 and Cyclin H. TFIIH forms an open bubble structure in the DNA helix (Giglia-Mari et al.,2004; Goosen,2010). The DNA helicases XPB and XPD facilitate the partial unwinding of the DNA duplex in an ATP-dependent manner, allowing the preincision complex to enter the site of the lesion (Figure 2) (Oksenych et al.,2010). The preincision complex consists of the XPA, RPA and XPG proteins and is assembled at the damage site (Zotter et al.,2006) (Figure 2). The function of XPA is verification of the lesion; in addition, XPA acts, together with the single strand DNA binding complex RPA, as an organizational orchestrator, so that the repair machinery is positioned around the lesion. The arrival of XPA and RPA leads to complete opening of the damaged DNA and catalyzes the release of the CAK complex from the TFIIH complex. Data suggest this step is essential for the initiation of incision/excision of the damaged DNA (Andressoo et al.,2006; Coin et al.,2008).

XPA and RPA in the preincision complex bind to the damaged DNA. Specific binding properties for certain structural DNA distortions have been reported for XPA, which suggests the protein recognizes conformations of the DNA and is able to verify the damage (Lao et al.,2000; Krasikova et al.,2010). XPA has no enzymatic activity to attribute to the incision step, but nevertheless is indispensable for DNA incision (Miyamoto et al.,1992). Through zinc finger motifs of XPA interaction with RPA is established (Ikegami et al.,1998). RPA consists of 3 subunits and with high affinity binds to the undamaged strand (de Laat et al.,1998b) (Figure 2). The protein roughly covers 30 nucleotides (corresponding in size to the excised product later in NER) and acts as a wedge between the DNA strands. It is also believed to protect the undamaged intact strand from inappropriate nuclease activity (de Laat et al.,1998a; Hermanson-Miller et al.,2002). RPA is concerned as the major component in the preincision complex, thereby also protecting the native template strand. Furthermore, RPA interacts with several other factors of the nucleotide excision repair pathway, like the endonucleases XPG and the ERCC1-XPF dimer, which are required for the dual incision of the damaged strand (Figure 2). RPA hereby facilitates the correct positioning of the endonucleases and orchestrates the open complex formation (Krasikova et al.,2010; Park et al.,2006). Besides that, RPA later plays a role in the DNA repair synthesis and ligation steps (Shivji et al.,1995). XPA exhibits a moderate preference for binding to damaged DNA, as do other NER factors. Individually, the proteins XPA and RPA do not show sufficient selectivity to explain the high efficiency of NER lesion removal, which is most likely due to a discrimination cascade of recognition and verification steps (Lin et al.,1992). XPA is thought to play a major role in verification, possibly by acting as a molecular sensor of aberrant electrostatic potential along the DNA substrate (Camenisch et al.,2008). Structural changes, like kinked backbones, in damaged DNA can induce deviant electrostatic potentials. Bulky adducts often result in sharply bent backbones due to the decrease of rigidity. Normally, base stacking supplies the DNA helix with strength and structure, but bulky lesions and hence loss of base stacking can weaken the sturdiness of the backbone. It is known that XPA has a higher affinity for kinked backbones. However how the exact recognition of the lesion is executed remains to be elucidated. But it is clear that the XPA-RPA complex is indispensable for the high efficiency of NER (Camenisch et al.,2008).

3.4 Incision, DNA repair synthesis and ligation

When the preincision complex is accurately positioned in relation to the damaged site by the XPA-RPA complex, single strand breaks are introduced by XPG and ERCC1-XPF (Figure 2). Several mechanistic theories were postulated over the years. A general consensus is that the combined actions of XPG and ERCC1-XPF result in excision of a 24-32 nucleotide long single strand fragment including the damaged site (Hess et al.,1997). XPG is responsible for the 3' incision and is putatively recruited by the TFIIH complex (Zotter et al.,2006). According to some studies its presence appears to be necessary for ERCC1-XPF activity, which is responsible for carrying out the 5' incision (Friedberg et al.,2006b; Wakasugi et al.,1997). Others propose a 'cut-patch-cut-patch' mechanism for the incision and resynthesis process within NER, where the 5' incision possibly precedes the 3' incision (Staresincic et al.,2009).

XPG is expected to have additional stabilization features, because of its ability to interact with XPB, XPD and several other subunits of the TFIIH complex(Friedberg et al.,2006b). Since loss of XPG results in very early death(Wijnhoven et al.,2007) the protein might be involved in systemic and important additional mechanisms, like transcription (Bessho,1999; Lee et al.,2002). Furthermore, XPG is suggested to have a role in oxidative damage removal (Dianov et al.,2000). The ERCC1-XPF seems to be a multifunctional complex as well, since it is also involved in interstand crosslink repair and homologous recombination (Niedernhofer et al.,2001; Al Minawi et al.,2009).

The excision of the damaged fragment is restored in original (undamaged) state by DNA synthesis and ligation steps (either by cut-patch-cut-patch mechanism or full excision followed by resynthesis and ligation). Both XPG and RPA are thought to be required for the transition between (pre)incision and post-incision events (Mocquet et al.,2008). XPG is thought to be involved in the recruitment of PCNA (Staresincic et al.,2009; Mocquet et al.,2008). Resynthesis of DNA requires PCNA because of its ability to interact with DNA polymerases (Mocquet et al.,2008). The mechanism of involvement of these polymerases in DNA resynthesis is not yet fully elucidated. Recent studies show at least three DNA polymerases are involved. Pol δ, Pol κ and Pol ϵ are recruited to damage sites (Figure 2). Recent *in vivo* studies show Pol β most likely plays no major role in NER (Ogi et al.,2010; Moser et al.,2007). To complete the repair of the damaged DNA site the resynthesized strand needs to be ligated. The primary participant in the subsequent ligation process of NER appears to be the XRCC1-Ligase 3 complex, which is shown to accumulate in both quiescent as well as proliferating cells after local UV irradiation (Moser et al.,2007). Ligase 1 appears to be involved in the ligation step in proliferating cells only (Moser et al.,2007). To date, the cross play of over 30 proteins in total is involved in NER to counteract DNA damage in the error free manner described above.

4. NER in cancer

DNA repair is vital to humans and other organisms and a defect in one of the genes can result in some severe syndromes or diseases by loss of genomic stability. Essential consequences of genomic instability can be cancer and other age-related diseases, such as neurological disorders as Huntington's disease and ataxias (Friedberg et al.,2006b). DNA damage for example can cause mutations that trigger (pre-)oncogenes, inactivate tumor suppressor genes or other indispensable genes which cause loss of homeostasis. Defects in the DNA repair machinery will inflate the mutational load, since DNA damage will be left unattended and subsequently gene mutations will accumulate. Therefore, organisms that harbor defective DNA repair are often more prone to develop cancer or (segmental) age-related diseases.

In humans, several syndromes have been identified which are the result of an impaired nucleotide excision repair pathway, of which Xeroderma Pigmentosum (XP), Cockayne syndrome (CS) and Trichothiodystrophy (TTD) are the most well-known. Since NER is the major defense against UV-induced DNA damage, all three syndromes are hallmarked by an extreme UV-sensitivity, of which XP ensues a highly elevated risk of developing skin cancer (Friedberg et al.,2006b; Cleaver et al.,2009).

The involvement of NER genes in rare and severe syndromes underscores the vital importance of this repair pathway. It is known that accumulative DNA damage is one of the most important causes in cancer development and loss of homeostasis in organisms (Mullaart et al.,1990; Lindahl,1993; Friedberg et al.,2006b; de Boer et al.,2000; Cleaver et al.,2009). Defects in DNA repair pathways are therefore also considered to accelerate aging and tumorigenesis. In defective NER both types of endpoints occur, XP patients are predisposed to cancer development while CS and TTD patients are not. The latter exhibit premature aging features which XP patients lack (Friedberg et al.,2006b; de Boer et al.,2000; Cleaver et al.,2009). Reason for this might be the involvement of several NER proteins in other significant cellular mechanisms. CSB is believed to be involved in (TC-)BER, while XPD is also associated with replication and transcription. Some of these affected mechanisms could overshadow the NER deficiency and ever increasing mutational load eventually predisposing an individual to cancer. Severely affected developmental and neurological systems could be more life threatening on the shorter term than tumor development is. This could be the rationale behind the fact that CS and TTD patients are extremely short-lived and not cancer prone.

5. Xeroderma pigmentosum

Xeroderma pigmentosum (XP), meaning parchment pigmented skin, was the first human causal NER-deficient disease identified (Cleaver et al.,2009). It is a rare, autosomal inherited neurodegenerative and skin disease in which exposure to sunlight (UV) can lead to skin cancer. In Western Europe and the USA the incidence frequency is approximately 1:250,000, rates are higher in Japan (1:40,000). XP-C and XP-A are the most common complementation forms of XP (Bhutto et al.,2008).

Early malignancies (from 1-2 years of age) in parts of the skin, eyes and the tip of the tongue develop due to sun-exposure (Table 1). Additionally, benign lesions like blistering, hyperpigmented spots and freckles are abundant (Figure 3). XP is associated with a more than 1,000-fold increase in risk of developing skin cancer. These cancers are mainly basal

Feature	%/age	Feature	%/age
Cutaneous abnormalities		*Neurological abnormalities*	
Median age of onset of symptoms	1.5 yr	Median age of onset	6 mo
Median age of onset of freckling	1.5 yr	Association with skin problems	33%
Photosensitivity	19%	Association with ocular abnormalities	36%
Cutaneous atrophy	23%	Low intelligence	80%
Cutaneous telangiectasia	17%	Abnormal motor activity	30%
Actinic keratoses	19%	Areflexia	20%
Malignant skin neoplasms	45%	Impaired hearing	18%
Median age of first cutaneous neoplasm	8 yr	Abnormal speech	13%
Ocular abnormalities		Abnormal EEG	11%
Frequency	40%	Microcephaly	24%
Median age of onset	4 yr	*Abnormalities associated with neurological defects*	
Conjunctival injection	18%	Slow growth	23%
Corneal abnormalities	17%	Delayed secondary sexual development	12%
Impaired vision	12%		
Photophobia	2%		
Ocular neoplasms	11%		
Median age of first ocular neoplasm	11 yr		

Adapted from Friedberg, E.C *et al.* 2006b

Table 1. Overview of some XP features and their average age of onset or frequency

and squamous cell carcinomas (45% of the XP patients) and to a lesser extent melanomas (Friedberg et al.,2006b) (Table 1). Besides skin cancers, XP patients have a 10-20 fold increased risk to develop internal cancers (Kraemer et al.,1984). The disease is mostly symptomatic during childhood. The mean latency time for cutaneous neoplasms is 8 years, this is in comparison to the general population in which the mean latency time is 50 years later (Kraemer,1997). Progressive neurological degeneration occurs in approximately 20% of the XP cases and can be correlated to deficiencies in specific XP genes (XPA, XPB, XPD and XPG) (Cleaver et al.,2009). XP-C and XP-F patients rarely develop neurological degeneration and if so with a later onset when compared for example to XP-A and XP-D patients (Kraemer,1997; Friedberg et al.,2006b). The heterogeneity in exhibited symptoms is correlated to the genetic heterogeneity in XP patients. XP-A, XP-B, XP-D and XP-G patients are in general the most severely affected and all these patients are defective in both GG-NER and TC-NER. Solely GG-NER is defective in XP-C and XP-E patients. XP-C and XP-E cells show higher survival rate after UV exposure than XP-A and XP-D cells for example (Friedberg et al.,2006b). This could be the reason that XP-C patients suffer less from sunburn. Most abundant XP variants in human are XP-A and XP-C (~50% of all XP cases) (Zeng et al.,1997).

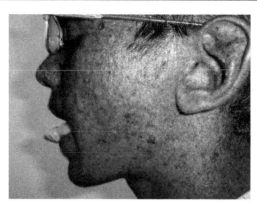

Fig. 3. Xeroderma pigmentosum.

Photo of a 19 year old Xeroderma pigmentosum patient suffering from hyperpigment skin lesions and a tongue carcinoma (IARC).

6. NER mouse models in cancer research

To investigate the role of the proteins involved in NER on survival and cancer development several transgenic mouse models were created, mimicking the existing NER mutations or deletions in humans. Table 2 shows an overview of NER mouse models and their accompanying spontaneous phenotypes. Selected knockout mouse models (*Xpa, Xpc* and *Xpe*) are described in more detail further below. These three models show a decreased lifespan in comparison to their concurrent wild type controls, but not as extreme as several other NER-deficient mouse models in Table 2. Therefore the mouse models survive long enough to study the effect of impaired NER on cancer development. Others, like *Xpb, Xpf, Xpg* and *Ercc1* deficient models are too short- lived to study carcinogenesis.

6.1 *Xpa* deficient mouse model
The first DNA repair defective models were the *Xpa*-deficient mouse models, generated by de Vries et al. (de Vries et al.,1995) and independently by Nakane et al (Nakane et al.,1995). *Xpa*-deficient mice appeared more cancer prone compared to their heterozygous and wild type littermates when exposed to carcinogenic and genotoxic compounds (de Vries et al.,1997b; Takahashi et al.,2002; Ide et al.,2001; Hoogervorst et al.,2005; Hoogervorst et al.,2004). As in humans, the mouse model exhibited a marked predisposition to skin cancer upon UV treatment of shaved dorsal skin (de Vries et al.,1995).
Survival studies without directed exposure were performed initially but always in a mixed genetic background, C57BL/6J/Ola129 (de Vries et al.,1997b) and C3H/heN strains(Takahashi et al.,2002) and fairly small numbers. However, both studies indicated that *Xpa-/-* mice (from here mentioned as *Xpa* mice) developed a significant number of spontaneous liver tumors. The C3H/heN strain wild type mice already showed 47% liver tumor incidence in the male mice within 16 months. The C57BL/6J/Ola129 mice were more resilient, no enhanced mortality was observed until the age of 1.5 years. The *Xpa* mice showed a 15% hepatocellular adenoma tumor incidence after 20 months, while there were no tumors in the wild type and heterozygous littermates. The lack of a pure genetic

Mouse model	Affected repair pathway	Enhanced spontaneous tumor response	Reference	Accelerated aging/developmental problems	Reference
$Xpa^{-/-}$	GG-NER/TC-NER	Yes, liver	(de Vries et al.,1997b; Melis et al.,2008; Tanaka et al.,2001)	Shorter life span, no pathology	(Melis et al.,2008)
$Xpb^{-/-}$	NER/transcription	n.a.		Impaired embryonic development	(Friedberg et al.,2006a)
$Xpc^{-/-}$	GG-NER	Yes, lung	(Hollander et al.,2005; Melis et al.,2008)	Shorter life span	(Melis et al.,2008)
Xpd^{TTD}	NER/transcription	No	(de Boer et al.,2002; Wijnhoven et al.,2005)	Shorter life span, aging and CR pathology	(de Boer et al.,2002; Wijnhoven et al.,2005)
Xpd^{XPCS}	NER/transcription	n.d.			
$Xpe (DDB2)^{-/-}$	GG-NER	Yes, various	(Ng et al.,2003; Yoon et al.,2005)		
$Xpf^{m/m}$	NER/ICL	n.a.		Very short life span, maximum 3 weeks	(Tian et al.,2004)
$Xpg^{-/-}$	TC-NER/transcription	n.a.		Very short life span, maximum 3 weeks	(Harada et al.,1999)
$mHR23B^{-/-}$	GG-NER	n.a.		Very short life span/embroynic lethality	(Ng et al.,2002)
$Csa^{-/-}$	TC-NER	No	(van der Horst et al.,2002)		
$Csb^{-/-}$	TC-NER/transcription	No	(van der Horst et al.,1997)	Normal life span, mild pathology	(van der Horst et al.,1997), unpublished results
$Ercc1^{-/-}$	NER/ICL	n.a.		Very short life span, maximum 4 weeks	(McWhir et al.,1993; Weeda et al.,1997)
$Ercc1^{\Delta7/-}$	NER/ICL	No	Personal communication van Steeg/Dollé	Short life span of 4–6 months	(Weeda et al.,1997)

ICL = interstrand cross link, CR = caloric restriction
n.a.: not applicable, mouse models are too short lived to develop tumors
n.d.: not determined

Table 2. Overview of spontaneous phenotypes of NER-deficient mouse models

background for this and other mouse models made it harder to investigate the underlying cause of the phenotypic responses in these mice. An *Xpa* mouse model in a pure genetic

C57BL/6J background more recently was investigated (Melis et al.,2008). C57BL/6J mice showed a low baseline tumor response and appear therefore suitable for studying mutagenesis and tumorigenesis. In a pure genetic background a significant increase in liver tumors was observed (10%). A small (but not significant) increase in lung tumors was also observed (6.6% of the *Xpa* mice) (Melis et al.,2008). Correspondingly, mutation accumulation in the C57BL/6J *Xpa* mice was significantly increased during survival compared to wild type mice in liver, implicating an *Xpa* repair defect and subsequent mutation induction in carcinogenesis (Melis et al.,2008).

Like human XP-A patients, *Xpa* mice appeared predisposed to skin cancer after UV light exposure to shaved dorsal skin of the mice (de Vries et al.,1995; Tanaka et al.,2001). Heterozygous *Xpa* mice did not show this cancer prone phenotype after UV exposure, not even when the *Xpa* mutation was crossed in in hairless mice (Berg et al.,1997). Skin cancer predisposition in XP mice might not only involve NER deficiency, but several reports indicate enhanced immunosuppression and impaired natural killer cell function are involved (Gaspari et al.,1993; Horio et al.,2001; Miyauchi-Hashimoto et al.,2001). *Xpa* mice were also predisposed to tumors of the cornea when exposed to UV radiation, see Table 3 (de Vries et al.,1998).

Chemical exposure of *Xpa* mice to 7,12-dimethyl-1,2-benz[a]anthracene (DMBA) also resulted in skin cancer (de Vries et al.,1995). Several chemical exposures in *Xpa* mice however shed some more light on the cancer development other than skin cancer, which in humans is the predominant tumor phenotype (Table 3). For example, oral treatment of *Xpa* deficient mice with genotoxic carcinogens like benzo[a]pyrene (B[a]P), 2-acetylaminofluorene (2-AAF), and 2-amino-1-methyl-6-phenylimidazo [4,5-b]-pyridine (PhIP) resulted in lung tumors and lymphomas (B[a]P), liver and bladder tumors (2-AAF) and intestinal adenomas plus lymphomas (PhIP) (de Vries et al.,1997b; van Steeg et al.,1998; van Steeg et al.,2000; Ide et al.,2000). Other human carcinogens like cyclosporin A (CsA) and diethylstilbestrol (DES), although not directly mutagenic, showed to be carcinogenic in *Xpa* mice after 39 week exposure, but in contrary the low potent human carcinogen phenacetin did not result in a significant increase in tumors.

LacZ and *Hprt* mutation measurements in *Xpa* mice after B[a]P and 2-AAF treatment showed a 2-3 fold increase in mutations compared to wild type mice after only 12-13 weeks of exposure (Hoogervorst et al.,2005; van Oostrom et al.,1999; Bol et al.,1998; de Vries et al.,1997b). This increase in mutational load in comparison to wild type indicates *Xpa* mice are more sensitive to mutation accumulation, which consequently corresponds to the increased cancer susceptibility of *Xpa* mice.

The increased sensitivity towards cancer development of *Xpa* mice made it possible to identify genotoxic carcinogens even more accurate and faster when combined with heterozygosity for p53. This latter mouse model could be beneficial in reducing and refining *in vivo* carcinogenicity testing of compounds.

6.2 *Xpc* deficient mouse model

Two independent *Xpc*-deficient mouse models were also created in the mid-nineties (Cheo et al.,1997; Sands et al.,1995). As the *Xpa* mouse model, this model is informative for human XP and cancer development in general. The model is especially interesting since it is only defective for GG-NER and not for TC-NER. Hereby, differences between pathways can be investigated.

Mouse model	Treatment	Target	Enhanced tumor response*	References
Xpa	UV-B radiation	Skin	Yes	(de Vries et al.,1995; Nakane et al.,1995)
	DMBA paint + TPA	Skin	Yes	(de Vries et al.,1995; Nakane et al.,1995)
	B[a]P gavage	Multiple, lymphomas	Yes	(de Vries et al.,1997a; van Oostrom et al.,1999)
	B[a]P diet	Stomach, esophagus	Yes	(Hoogervorst et al.,2003)
	B[a]P intratracheal instillation	Lung	Yes	(Ide et al.,2000)
	AFB1 i.p. injection	Liver	Yes	(Takahashi et al.,2002)
	PhIP diet	Lymphoma, small intestine	No	(Klein et al.,2001)
	4NQO drinking water	Tongue	Yes	(Ide et al.,2001)
	2-AAF diet	Liver, bladder, gall bladder	Yes	(Hoogervorst et al.,2005; van Kreijl et al.,2001)
	CsA	Lymphoma	Yes	(van Kesteren et al.,2009)
	DES	Osteosarcoma, lymphoma	Yes	(McAnulty et al.,2005)
	Wy	Liver	Yes	(van Kreijl et al.,2001)
	DEHP	Liver	No	Unpublished results
	p-cres	Liver	Yes	Unpublished results
Xpc	UV-B radiation	Skin	Yes	(Sands et al.,1995; Berg et al.,1998)
	2-AAF diet	Liver, bladder	Yes	(Hoogervorst et al.,2005)
	AAF i.p. injection	Liver, lung	Yes	(Cheo et al.,1999)
	NOH-AAF i.p. injection	Liver, lung	Yes	(Cheo et al.,1999)
	DEHP	Liver	No	Unpublished results
	p-cres	Liver	Yes	Unpublished results
Xpe/ DDB2	UV-B radiation	Skin	Yes	(Itoh et al.,2004)
	DMBA paint	Skin	No	(Itoh et al.,2004)

* in comparison to the untreated controls
DEHP = Di(2-ethylhexyl) phthalate
AFB1 = Aflatoxin B1
4NQO = 4-Nitroquinoline 1-oxide
WY = Wyeth-14643
p-cres = p-cresidine
NOH-AAF = N-hydroxyacetylaminofluorene

Table 3. Tumor responses in *Xpa, Xpc* and *Xpe* mice upon exposure

As in human XP-C patients, *Xpc* mice are highly predisposed to UV radiation-induced skin cancer (Table 3) (Berg et al.,1998; Cheo et al.,1996; Cheo et al.,2000; Friedberg et al.,1999; Sands et al.,1995). Contrasting to *Xpa*+/- mice the heterozygous *Xpc* mice are more susceptible to UV-induced skin cancer (but only at approximately from 1 year old) when compared to their wild type littermates. The haploinsufficient sensitivity could mean that XPC is a rate limiting factor in NER and since XPC is involved in damage recognition might explain the difference with *Xpa* heterozygous mice. Exposure studies with 2-AAF using *Xpc* mice showed a significant predisposition to liver and lung tumors compared to the heterozygous *Xpc* and wild type mice (Table 3) (Cheo et al.,1999; Friedberg et al.,2006b). Internal tumor incidence is higher in XP mice than in human XP, since patients normally develop skin cancer at a faster rate and die of resulting metastatic complications. NER is believed to be the sole pathway to remove CPD and 6-4PP lesions, while for chemical carcinogenic exposure other repair mechanisms are also present in the cell. In human, other types of cancer generally do not develop fast enough and are possibly overshadowed by skin cancers in XP.

In a mixed genetic background (C57BL/6J/129) no decrease in survival was found in relation to wild type mice, even though *Xpc* mice showed an extremely high and significantly increased lung tumor incidence (100%). However, in this study the wild type mice were not genetically related to the *Xpc* mice (Hollander et al.,2005). The spontaneous survival characteristics of *Xpc* mice in a pure genetic C57BL/6J background together with their related wild type littermates were also investigated. *Xpc* mice showed a significant decrease in survival, again exhibited a significant increase in lung and liver tumors and an increased mutation accumulation in these tissues compared to wild type mice (Melis et al., 2008). Here, *Xpc* mice showed a divergent tumor spectrum from *Xpa* mice in the same genetic C57BL/6J background. The additional increase in lung tumor development in two independent spontaneous survival studies indicate XPC is involved in other pathways besides NER. A corresponding strong increase in mutational load during aging was found in lungs of the C57BL/6J *Xpc* mice, which was not the case in *Xpa* mice (Melis et al.,2008). Uehara *et al.* have shown that enhanced spontaneous age-related mutation accumulation in *Xpc* mice is tissue dependent. Liver, lung, heart and spleen exhibited an increase in mutant frequency compared to wild type, while this difference was not visible in brain and small intestine. Mutant frequencies of liver, lung and spleen are higher in *Xpc* mice compared to *Xpa* mice, just as the tumor incidence in this study (Melis et al.,2008). The additional increase in mutational load in *Xpc* mice might be caused by increased sensitivity towards oxidative DNA damage. XPC functioning has been implied in other DNA repair pathways like base excision repair and non-homologous end joining or might be involved in redox homeostasis (D'Errico et al.,2006; Despras et al.,2007; Liu et al.,2010; Okamoto et al.,2008; Rezvani et al.,2010; Shimizu et al.,2003; Uehara et al.,2009).

Chemical exposures to B[a]P (Wickliffe et al.,2006), 3,4-epoxy-1-butene (EB) (Wickliffe et al.,2006), DMBA (Wijnhoven et al.,2001) and UV-B (Ikehata et al.,2007) also showed significantly enhanced mutant frequencies compared to wild type mice in several tissues. Direct comparisons to *Xpa* mice in these studies have not been made, however when *Xpa* and *Xpc* mice were exposed to pro-oxidants (DEHP and paraquat) for 39 weeks, *Xpc* again exhibited a higher mutant frequency than *Xpa*.

6.3 *Xpe* deficient mouse model

In 2004 and 2005 Itoh *et al.* and Yoon *et al.* independently generated a strain of *DDB2*-/- mice (Itoh,2006; Itoh et al.,2004; Yoon et al.,2005). The latter group reported that *DDB2*-/- mice show a decrease in spontaneous survival (n=10) compared to wild type (Yoon et al.,2005). Also the heterozygous *DDB2*[+/-] mice showed a decreased lifespan, although not as severe as the *DDB2*[-/-] mice. Six out of 10 *DDB2*[-/-] mice harbored tumors at the end of life, while 3 out of 10 *DDB2*[+/-] mice were tumor bearing (Yoon et al.,2005). *DDB2*[-/-] mice additionally showed to be cancer prone upon UV-B exposure, resulting in a significant increase in skin tumors (Table 3) (Itoh,2006; Itoh et al.,2004; Yoon et al.,2005). DMBA treatment however did not enhance tumor incidence compared to wild type (Table 3) (Itoh,2006; Itoh et al.,2004). DDB2 deficiency is, due to these and other studies, since being classified as a XPE phenotype. Besides UV-B and DMBA exposure, other *in vivo* carcinogen exposures have not been reported in these models so far. DDB2 is well conserved between humans and mice and appears to function as a tumor suppressor, at least in part, by controlling p53-mediated apoptosis after UV-irradiation (Itoh et al.,2004).

7. Conclusion

DNA repair has proven to be of vital importance and protects or at least delays cancer development and several age-related diseases. DNA damage accumulation and consequent mutation accumulation is considered pathogenic. NER has been shown to be a highly versatile and important DNA repair pathway, removing helix distorting DNA damages. Mutations in the XP genes of NER in human can result in the severe syndrome Xeroderma pigmentosum, which is accompanied by a cancer predisposition and severe UV sensitivity. Mouse models mimicking this human syndrome are important to study cancer development and the consequences of persistent DNA damage. Novel functionality of DNA repair proteins and implications of their deficiency in mutagenesis, cell cycle regulation, carcinogenesis and aging were discovered using NER-deficient models. Besides mechanistic insight these models can be used as a refined model in carcinogenicity testing, especially in combination with p53 heterozygosity. The increased cancer susceptibility can be beneficial towards a decrease in the number of animals used and the duration of carcinogenicity testing.

8. References

Al Minawi, A. Z., Lee, Y. F., Hakansson, D., Johansson, F., Lundin, C., Saleh-Gohari, N., Schultz, N., Jenssen, D., Bryant, H. E., Meuth, M., Hinz, J. M., and Helleday, T. (2009). The ERCC1/XPF endonuclease is required for completion of homologous recombination at DNA replication forks stalled by inter-strand cross-links. *Nucleic Acids Res.* 37, 6400-6413.

Alekseev, S., Luijsterburg, M. S., Pines, A., Geverts, B., Mari, P. O., Giglia-Mari, G., Lans, H., Houtsmuller, A. B., Mullenders, L. H., Hoeijmakers, J. H., and Vermeulen, W. (2008). Cellular concentrations of DDB2 regulate dynamic binding of DDB1 at UV-induced DNA damage. *Mol.Cell Biol.* 28, 7402-7413.

Anand, P., Kunnumakkara, A. B., Sundaram, C., Harikumar, K. B., Tharakan, S. T., Lai, O. S., Sung, B., and Aggarwal, B. B. (2008). Cancer is a preventable disease that requires major lifestyle changes. *Pharm.Res.* 25, 2097-2116.

Andressoo, J. O., Hoeijmakers, J. H., and Mitchell, J. R. (2006). Nucleotide excision repair disorders and the balance between cancer and aging. *Cell Cycle* 5, 2886-2888.

Araki, M., Masutani, C., Takemura, M., Uchida, A., Sugasawa, K., Kondoh, J., Ohkuma, Y., and Hanaoka, F. (2001). Centrosome protein centrin 2/caltractin 1 is part of the xeroderma pigmentosum group C complex that initiates global genome nucleotide excision repair. *J.Biol.Chem.* 276, 18665-18672.

Araujo, S. J., Nigg, E. A., and Wood, R. D. (2001). Strong functional interactions of TFIIH with XPC and XPG in human DNA nucleotide excision repair, without a preassembled repairosome. *Mol.Cell Biol.* 21, 2281-2291.

Berg, R. J., de Vries, A., van Steeg, H., and de Gruijl, F. R. (1997). Relative susceptibilities of XPA knockout mice and their heterozygous and wild-type littermates to UVB-induced skin cancer. *Cancer Res.* 57, 581-584.

Berg, R. J., Ruven, H. J., Sands, A. T., de Gruijl, F. R., and Mullenders, L. H. (1998). Defective global genome repair in XPC mice is associated with skin cancer susceptibility but not with sensitivity to UVB induced erythema and edema. *J.Invest Dermatol.* 110, 405-409.

Bessho, T. (1999). Nucleotide excision repair 3' endonuclease XPG stimulates the activity of base excision repairenzyme thymine glycol DNA glycosylase. *Nucleic Acids Res.* 27, 979-983.

Bhutto, A. M. and Kirk, S. H. (2008). Population distribution of xeroderma pigmentosum. *Adv.Exp.Med.Biol.* 637, 138-143.

Bol, S. A., van Steeg, H., Jansen, J. G., Van Oostrom, C., de Vries, A., de Groot, A. J., Tates, A. D., Vrieling, H., van Zeeland, A. A., and Mullenders, L. H. (1998). Elevated frequencies of benzo(a)pyrene-induced Hprt mutations in internal tissue of XPA-deficient mice. *Cancer Res.* 58, 2850-2856.

Cadet, J., Douki, T., Gasparutto, D., and Ravanat, J. L. (2003). Oxidative damage to DNA: formation, measurement and biochemical features. *Mutat.Res.* 531, 5-23.

Camenisch, U. and Nageli, H. (2008). XPA gene, its product and biological roles. *Adv.Exp.Med.Biol.* 637, 28-38.

Chen, X., Zhang, Y., Douglas, L., and Zhou, P. (2001). UV-damaged DNA-binding proteins are targets of CUL-4A-mediated ubiquitination and degradation. *J.Biol.Chem.* 276, 48175-48182.

Cheo, D. L., Burns, D. K., Meira, L. B., Houle, J. F., and Friedberg, E. C. (1999). Mutational inactivation of the xeroderma pigmentosum group C gene confers predisposition to 2-acetylaminofluorene-induced liver and lung cancer and to spontaneous testicular cancer in Trp53-/- mice. *Cancer Res.* 59, 771-775.

Cheo, D. L., Meira, L. B., Burns, D. K., Reis, A. M., Issac, T., and Friedberg, E. C. (2000). Ultraviolet B radiation-induced skin cancer in mice defective in the Xpc, Trp53, and Apex (HAP1) genes: genotype-specific effects on cancer predisposition and pathology of tumors. *Cancer Res.* 60, 1580-1584.

Cheo, D. L., Meira, L. B., Hammer, R. E., Burns, D. K., Doughty, A. T., and Friedberg, E. C. (1996). Synergistic interactions between XPC and p53 mutations in double-mutant mice: neural tube abnormalities and accelerated UV radiation-induced skin cancer. *Curr.Biol.* 6, 1691-1694.

Cheo, D. L., Ruven, H. J., Meira, L. B., Hammer, R. E., Burns, D. K., Tappe, N. J., van Zeeland, A. A., Mullenders, L. H., and Friedberg, E. C. (1997). Characterization of defective nucleotide excision repair in XPC mutant mice. *Mutat.Res.* 374, 1-9.

Cleaver, J. E., Lam, E. T., and Revet, I. (2009). Disorders of nucleotide excision repair: the genetic and molecular basis of heterogeneity. *Nat.Rev.Genet.* 10, 756-768.

Coin, F., Oksenych, V., Mocquet, V., Groh, S., Blattner, C., and Egly, J. M. (2008). Nucleotide excision repair driven by the dissociation of CAK from TFIIH. *Mol.Cell* 31, 9-20.

D'Errico, M., Parlanti, E., Teson, M., de Jesus, B. M., Degan, P., Calcagnile, A., Jaruga, P., Bjoras, M., Crescenzi, M., Pedrini, A. M., Egly, J. M., Zambruno, G., Stefanini, M., Dizdaroglu, M., and Dogliotti, E. (2006). New functions of XPC in the protection of human skin cells from oxidative damage. *EMBO J.* 25, 4305-4315.

de Boer, J., Andressoo, J. O., de Wit, J., Huijmans, J., Beems, R. B., van Steeg, H., Weeda, G., van der Horst, G. T., van Leeuwen, W., Themmen, A. P., Meradji, M., and Hoeijmakers, J. H. (2002). Premature aging in mice deficient in DNA repair and transcription. *Science* 296, 1276-1279.

de Boer, J. and Hoeijmakers, J. H. (2000). Nucleotide excision repair and human syndromes. *Carcinogenesis* 21, 453-460.

de Laat, W. L., Appeldoorn, E., Jaspers, N. G., and Hoeijmakers, J. H. (1998a). DNA structural elements required for ERCC1-XPF endonuclease activity. *J.Biol.Chem.* 273, 7835-7842.

de Laat, W. L., Appeldoorn, E., Sugasawa, K., Weterings, E., Jaspers, N. G., and Hoeijmakers, J. H. (1998b). DNA-binding polarity of human replication protein A positions nucleases in nucleotide excision repair. *Genes Dev.* 12, 2598-2609.

de Vries, A., Dolle, M. E., Broekhof, J. L., Muller, J. J., Kroese, E. D., van Kreijl, C. F., Capel, P. J., Vijg, J., and van Steeg, H. (1997a). Induction of DNA adducts and mutations in spleen, liver and lung of XPA-deficient/lacZ transgenic mice after oral treatment with benzo[a]pyrene: correlation with tumour development. *Carcinogenesis* 18, 2327-2332.

de Vries, A., Gorgels, T. G., Berg, R. J., Jansen, G. H., and van Steeg, H. (1998). Ultraviolet-B induced hyperplasia and squamous cell carcinomas in the cornea of XPA-deficient mice. *Exp.Eye Res.* 67, 53-59.

de Vries, A., van Oostrom, C. T., Dortant, P. M., Beems, R. B., van Kreijl, C. F., Capel, P. J., and van Steeg, H. (1997b). Spontaneous liver tumors and benzo[a]pyrene-induced lymphomas in XPA-deficient mice. *Mol.Carcinog.* 19, 46-53.

de Vries, A., van Oostrom, C. T., Hofhuis, F. M., Dortant, P. M., Berg, R. J., de Gruijl, F. R., Wester, P. W., van Kreijl, C. F., Capel, P. J., van Steeg, H., and . (1995). Increased susceptibility to ultraviolet-B and carcinogens of mice lacking the DNA excision repair gene XPA. *Nature* 377, 169-173.

Despras, E., Pfeiffer, P., Salles, B., Calsou, P., Kuhfittig-Kulle, S., Angulo, J. F., and Biard, D. S. (2007). Long-term XPC silencing reduces DNA double-strand break repair. *Cancer Res.* 67, 2526-2534.

Dianov, G. L., Thybo, T., Dianova, I. I., Lipinski, L. J., and Bohr, V. A. (2000). Single nucleotide patch base excision repair is the major pathway for removal of thymine glycol from DNA in human cell extracts. *J.Biol.Chem.* 275, 11809-11813.

Dip, R., Camenisch, U., and Naegeli, H. (2004). Mechanisms of DNA damage recognition and strand discrimination in human nucleotide excision repair. *DNA Repair (Amst)* 3, 1409-1423.

El Mahdy, M. A., Zhu, Q., Wang, Q. E., Wani, G., Praetorius-Ibba, M., and Wani, A. A. (2006). Cullin 4A-mediated proteolysis of DDB2 protein at DNA damage sites regulates in vivo lesion recognition by XPC. *J.Biol.Chem.* 281, 13404-13411.

Fitch, M. E., Nakajima, S., Yasui, A., and Ford, J. M. (2003). In vivo recruitment of XPC to UV-induced cyclobutane pyrimidine dimers by the DDB2 gene product. *J.Biol.Chem.* 278, 46906-46910.

Fousteri, M. and Mullenders, L. H. (2008). Transcription-coupled nucleotide excision repair in mammalian cells: molecular mechanisms and biological effects. *Cell Res.* 18, 73-84.

Fousteri, M., Vermeulen, W., van Zeeland, A. A., and Mullenders, L. H. (2006). Cockayne syndrome A and B proteins differentially regulate recruitment of chromatin remodeling and repair factors to stalled RNA polymerase II in vivo. *Mol.Cell* 23, 471-482.

Friedberg, E. C. (1995). Out of the shadows and into the light: the emergence of DNA repair. *Trends Biochem.Sci.* 20, 381.

Friedberg, E. C., Cheo, D. L., Meira, L. B., and Reis, A. M. (1999). Cancer predisposition in mutant mice defective in the XPC DNA repair gene. *Prog.Exp.Tumor Res.* 35, 37-52.

Friedberg, E. C. and Meira, L. B. (2006a). Database of mouse strains carrying targeted mutations in genes affecting biological responses to DNA damage Version 7. *DNA Repair (Amst)* 5, 189-209.

Friedberg, E. C., Walker, G. C., Siede, W., Wood, R. D., Schultz, R. A, and Ellenberger, T. (2006b). DNA Repair and Mutagenesis. ASM Press).

Garinis, G. A., Jans, J., and van der Horst, G. T. (2006). Photolyases: capturing the light to battle skin cancer. *Future.Oncol.* 2, 191-199.

Gaspari, A. A., Fleisher, T. A., and Kraemer, K. H. (1993). Impaired interferon production and natural killer cell activation in patients with the skin cancer-prone disorder, xeroderma pigmentosum. *J.Clin.Invest* 92, 1135-1142.

Giglia-Mari, G., Coin, F., Ranish, J. A., Hoogstraten, D., Theil, A., Wijgers, N., Jaspers, N. G., Raams, A., Argentini, M., van der Spek, P. J., Botta, E., Stefanini, M., Egly, J. M., Aebersold, R., Hoeijmakers, J. H., and Vermeulen, W. (2004). A new, tenth subunit of TFIIH is responsible for the DNA repair syndrome trichothiodystrophy group A. *Nat.Genet.* 36, 714-719.

Goosen, N. (2010). Scanning the DNA for damage by the nucleotide excision repair machinery. *DNA Repair (Amst)* 9, 593-596.

Groisman, R., Polanowska, J., Kuraoka, I., Sawada, J., Saijo, M., Drapkin, R., Kisselev, A. F., Tanaka, K., and Nakatani, Y. (2003). The ubiquitin ligase activity in the DDB2 and CSA complexes is differentially regulated by the COP9 signalosome in response to DNA damage. *Cell* 113, 357-367.

Guarente, L. P., Partridge, L., and Wallace, D. C. (2008). Molecular Biology of Aging. Cold Spring Harbor Laboratory Press).

Harada, Y. N., Shiomi, N., Koike, M., Ikawa, M., Okabe, M., Hirota, S., Kitamura, Y., Kitagawa, M., Matsunaga, T., Nikaido, O., and Shiomi, T. (1999). Postnatal growth failure, short life span, and early onset of cellular senescence and subsequent immortalization in mice lacking the xeroderma pigmentosum group G gene. *Mol.Cell Biol.* 19, 2366-2372.

Henning, K. A., Li, L., Iyer, N., McDaniel, L. D., Reagan, M. S., Legerski, R., Schultz, R. A., Stefanini, M., Lehmann, A. R., Mayne, L. V., and Friedberg, E. C. (1995). The Cockayne syndrome group A gene encodes a WD repeat protein that interacts with CSB protein and a subunit of RNA polymerase II TFIIH. *Cell* 82, 555-564.

Hermanson-Miller, I. L. and Turchi, J. J. (2002). Strand-specific binding of RPA and XPA to damaged duplex DNA. *Biochemistry* 41, 2402-2408.

Hess, M. T., Schwitter, U., Petretta, M., Giese, B., and Naegeli, H. (1997). Bipartite substrate discrimination by human nucleotide excision repair. *Proc.Natl.Acad.Sci.U.S.A* 94, 6664-6669.

Hollander, M. C., Philburn, R. T., Patterson, A. D., Velasco-Miguel, S., Friedberg, E. C., Linnoila, R. I., and Fornace, A. J., Jr. (2005). Deletion of XPC leads to lung tumors in mice and is associated with early events in human lung carcinogenesis. *Proc.Natl.Acad.Sci.U.S.A* 102, 13200-13205.

Hoogervorst, E. M., de Vries, A., Beems, R. B., van Oostrom, C. T., Wester, P. W., Vos, J. G., Bruins, W., Roodbergen, M., Cassee, F. R., Vijg, J., van Schooten, F. J., and van Steeg, H. (2003). Combined oral benzo[a]pyrene and inhalatory ozone exposure have no effect on lung tumor development in DNA repair-deficient Xpa mice. *Carcinogenesis* 24, 613-619.

Hoogervorst, E. M., van Oostrom, C. T., Beems, R. B., van Benthem, J., Gielis, S., Vermeulen, J. P., Wester, P. W., Vos, J. G., de Vries, A., and van Steeg, H. (2004). p53 heterozygosity results in an increased 2-acetylaminofluorene-induced urinary bladder but not liver tumor response in DNA repair-deficient Xpa mice. *Cancer Res.* 64, 5118-5126.

Hoogervorst, E. M., van Oostrom, C. T., Beems, R. B., van Benthem, J., van den, Berg J., van Kreijl, C. F., Vos, J. G., de Vries, A., and van Steeg, H. (2005). 2-AAF-induced tumor development in nucleotide excision repair-deficient mice is associated with a defect in global genome repair but not with transcription coupled repair. *DNA Repair (Amst)* 4, 3-9.

Hoogstraten, D., Bergink, S., Ng, J. M., Verbiest, V. H., Luijsterburg, M. S., Geverts, B., Raams, A., Dinant, C., Hoeijmakers, J. H., Vermeulen, W., and Houtsmuller, A. B. (2008). Versatile DNA damage detection by the global genome nucleotide excision repair protein XPC. *J.Cell Sci.* 121, 2850-2859.

Horio, T., Miyauchi-Hashimoto, H., Kuwamoto, K., Horiki, S., Okamoto, H., and Tanaka, K. (2001). Photobiologic and photoimmunologic characteristics of XPA gene-deficient mice. *J.Investig.Dermatol.Symp.Proc.* 6, 58-63.

Ide, F., Iida, N., Nakatsuru, Y., Oda, H., Tanaka, K., and Ishikawa, T. (2000). Mice deficient in the nucleotide excision repair gene XPA have elevated sensitivity to benzo[a]pyrene induction of lung tumors. *Carcinogenesis* 21, 1263-1265.

Ide, F., Oda, H., Nakatsuru, Y., Kusama, K., Sakashita, H., Tanaka, K., and Ishikawa, T. (2001). Xeroderma pigmentosum group A gene action as a protection factor against 4-nitroquinoline 1-oxide-induced tongue carcinogenesis. *Carcinogenesis* 22, 567-572.

Ikegami, T., Kuraoka, I., Saijo, M., Kodo, N., Kyogoku, Y., Morikawa, K., Tanaka, K., and Shirakawa, M. (1998). Solution structure of the DNA- and RPA-binding domain of the human repair factor XPA. *Nat.Struct.Biol.* 5, 701-706.

Ikehata, H., Saito, Y., Yanase, F., Mori, T., Nikaido, O., and Ono, T. (2007). Frequent recovery of triplet mutations in UVB-exposed skin epidermis of Xpc-knockout mice. *DNA Repair (Amst)* 6, 82-93.

Itoh, T. (2006). Xeroderma pigmentosum group E and DDB2, a smaller subunit of damage-specific DNA binding protein: proposed classification of xeroderma pigmentosum, Cockayne syndrome, and ultraviolet-sensitive syndrome. *J.Dermatol.Sci.* 41, 87-96.

Itoh, T., Cado, D., Kamide, R., and Linn, S. (2004). DDB2 gene disruption leads to skin tumors and resistance to apoptosis after exposure to ultraviolet light but not a chemical carcinogen. *Proc.Natl.Acad.Sci.U.S.A* 101, 2052-2057.

Kamiuchi, S., Saijo, M., Citterio, E., de Jager, M., Hoeijmakers, J. H., and Tanaka, K. (2002). Translocation of Cockayne syndrome group A protein to the nuclear matrix: possible relevance to transcription-coupled DNA repair. *Proc.Natl.Acad.Sci.U.S.A* 99, 201-206.

Kinzler KW and Vogelstein B (2002). The genetic basis of human cancer. (New York: McGraw-Hill).

Klein, J. C., Beems, R. B., Zwart, P. E., Hamzink, M., Zomer, G., van Steeg, H., and van Kreijl, C. F. (2001). Intestinal toxicity and carcinogenic potential of the food mutagen 2-amino-1-methyl-6-phenylimidazo[4,5-b]pyridine (PhIP) in DNA repair deficient XPA-/- mice. *Carcinogenesis* 22, 619-626.

Kraemer, K. H. (1997). Sunlight and skin cancer: another link revealed. *Proc.Natl.Acad.Sci.U.S.A* 94, 11-14.

Kraemer, K. H., Lee, M. M., and Scotto, J. (1984). DNA repair protects against cutaneous and internal neoplasia: evidence from xeroderma pigmentosum. *Carcinogenesis* 5, 511-514.

Krasikova, Y. S., Rechkunova, N. I., Maltseva, E. A., Petruseva, I. O., and Lavrik, O. I. (2010). Localization of xeroderma pigmentosum group A protein and replication protein A on damaged DNA in nucleotide excision repair. *Nucleic Acids Res.*

Lao, Y., Gomes, X. V., Ren, Y., Taylor, J. S., and Wold, M. S. (2000). Replication protein A interactions with DNA. III. Molecular basis of recognition of damaged DNA. *Biochemistry* 39, 850-859.

Lee, S. K., Yu, S. L., Prakash, L., and Prakash, S. (2002). Requirement of yeast RAD2, a homolog of human XPG gene, for efficient RNA polymerase II transcription. implications for Cockayne syndrome. *Cell* 109, 823-834.

Lin, J. J. and Sancar, A. (1992). (A)BC excinuclease: the Escherichia coli nucleotide excision repair enzyme. *Mol.Microbiol.* 6, 2219-2224.

Lindahl, T. (1993). Instability and decay of the primary structure of DNA. *Nature* 362, 709-715.

Liu, S. Y., Wen, C. Y., Lee, Y. J., and Lee, T. C. (2010). XPC silencing sensitizes glioma cells to arsenic trioxide via increased oxidative damage. *Toxicol.Sci.* 116, 183-193.

Lo, H. L., Nakajima, S., Ma, L., Walter, B., Yasui, A., Ethell, D. W., and Owen, L. B. (2005). Differential biologic effects of CPD and 6-4PP UV-induced DNA damage on the induction of apoptosis and cell-cycle arrest. *BMC.Cancer* 5, 135.

Lodish, H., Berk, A., Matsudaira, P., Kaiser, C. A., Krieger, M., Scott, M. P., Zipurksy, S. L., and Darnell, J. (2004). Molecular Biology of the Cell. WH Freeman).

Matsuda, N., Azuma, K., Saijo, M., Iemura, S., Hioki, Y., Natsume, T., Chiba, T., Tanaka, K., and Tanaka, K. (2005). DDB2, the xeroderma pigmentosum group E gene product, is directly ubiquitylated by Cullin 4A-based ubiquitin ligase complex. *DNA Repair (Amst)* 4, 537-545.

McAnulty, P. A. and Skydsgaard, M. (2005). Diethylstilbestrol (DES): carcinogenic potential in Xpa-/-, Xpa-/- / p53+/-, and wild-type mice during 9 months' dietary exposure. *Toxicol.Pathol.* 33, 609-620.

McWhir, J., Selfridge, J., Harrison, D. J., Squires, S., and Melton, D. W. (1993). Mice with DNA repair gene (ERCC-1) deficiency have elevated levels of p53, liver nuclear abnormalities and die before weaning. *Nat.Genet.* 5, 217-224.

Melis, J. P., Wijnhoven, S. W., Beems, R. B., Roodbergen, M., van den, Berg J., Moon, H., Friedberg, E., van der Horst, G. T., Hoeijmakers, J. H., Vijg, J., and van Steeg, H. (2008). Mouse models for xeroderma pigmentosum group A and group C show divergent cancer phenotypes. *Cancer Res.* 68, 1347-1353.

Min, J. H. and Pavletich, N. P. (2007). Recognition of DNA damage by the Rad4 nucleotide excision repair protein. *Nature* 449, 570-575.

Miyamoto, I., Miura, N., Niwa, H., Miyazaki, J., and Tanaka, K. (1992). Mutational analysis of the structure and function of the xeroderma pigmentosum group A complementing protein. Identification of essential domains for nuclear localization and DNA excision repair. *J.Biol.Chem.* 267, 12182-12187.

Miyauchi-Hashimoto, H., Kuwamoto, K., Urade, Y., Tanaka, K., and Horio, T. (2001). Carcinogen-induced inflammation and immunosuppression are enhanced in xeroderma pigmentosum group A model mice associated with hyperproduction of prostaglandin E2. *J.Immunol.* 166, 5782-5791.

Mocquet, V., Laine, J. P., Riedl, T., Yajin, Z., Lee, M. Y., and Egly, J. M. (2008). Sequential recruitment of the repair factors during NER: the role of XPG in initiating the resynthesis step. *EMBO J.* 27, 155-167.

Moser, J., Kool, H., Giakzidis, I., Caldecott, K., Mullenders, L. H., and Fousteri, M. I. (2007). Sealing of chromosomal DNA nicks during nucleotide excision repair requires XRCC1 and DNA ligase III alpha in a cell-cycle-specific manner. *Mol.Cell* 27, 311-323.

Mullaart, E., Lohman, P. H., Berends, F., and Vijg, J. (1990). DNA damage metabolism and aging. *Mutat.Res.* 237, 189-210.

Nag, A., Bondar, T., Shiv, S., and Raychaudhuri, P. (2001). The xeroderma pigmentosum group E gene product DDB2 is a specific target of cullin 4A in mammalian cells. *Mol.Cell Biol.* 21, 6738-6747.

Nakane, H., Takeuchi, S., Yuba, S., Saijo, M., Nakatsu, Y., Murai, H., Nakatsuru, Y., Ishikawa, T., Hirota, S., Kitamura, Y., and . (1995). High incidence of ultraviolet-B-or chemical-carcinogen-induced skin tumours in mice lacking the xeroderma pigmentosum group A gene. *Nature* 377, 165-168.

Nakatsu, Y., Asahina, H., Citterio, E., Rademakers, S., Vermeulen, W., Kamiuchi, S., Yeo, J. P., Khaw, M. C., Saijo, M., Kodo, N., Matsuda, T., Hoeijmakers, J. H., and Tanaka, K. (2000). XAB2, a novel tetratricopeptide repeat protein involved in transcription-coupled DNA repair and transcription. *J.Biol.Chem.* 275, 34931-34937.

Ng, J. M., Vermeulen, W., van der Horst, G. T., Bergink, S., Sugasawa, K., Vrieling, H., and Hoeijmakers, J. H. (2003). A novel regulation mechanism of DNA repair by damage-induced and RAD23-dependent stabilization of xeroderma pigmentosum group C protein. *Genes Dev.* 17, 1630-1645.

Ng, J. M., Vrieling, H., Sugasawa, K., Ooms, M. P., Grootegoed, J. A., Vreeburg, J. T., Visser, P., Beems, R. B., Gorgels, T. G., Hanaoka, F., Hoeijmakers, J. H., and van der Horst, G. T. (2002). Developmental defects and male sterility in mice lacking the ubiquitin-like DNA repair gene mHR23B. *Mol.Cell Biol.* 22, 1233-1245.

Nichols, A. F., Itoh, T., Graham, J. A., Liu, W., Yamaizumi, M., and Linn, S. (2000). Human damage-specific DNA-binding protein p48. Characterization of XPE mutations and regulation following UV irradiation. *J.Biol.Chem.* 275, 21422-21428.

Niedernhofer, L. J., Essers, J., Weeda, G., Beverloo, B., de Wit, J., Muijtjens, M., Odijk, H., Hoeijmakers, J. H., and Kanaar, R. (2001). The structure-specific endonuclease Ercc1-Xpf is required for targeted gene replacement in embryonic stem cells. *EMBO J.* 20, 6540-6549.

Nishi, R., Okuda, Y., Watanabe, E., Mori, T., Iwai, S., Masutani, C., Sugasawa, K., and Hanaoka, F. (2005). Centrin 2 stimulates nucleotide excision repair by interacting with xeroderma pigmentosum group C protein. *Mol.Cell Biol.* 25, 5664-5674.

Ogi, T., Limsirichaikul, S., Overmeer, R. M., Volker, M., Takenaka, K., Cloney, R., Nakazawa, Y., Niimi, A., Miki, Y., Jaspers, N. G., Mullenders, L. H., Yamashita, S., Fousteri, M. I., and Lehmann, A. R. (2010). Three DNA polymerases, recruited by different mechanisms, carry out NER repair synthesis in human cells. *Mol.Cell* 37, 714-727.

Okamoto, Y., Chou, P. H., Kim, S. Y., Suzuki, N., Laxmi, Y. R., Okamoto, K., Liu, X., Matsuda, T., and Shibutani, S. (2008). Oxidative DNA damage in XPC-knockout and its wild mice treated with equine estrogen. *Chem.Res.Toxicol.* 21, 1120-1124.

Oksenych, V. and Coin, F. (2010). The long unwinding road: XPB and XPD helicases in damaged DNA opening. *Cell Cycle* 9, 90-96.

Ortolan, T. G., Chen, L., Tongaonkar, P., and Madura, K. (2004). Rad23 stabilizes Rad4 from degradation by the Ub/proteasome pathway. *Nucleic Acids Res.* 32, 6490-6500.

Park, C. J. and Choi, B. S. (2006). The protein shuffle. Sequential interactions among components of the human nucleotide excision repair pathway. *FEBS J.* 273, 1600-1608.

Rapic-Otrin, V., McLenigan, M. P., Bisi, D. C., Gonzalez, M., and Levine, A. S. (2002). Sequential binding of UV DNA damage binding factor and degradation of the p48 subunit as early events after UV irradiation. *Nucleic Acids Res.* 30, 2588-2598.

Rezvani, H. R., Kim, A. L., Rossignol, R., Ali, N., Daly, M., Mahfouf, W., Bellance, N., Taieb, A., de Verneuil, H., Mazurier, F., and Bickers, D. R. (2010). XPC silencing in normal human keratinocytes triggers metabolic alterations that drive the formation of squamous cell carcinomas. *J.Clin.Invest.*

Sands, A. T., Abuin, A., Sanchez, A., Conti, C. J., and Bradley, A. (1995). High susceptibility to ultraviolet-induced carcinogenesis in mice lacking XPC. *Nature* 377, 162-165.

Shimizu, Y., Iwai, S., Hanaoka, F., and Sugasawa, K. (2003). Xeroderma pigmentosum group C protein interacts physically and functionally with thymine DNA glycosylase. *EMBO J.* 22, 164-173.

Shivji, M. K., Podust, V. N., Hubscher, U., and Wood, R. D. (1995). Nucleotide excision repair DNA synthesis by DNA polymerase epsilon in the presence of PCNA, RFC, and RPA. *Biochemistry* 34, 5011-5017.

Staresincic, L., Fagbemi, A. F., Enzlin, J. H., Gourdin, A. M., Wijgers, N., Dunand-Sauthier, I., Giglia-Mari, G., Clarkson, S. G., Vermeulen, W., and Scharer, O. D. (2009). Coordination of dual incision and repair synthesis in human nucleotide excision repair. *EMBO J.* 28, 1111-1120.

Sugasawa, K. (2008). XPC: its product and biological roles. *Adv.Exp.Med.Biol.* 637, 47-56.

Sugasawa, K., Okamoto, T., Shimizu, Y., Masutani, C., Iwai, S., and Hanaoka, F. (2001). A multistep damage recognition mechanism for global genomic nucleotide excision repair. *Genes Dev.* 15, 507-521.

Sugasawa, K., Okuda, Y., Saijo, M., Nishi, R., Matsuda, N., Chu, G., Mori, T., Iwai, S., Tanaka, K., Tanaka, K., and Hanaoka, F. (2005). UV-induced ubiquitylation of XPC protein mediated by UV-DDB-ubiquitin ligase complex. *Cell* 121, 387-400.

Sugasawa, K., Shimizu, Y., Iwai, S., and Hanaoka, F. (2002). A molecular mechanism for DNA damage recognition by the xeroderma pigmentosum group C protein complex. *DNA Repair (Amst)* 1, 95-107.

Sunesen, M., Stevnsner, T., Brosh, R. M., Jr., Dianov, G. L., and Bohr, V. A. (2002). Global genome repair of 8-oxoG in hamster cells requires a functional CSB gene product. *Oncogene* 21, 3571-3578.

Takahashi, Y., Nakatsuru, Y., Zhang, S., Shimizu, Y., Kume, H., Tanaka, K., Ide, F., and Ishikawa, T. (2002). Enhanced spontaneous and aflatoxin-induced liver tumorigenesis in xeroderma pigmentosum group A gene-deficient mice. *Carcinogenesis* 23, 627-633.

Tanaka, K., Kamiuchi, S., Ren, Y., Yonemasu, R., Ichikawa, M., Murai, H., Yoshino, M., Takeuchi, S., Saijo, M., Nakatsu, Y., Miyauchi-Hashimoto, H., and Horio, T. (2001).

UV-induced skin carcinogenesis in xeroderma pigmentosum group A (XPA) gene-knockout mice with nucleotide excision repair-deficiency. *Mutat.Res.* 477, 31-40.

Tang, J. Y., Hwang, B. J., Ford, J. M., Hanawalt, P. C., and Chu, G. (2000). Xeroderma pigmentosum p48 gene enhances global genomic repair and suppresses UV-induced mutagenesis. *Mol.Cell* 5, 737-744.

Tantin, D. (1998). RNA polymerase II elongation complexes containing the Cockayne syndrome group B protein interact with a molecular complex containing the transcription factor IIH components xeroderma pigmentosum B and p62. *J.Biol.Chem.* 273, 27794-27799.

Tantin, D., Kansal, A., and Carey, M. (1997). Recruitment of the putative transcription-repair coupling factor CSB/ERCC6 to RNA polymerase II elongation complexes. *Mol.Cell Biol.* 17, 6803-6814.

Tian, M., Shinkura, R., Shinkura, N., and Alt, F. W. (2004). Growth retardation, early death, and DNA repair defects in mice deficient for the nucleotide excision repair enzyme XPF. *Mol.Cell Biol.* 24, 1200-1205.

Uehara, Y., Ikehata, H., Furuya, M., Kobayashi, S., He, D., Chen, Y., Komura, J., Ohtani, H., Shimokawa, I., and Ono, T. (2009). XPC is involved in genome maintenance through multiple pathways in different tissues. *Mutat.Res.* 670, 24-31.

van der Horst, G. T., Meira, L., Gorgels, T. G., de Wit, J., Velasco-Miguel, S., Richardson, J. A., Kamp, Y., Vreeswijk, M. P., Smit, B., Bootsma, D., Hoeijmakers, J. H., and Friedberg, E. C. (2002). UVB radiation-induced cancer predisposition in Cockayne syndrome group A (Csa) mutant mice. *DNA Repair (Amst)* 1, 143-157.

van der Horst, G. T., van Steeg, H., Berg, R. J., van Gool, A. J., de Wit, J., Weeda, G., Morreau, H., Beems, R. B., van Kreijl, C. F., de Gruijl, F. R., Bootsma, D., and Hoeijmakers, J. H. (1997). Defective transcription-coupled repair in Cockayne syndrome B mice is associated with skin cancer predisposition. *Cell* 89, 425-435.

van Kesteren, P. C., Beems, R. B., Luijten, M., Robinson, J., de Vries, A., and van Steeg, H. (2009). DNA repair-deficient Xpa/p53 knockout mice are sensitive to the non-genotoxic carcinogen cyclosporine A: escape of initiated cells from immunosurveillance? *Carcinogenesis* 30, 538-543.

van Kreijl, C. F., McAnulty, P. A., Beems, R. B., Vynckier, A., van Steeg, H., Fransson-Steen, R., Alden, C. L., Forster, R., van der Laan, J. W., and Vandenberghe, J. (2001). Xpa and Xpa/p53+/- knockout mice: overview of available data. *Toxicol.Pathol.* 29 Suppl, 117-127.

van Oostrom, C. T., Boeve, M., van den, Berg J., de Vries, A., Dolle, M. E., Beems, R. B., van Kreijl, C. F., Vijg, J., and van Steeg, H. (1999). Effect of heterozygous loss of p53 on benzo[a]pyrene-induced mutations and tumors in DNA repair-deficient XPA mice. *Environ.Mol.Mutagen.* 34, 124-130.

van Steeg, H., Klein, H., Beems, R. B., and van Kreijl, C. F. (1998). Use of DNA repair-deficient XPA transgenic mice in short-term carcinogenicity testing. *Toxicol.Pathol.* 26, 742-749.

van Steeg, H., Mullenders, L. H., and Vijg, J. (2000). Mutagenesis and carcinogenesis in nucleotide excision repair-deficient XPA knock out mice. *Mutat.Res.* 450, 167-180.

Wakasugi, M., Reardon, J. T., and Sancar, A. (1997). The non-catalytic function of XPG protein during dual incision in human nucleotide excision repair. *J.Biol.Chem.* 272, 16030-16034.

Weeda, G., Donker, I., de Wit, J., Morreau, H., Janssens, R., Vissers, C. J., Nigg, A., van Steeg, H., Bootsma, D., and Hoeijmakers, J. H. (1997). Disruption of mouse ERCC1 results in a novel repair syndrome with growth failure, nuclear abnormalities and senescence. *Curr.Biol.* 7, 427-439.

Wickliffe, J. K., Galbert, L. A., Ammenheuser, M. M., Herring, S. M., Xie, J., Masters, O. E., III, Friedberg, E. C., Lloyd, R. S., and Ward, J. B., Jr. (2006). 3,4-Epoxy-1-butene, a reactive metabolite of 1,3-butadiene, induces somatic mutations in Xpc-null mice. *Environ.Mol.Mutagen.* 47, 67-70.

Wijnhoven, S. W., Beems, R. B., Roodbergen, M., van den, Berg J., Lohman, P. H., Diderich, K., van der Horst, G. T., Vijg, J., Hoeijmakers, J. H., and van Steeg, H. (2005). Accelerated aging pathology in ad libitum fed Xpd(TTD) mice is accompanied by features suggestive of caloric restriction. *DNA Repair (Amst)* 4, 1314-1324.

Wijnhoven, S. W., Hoogervorst, E. M., de Waard, H., van der Horst, G. T., and van Steeg, H. (2007). Tissue specific mutagenic and carcinogenic responses in NER defective mouse models. *Mutat.Res.* 614, 77-94.

Wijnhoven, S. W., Kool, H. J., Mullenders, L. H., Slater, R., van Zeeland, A. A., and Vrieling, H. (2001). DMBA-induced toxic and mutagenic responses vary dramatically between NER-deficient Xpa, Xpc and Csb mice. *Carcinogenesis* 22, 1099-1106.

Wittschieben, B. O., Iwai, S., and Wood, R. D. (2005). DDB1-DDB2 (xeroderma pigmentosum group E) protein complex recognizes a cyclobutane pyrimidine dimer, mismatches, apurinic/apyrimidinic sites, and compound lesions in DNA. *J.Biol.Chem.* 280, 39982-39989.

Yokoi, M., Masutani, C., Maekawa, T., Sugasawa, K., Ohkuma, Y., and Hanaoka, F. (2000). The xeroderma pigmentosum group C protein complex XPC-HR23B plays an important role in the recruitment of transcription factor IIH to damaged DNA. *J.Biol.Chem.* 275, 9870-9875.

Yoon, T., Chakrabortty, A., Franks, R., Valli, T., Kiyokawa, H., and Raychaudhuri, P. (2005). Tumor-prone phenotype of the DDB2-deficient mice. *Oncogene* 24, 469-478.

Zeng, L., Quilliet, X., Chevallier-Lagente, O., Eveno, E., Sarasin, A., and Mezzina, M. (1997). Retrovirus-mediated gene transfer corrects DNA repair defect of xeroderma pigmentosum cells of complementation groups A, B and C. *Gene Ther.* 4, 1077-1084.

Zotter, A., Luijsterburg, M. S., Warmerdam, D. O., Ibrahim, S., Nigg, A., van Cappellen, W. A., Hoeijmakers, J. H., van Driel, R., Vermeulen, W., and Houtsmuller, A. B. (2006). Recruitment of the nucleotide excision repair endonuclease XPG to sites of UV-induced dna damage depends on functional TFIIH. *Mol.Cell Biol.* 26, 8868-8879.

6

Recombinant Viral Vectors for Investigating DNA Damage Responses and Gene Therapy of Xeroderma Pigmentosum

Carolina Quayle[1], Carlos Frederico Martins Menck[1]
and Keronninn Moreno Lima-Bessa[2]
[1]Dept. of Microbiology, Institute of Biomedical Sciences, University of Sao Paulo
[2]Dept. of Cellular Biology and Genetics, Institute of Biosciences
Federal University of Rio Grande do Norte
Brazil

1. Introduction

1.1 The dark side of the sun

The genome of all living organisms is constantly threatened by a number of endogenous and exogenous DNA damaging agents. Such damage may disturb essential cellular processes, such as DNA replication and transcription, thereby resulting in double-strand breaks (referred to as 'replication fork collapse'), which can lead to chromosomal aberrations and/or cell death, ultimately contributing to mutagenesis, early aging and tumorigenesis (Ciccia & Elledge, 2010). One of the most important exogenous sources of DNA damage is the ultraviolet radiation (UV) component of sunlight, since it is responsible for a wide range of biological effects, including alteration in the structure of biologically essential molecules, such as proteins and nucleic acids. Indeed, UV is one of the most effective and carcinogenic exogenous agents that act on DNA, threatening the genome integrity and affecting normal life processes in different aquatic and terrestrial organisms, ranging from prokaryotes to mammals (Rastogi et al., 2010). In addition, UV is the major etiologic agent in the development of human skin cancers (Narayanan et al., 2010).

Sunlight is the primary UV source, whose spectrum is usually classified according to its wavelength in UVA (320-400 nm; lowest energy), UVB (280-320 nm) and UVC (200-280 nm; highest energy). Although these three UV bands are present in sunlight, the stratospheric ozone layer entirely blocks the UVC and most of UVB, thus the solar UV spectrum that reaches the Earth's ground is composed by UVA and some UVB, even though ozone layer depletion can cause changes in this spectral distribution (Kuluncsics et al., 1999).

The chemical nature and efficiency in the formation of DNA lesions greatly depend on the wavelength of the incident photons. Despite its lowest energy, UVA light can deeply penetrate into the cells, mostly damaging DNA by indirect effects caused by the generation of reactive oxygen species which may react with nitrogen bases, resulting in base alterations and breaks in the DNA molecule. On the other hand, UVB can be directly absorbed by DNA bases, producing two main types of DNA damage, the cyclobutane pyrimidine dimers (CPDs) and pyrimidine-pyrimidone-(6-4)-photoproducts (6-4PPs), both resulting from covalent linkages between adjacent pyrimidines located on the same DNA strand, which leads to severe structural distortions in the DNA double helix. Interestingly, it has been recently demonstrated that UVA can also be directly absorbed by the DNA molecule, efficiently generating both CPDs and 6-4PPs (Schuch et al, 2009).

CPDs correspond to the formation of a four-member ring structure involving carbons C5 and C6 of both neighboring bases, whereas 6-4PPs are formed by a non-cyclic bond between C6 (of the 5'-end) and C4 (of the 3'-end) of the involved pyrimidines. Since those lesions induce strong distortions in the DNA molecule, they may lead to severe consequences to the cell if not properly removed, such as transcription arrest and replication blockage, thus disturbing cell metabolism, interfering with the cell cycle and, eventually, inducing cell death. DNA mutations can also result from misleading DNA processing. Long term consequences may include even more deleterious events, such as photoaging and cancer (Sinha & Häder, 2002; Narayanan et al., 2010; Rastogi et al., 2010).

1.2 DNA repair of UV lesions and related human syndromes

To ensure the maintenance of the genome integrity, several mechanisms that counteract DNA damage have emerged very early in evolution, including an intricate machinery of DNA repair, damage tolerance, and checkpoint pathways (Figure 1).

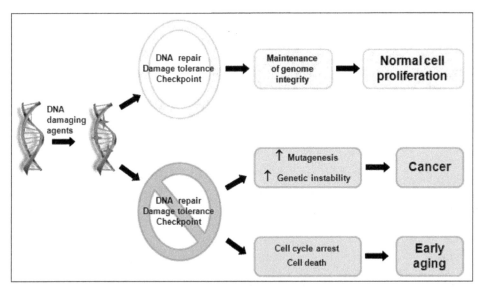

Fig. 1. Main consequences of DNA damage. DNA damage can be induced by a variety of endogenous and exogenous agents. Several mechanisms, including an intricate machinery of DNA repair, damage tolerance, and checkpoint pathways, counteract DNA damage, aiming for the maintenance of genome stability, and guaranteeing normal cell proliferation. When these mechanisms fail, errors in DNA replication and/or aberrant chromosomal segregations take place, increasing mutagenesis and genetic instability and contributing to a higher risk of cancer development. Alternatively, these damages may disturb the transcription and/or cause replication blockage, leading to cell death , thus contributing to early aging.

The nucleotide excision repair (NER) is one of the most versatile and flexible DNA repair systems, removing a wide range of structurally unrelated DNA double-helix distorting lesions, including UV photoproducts, bulky chemical adducts, DNA-intrastrand crosslinks, and some forms of oxidatively generated damage by orchestrating the concerted action of over 30 proteins, including the seven that are functionally impaired in xeroderma pigmentosum patients (XPA to XPG) (Costa et al., 2003; de Boer & Hoeijmakers, 2000). The NER pathway has been extensively studied at the molecular level in both prokaryotic and eukaryotic organisms. Depending on whether the damage is located in a transcriptionally active or inactive domain in the genome, its repair will be processed by one of two NER subpathways: global genome repair (GG-NER) or transcription-coupled repair (TC-NER). Indeed, while GG-NER is a random process, removing distorting lesions over the entire genome, TC-NER focus on those lesions which block RNA polymerases elongation, thus being highly specific and efficient (Fousteri & Mullenders, 2008; Hanawalt, 2002).

Briefly, the NER pathway involves a sequential cascade of events that starts with damage recognition, which defines the major difference between GG-NER and TC-NER. The latter is triggered upon blockage of RNA polymerase translocation at the DNA damage site, whereas GG-NER is evoked by specialized damage recognition factors, including the XPC-hHR23B heterodimer, and also XPE for certain lesions. The subsequent steps are carried out by a common set of NER factors that are shared by both subpathways and involve opening of the DNA helix around the lesion site by the concerted action of two helicases; dual incision of the damaged strand at both sides of the lesion by two endonucleases; removal of the damaged oligonucleotide (24-32 mer); gap filling of the excised patch using the undamaged strand as a template by the action of the replication machinery; and ligation of the new fragment to the chromatin by DNA ligase (Cleaver et al., 2009; Costa et al., 2003). Even though the core NER proteins that carry out damage recognition, excision, and repair reactions have been identified and extensively characterized, the regulatory pathways which govern the threshold levels of NER have not been fully elucidated (Liu et al., 2010). A schematic representation of this repair mechanism in humans is illustrated in Figure 2.

Several human autosomal recessive diseases are caused by dysfunction of the NER pathway, xeroderma pigmentosum (XP) being the prototype. Although this chapter will mainly focus on the XP syndrome, deficiencies in NER can also lead to other genetic diseases, such as trichothiodystrophy (TTD), Cockayne syndrome (CS), cerebro–oculo–facial–skeletal syndrome (COFS) and UV-sensitive syndrome (UVsS), all of which have photosensitivity as a common feature.

Xeroderma pigmentosum (XP) is a rare human disorder transmitted in an autosomal recessive fashion characterized by severe UV light photosensitivity, pigmentary changes, premature skin aging and a greater than 1,000-fold increase incidence of skin and mucous membrane cancer, including squamous and basal cell carcinomas and melanomas, with a 30-year reduction in life span (Cleaver et al., 2009; Karalis et al., 2011; Narayanan et al., 2010). In addition to cutaneous features, patients often develop ocular abnormalities, including neoplasms which may cause blindness. For most patients, often referred to as classical XP, this syndrome is caused by an impaired GG-NER activity, with or without deficiencies in TC-NER, determined by mutations in one of seven NER genes (*XPA* to *XPG*). When TC-NER is also affected (mutations in *XPA*, *XPB*, *XPD* and *XPG* genes), accelerated neurodegeneration may also occur in a substantial number of patients, suggesting increased neuronal cell death due to accumulated endogenous damage (Gerstenblith et al., 2010; Hoeijmakers, 2009). The eighth complementation group corresponds to the XP-variant

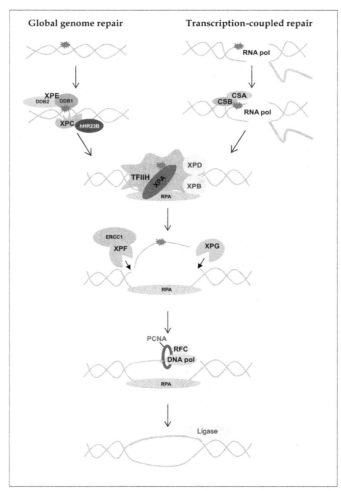

Fig. 2. Schematic representation of repair of DNA lesions by nucleotide excision repair (NER). Depending on where the DNA damage is located in the genome, it will be processed by one of the two NER subpathways: the global genome repair (GG-NER) or the transcription-coupled repair (TC-NER), that basically differ in the lesion recognition step. Lesions occurring randomly in the genome are recognized by the XPC-HR23B complex, with the participation of XPE (DDB1-DDB2) for certain lesions, both complexes are GG-NER-specific. On the other hand, lesions present in the transcribed strand of active genes that lead to the RNA polymerase arrest trigger the TC-NER subpathway, which involves the CSA and CSB proteins. The following steps are common to both subpathways. The DNA double helix around the lesion is opened by XPB and XPD (helicases belonging to the TFIIH complex) and the single strand region is stabilized by RPA, allowing damage verification by the XPA protein. The DNA around the damaged site is then cleaved by the XPF–ERCC1 and XPG endonucleases, excising an oligonucleotide of 24-32 mer, and this patch is resynthesized by the replication machinery using the undamaged strand as a template. Finally, the new fragment is sealed to the chromatin by the DNA ligase.

(XPV) patients, whose XP phenotype is related to mutations in the *POLH* gene, which encodes the translesion synthesis DNA polymerase eta responsible for the replication process on UV-irradiated DNA templates (Johnson et al., 1999; Masutani et al., 1999).

A list of NER genes, which are related to XP syndrome, with their specific functions is given in Table 1.

Gene	Protein	Protein size (A.A.)	Function	Pathway
XPA	XPA	273	Interacts with RPA and other NER proteins, stabilizing ssDNA regions and also facilitating the repair complex assembly.	GG-NER TC-NER
XPB	XPB	782	Belongs to TFIIH complex, working as a 3` → 5` helicase.	GG-NER TC-NER
XPC	XPC	940	Responsible for lesion recognition in GG-NER.	GG-NER
XPD	XPD	760	Belongs to the TFIIH complex, working as a 5` → 3` helicase.	GG-NER TC-NER
DDB2	XPE/p48 subunit	428	Forms a complex with XPE/p127 subunit, which is believed to facilitate the identification of lesions that are poorly recognized by XPC-hHR23B.	GG-NER
XPF	XPF	905	Found as a complex with ERCC1, which functions as an endonuclease 5' of the lesion.	GG-NER TC-NER
XPG	XPG	1186	Functions as an endonuclease 3' of the lesion.	GG-NER TC-NER

*GG-NER- global genome repair; TC-NER- transcription-coupled repair.

Table 1. List of NER genes related to xeroderma pigmentosum and their roles in human DNA repair.

The Cockayne syndrome (CS) is predominantly a developmental and neurological disorder, caused by mutations leading to a defective TC-NER, which prevents recovery from blocked transcription after DNA damage. CS patients are characterized by early growth and development cessation, severe and progressive neurodysfunction associated with demyelination, sensorineural hearing loss, cataracts, cachexia, and frailty (Weidenheim et al., 2009). Curiously, although severe photosensitivity is a common feature reported for most CS patients, it is not linked to an increased frequency of skin cancers, like it is in XP patients. Interestingly, specific mutations in one of three XP genes (*XPB*, *XPD* and *XPG*) may result in a clinical phenotype which reflects a combination of the traits associated with XP and CS (XP/CS patients). This observation indicates that simultaneous defects in GG-NER and TC-NER can cause mutagenesis and cancer in some tissues and accelerated cell death and premature aging in others (Hoeijmakers, 2009).

The hallmark of trichothiodystrophy (TTD) is sulfur-deficient brittle hair, caused by a greatly reduced content of cysteine-rich matrix proteins in the hair shafts. In severe cases, mental abilities are also affected. Abnormal characteristics at birth and pregnancy complications are also common features of TTD, which may imply a role for DNA repair genes in normal fetal development (Stefanini et al., 2010). As CS patients, TTD patients do not present a high incidence of skin cancers. Genetically, three genes were identified for this disease (*XPB*, *XPD* and *TTDA*), but most TTD patients exhibit mutations on the two alleles of the *XPD* gene (Itin et al., 2001).

Cerebro–oculo–facial–skeletal syndrome (COFS) is a disorder determined by mutations in *CSB*, *XPD*, *XPG* and *ERCC1* genes, leading to a defective TC-NER (Suzumura & Arisaka, 2010). It is characterized by congenital microcephaly, congenital cataracts and/or microphthalmia, arthrogryposis, severe developmental delay, an accentuated postnatal growth failure and facial dysmorphism.

Photosensitivity and freckling are the main features of patients with UV-sensitive syndrome (UVsS), but these patients have mild symptoms and no neurological or developmental abnormalities or skin tumors. Although other genes may be involved, mutations in the *CSB* gene were found in some of these patients, leading to defective TC-NER of UV damage (Horibata et al., 2004; Spivak, 2005).

Therefore, the general relationship between defects in NER genes and clinical disease phenotypes is complex, since mutations in several genes can cause the same phenotype, and different mutations in the same gene can cause different phenotypes (Kraemer et al., 2007).

Even though DNA repair malfunctions are autosomal recessive diseases and their incidence is therefore relatively low (~1/100,000), many of the individuals with DNA repair deficiencies die in early childhood since there is no effective treatment, only palliative care. Therefore, the search for a long-term treatment has been intense. Several strategies using recombinant viral vectors are being used in order to improve the resistance of cells from these patients to DNA damaging agents (Lima-Bessa et al., 2009; Menck et al., 2007). Also, the studies of DNA repair mechanisms have yielded a better understanding of specific cell processes which lead to human diseases such as cancer, neurodegeneration and aging (Hoeijmakers, 2009). This review will focus on the use of recombinant viral vectors for the purposes of investigating both the cellular responses to DNA damage and the perspectives of providing therapy for XP patients.

2. Recombinant viral vectors as gene delivery tools

An ideal gene delivery tool should have the ability to transduce proliferating and fully differentiated cells with high efficiency; mediate high-level, prolonged and controlled transgene expression; have little toxicity (both at cellular and organism levels); elicit small immune responses *in vivo*; and be able to accommodate large DNA fragments for transgene transduction (Howarth et al., 2010). Unfortunately, there is no single tool that fulfills all these criteria.

Viruses have had million of years to improve their capacity to infect cells with the aid of evolutionary pressures. Researchers have been trying to take advantage of this ability creating recombinant viral vectors. In general, for that purpose, the viral genome is manipulated and sequences needed to form the infective virion are deleted, opening space to insert the transgene of interest.

Several viral vectors have been created and the most widely used are: adenovirus, retrovirus (including lentivirus) and adeno-associated virus. The main characteristics of these vectors are presented in Table 2.

Virus	Nucleic acid	Genome size (Kb)	Envelope	Virion size (nm)	Integration	Transgene size (Kb)	Immune response	Transgene expression
Adenovirus	dsDNA linear	36		90	episomal	8 - 25	***	days - months
Adeno-associated virus	ssDNA linear	4.7		25	site-specific	4.7 - 9	*	months-years
Retrovirus	ssRNA (homodimer)	7 - 12	*	100	random	<10	**	years
Lentivirus	ssRNA (homodimer)	9	*	100	random	10 - 16	**	years

Table 2. Main features of viruses currently used as recombinant vectors for gene delivery.

Searching for the perfect gene delivery tool, intense modifications have been added to the vectors' genomes, nucleocapsid and envelopes, always searching for less immunogenic vectors, with higher and more specific transduction properties. Currently, recombinant viruses are the vector of choice for research and clinical trials worldwide, but still only few phase II or III trials are being conducted (Atkinson & Chalmers, 2010). All viral vectors cited here have already been used in *in vitro*, *ex vivo* and *in vivo* experiments and in clinical trials.

2.1 Recombinant adenoviral vectors

Adenoviruses (Ad) are non-enveloped double-stranded DNA viruses with tropism for the respiratory and ocular tissues. The first generation recombinant vector can carry up to 8 Kbp of DNA, while the last generation, in which the viral DNA sequence is completely deleted (also named gutless), is able to efficiently transduce over 25 Kbp of DNA (Atkinson & Chalmers, 2010).

Despite the fact that the gutless vector needs the aid of helper viral proteins supplied *in trans*, adenoviral vectors are easily produced in high titers. Once the transgene has been delivered inside the nucleus it remains episomal, reducing the risk of tumorigenesis induced by insertional mutagenesis. On the other hand, the episomal DNA is not replicated and its segregation in mitosis leads to the eventual loss of the transgene in the daughter cells. Thus, the transgene expression is short-lived. A possible solution is to add a site-specific integration sequence next to the transgene, leading to a prolonged transgene expression (Atkinson & Chalmers, 2010). Another advantage of the adenoviral vectors is their ability to transduce post mitotic cells since the transgene is already delivered in its active form, as a double-stranded DNA. This property is of particular interest when aiming for gene therapy in neurons (Atkinson & Chalmers, 2010).

The biggest challenge for the use of adenoviral vectors *in vivo* is the immunological response it elicits. This strong response is not only due to the natural immunogenicity of its components, but also to pre-existing immunity caused by previous contact with at least one of the over 50 serotypes of human infecting adenovirus (Seregin & Amalfitano, 2009). Taking into consideration that these vectors are only capable of a transient expression of the transgene and that repeated dosage might be necessary, a strong immune response is very undesirable. Possible alternatives to circumvent this issue are: manipulation of the viral capsid proteins and DNA, making them less immunogenic; the usage of a different serotype on each application; and the use of immunosuppressants (Atkinson & Chalmers, 2010; Seregin & Amalfitano, 2009).

The great importance of the immunological response against a gene therapy vector was brought to attention when, in 1999, a patient suffering from an ornithine transcarbamylase deficiency, died due to an unexpected inflammatory response reaction to the adenoviral vector used in a clinical trial (Edelstein et al., 2007). Still, adenoviral vectors are currently the most widely used viral vectors in clinical trials, accounting for approximately 24% of all vectors used in gene therapy clinical trials (Edelstein et al., 2007; Hall et al., 2010).

2.2 Recombinant adeno-associated viral (AAV) vectors

Adeno-associated viruses (AAV) are non enveloped, single-stranded DNA, with serotype-specific tropism viruses. To date, 12 serotypes have been identified in primate or human tissues (Schmidt et al., 2008) in a total of over 100 known serotypes (Wang et al., 2011). Their productive lytic infection depends on the presence of a helper virus, adeno or herpesvirus, that provide *in trans* the necessary genes for the AAV replication and virion production. In the absence of a helper virus, the AAV establishes its latent cycle integrating specifically in the 19q13.4 region of the human genome (Daya & Berns, 2008). The site-specific integration is mainly dependent on the virus internal terminal repeats (ITRs), the integration efficiency element (IEE) and Rep 68 and Rep 78 genes. In the 19q13.4 region, several muscle-related genes are present, including some responsible for actin organization. No significant side effects have been observed due to AAV genome integration in this chromosome region (Daya & Berns, 2008).

The onset of transgene expression delivered by an AAV vector is delayed, usually starting several days after the transduction, probably due to the time invested in the synthesis of the DNA second strand (Michelfelder & Trepel, 2009). Although late, the transgene expression is long lasting and there is a very low humoral response, mainly related to previous exposure to the viral antigens (Daya & Berns, 2008). Despite the small size of the AAV nucleocapsid and genome, it has been shown that transgenes up to 7.2 Kb can be delivered by AAV vectors, but the oversized genomes reduce at least 10 fold the transduction efficiency (Dong et al., 2010). Several strategies have been developed seeking to optimize the vector capacity, such as the *trans*-splicing vector. With the simultaneous usage of two AAV vectors, this technology takes advantage of the concatamers formed by the ITRs that can recombine to form the desired transgene inside the transduced cell. These trans-splicing vectors allow the final transgene to have up to 9 Kb (Daya & Berns, 2008).

Only recently adeno-associated viral vectors started being used in gene therapy research and account for less than 4% of all vectors used in gene therapy clinical trials (Edelstein et al., 2007; Hall et al., 2010). Although these vectors do not behave as the parental virus, since they do not integrate in the genome (due to the lack of the REP protein), gene expression can be very long and elicit low immunological responses, making AAV vectors promising in gene therapy investigations.

2.3 Recombinant retroviral vectors

The *Retroviridae* family is characterized by a single-stranded RNA genome which can only replicate inside the host cell with the aid of an RNA-dependent DNA polymerase, the reverse transcriptase. This enzyme transcribes the virus' RNA into a DNA sequence that the host cell machinery can transcribe and translate (Froelich et al., 2010).

Retroviral vectors are capable of transducing a wide range of cell types, are able to accommodate extensive changes in their genome, accept long transgenes, have low immunogenicity, can be produced in high titers, and promote a prolonged transgene expression due to their ability to integrate into the host cell genome (Froelich et al., 2010). On the other hand, most retroviral vectors can only transduce replicating cells since the transport of the transcribed viral DNA to the nucleus is mitosis-dependent. Additionally, there is always the risk of insertional mutagenesis due to the semi-random integration of the vector genome in the host cell's genome (Froelich et al., 2010). Nowadays, the most widely used retroviruses as gene therapy tools are the lentiviruses (LVs), such as the human immunodeficiency virus (HIV). These vectors have the same advantages as other retroviral vectors and are capable of transducing post mitotic cells. Moreover, the LVs tend not to integrate by transcription initiation sites, reducing the risk of insertional tumorigenesis (Froelich et al., 2010).

The retroviral vectors were the first vectors used in gene therapy clinical trials in 1989 (Edelstein et al., 2007, Rosenberg et al., 1990) and are extensively used in fundamental biological research, functional genomics and gene therapy (Mátrai et al., 2010). In 2004, 28% of the clinical trials involving viral vectors included retroviral vectors (Edelstein et al., 2007); in 2010 that number dropped to approximately 23% (Voigt et al., 2008). This drawback is due to the unfortunate events of the French severe combined immunodeficiency (SCID) trial in 2002, where two out of ten children died in consequence of a leukemia, which was related to the insertional mutagenesis of the retroviral vector used (Edelstein et al., 2007).

Since then, special attention has been paid to the safety of these vectors as many are known to derive from viruses that cause severe diseases, such as the acquired immunodeficiency syndrome (AIDS). Strategies are constantly developed to prevent the risk of insertional mutagenesis. For that purpose, in addition to the virions being replication-defective, generated by *trans*-complementation, several further manipulations of the viral genome were made. The development of a self-inactivating (SIN) vector (Iwakuma et al., 1999) prevents horizontal and vertical gene transfer and diminishes the probability of the production of a replicating virion or over-expression of a host cell oncogene (Edelstein et al., 2007).

3. Investigating DNA damage responses with adenoviral vectors in human cells

3.1 *In vitro* and *in vivo* adenoviral gene transduction for the correction of DNA repair defects

The knowledge of the molecular defects in XP cells was the starting point for understanding how human cells handle lesions in their genome. So far, different techniques have been used to study DNA repair mechanisms and reverse malfunctions in this essential system. One powerful tool employed in these studies has been the use of recombinant adenoviral vectors to transduce DNA repair genes directly into human skin cells, aiming to improve the knowledge of basic mechanisms that cells use to protect their genome.

Experiments using first generation recombinant adenoviral vectors have been successfully employed in the transduction of both SV40-transformed and primary fibroblasts derived from XP-A, XP-C, XP-D and XP-V patients (Armelini et al., 2007). The expression of the respective functional proteins in all transduced defective cell populations was significantly increased, reaching levels even higher than seen for wild type cells (Armelini et al., 2005;

Lima-Bessa et al., 2006; Muotri et al., 2002). Moreover, different phenotypical analyses, including cell cycle, apoptosis and cell survival assays, have been carried out, all indicating that the protein expression mediated by the recombinant adenoviruses was clearly accompanied by the recovery of the DNA repair ability and increased resistance to UV radiation, thereby demonstrating functional correction of the XP phenotype. It is worth mentioning that, even though transgene expression mediated by adenoviruses is typically short-lived, sustainable high expression of XPA and XPC proteins with parallel increased UV-irradiation resistance was obtained even two months after cell transduction (Muotri et al., 2002).

For XP-A, XP-C and XP-D transduced cell lines, phenotypic analyses also involved assays aiming to investigate their ability to perform DNA repair after UV irradiation. This has been measured through determination of unscheduled DNA repair synthesis (UDS), which corresponds to the incorporation of [methyl-^{3}H] thymidine in cells that are not in S-phase, and is visualized by autoradiography as the presence of radioactive grains inside nuclei. Interestingly, UDS activity in all transduced deficient cell lines was restored to levels comparable to NER proficient cell lines, indicating those cells became able to efficiently remove UV lesions by restoring NER activity.

It is well known that UV radiation promotes DNA elongation delay as a result of replication blockage by UV photolesions (Cleaver et al., 1983), which can be easily seen by running pulse-chase experiments in alkaline sucrose gradients. Using this approach, it has been possible to show that XP-V transduced cells were able to elongate nascent DNA on UV-damaged DNA templates as efficiently as wild type cells (Lima-Bessa et al., 2006), once again demonstrating the great potential of recombinant adenoviruses in the transduction and expression of functional proteins.

One interesting conclusion came from the observation that even though *XPA*, *XPC* and *XPD* genes were over-expressed in all transduced cell lines when compared to NER proficient cells, this had no impact in the UV-resistance or NER capability, suggesting that neither of these proteins is limiting for NER in human cells. Another possible explanation is that once the NER pathway requires a coordinated action of several proteins, increasing only one of these proteins does not result in speeding up removal of the DNA lesions. Similarly, the excess of polη (*XPV*) mediated by adenoviral transduction has not affected cell survival nor elongation of replication products in UV-treated XP-A human cells, suggesting not only that polη is not a limiting factor for the efficient replication of the UV-damaged DNA in XP-A cells, but also demonstrating that the deleterious effects caused by the remaining DNA lesions in the genome cannot be mitigated by an efficient bypass mediated by polη.

However, the potential of such vectors is not restricted to *in vitro* assays. Indeed, another real perspective is their use to investigate the molecular mechanisms of DNA repair and their consequences *in vivo*, thus opening new avenues for a better understanding of cellular and physiologic responses to DNA damage. *In vivo* experiments may also help to establish the relationship between DNA repair, cancer and aging, as mice models for different DNA repair syndromes have been developed by different groups worldwide. Despite the extensive use of these models to broaden the understanding of several DNA repair related disorders, little work has been done *in vivo* testing gene therapy strategies for these diseases. Indeed, up to the present moment, only one study showed an efficient *in vivo* gene therapy protocol for complementation of the XP phenotype (Marchetto et al., 2004).

Exciting results by Marchetto and co-workers showed that the administration of subcutaneous injections of an adenoviral vector carrying the *XPA* human gene directly into the dorsal region of XP-A knockout mice led to an extensive expression of the heterologous protein in different skin cells, including dermal fibroblasts, cells of the hair follicle and basal replicating keratinocytes, which are believed to be the starting point of most skin tumors. As a result, the repair capability of these transduced cells was restored, thus preventing UVB-induced deleterious skin effects, such as persistent scars, skin hyperkeratosis and, ultimately, avoiding the formation of squamous cell carcinomas (Marchetto et al., 2004).

Despite the promising results of this work, no others followed. Researchers are now aware of several possible limitations and complications of gene therapy after some unexpected severe events in clinical trials (Edelstein et al., 2007) and are spending more time improving gene targeting tools and techniques before risking *in vivo* approaches. In that sense, extreme progress has been made with experiments *in vitro,* as previously presented. A general panel showing the main uses of the recombinant adenoviral vectors carrying DNA repair genes is presented in Figure 3.

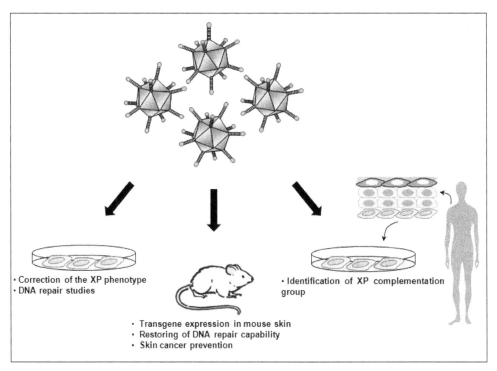

Fig. 3. DNA repair gene transduction by recombinant adenoviruses. Adenoviral vectors have been successfully employed to transduce human XP genes directly into established human cell lines (left), XP knockout mice skin (center), and fibroblasts from the skin of XP patients (right). Endpoints are indicated for each particular case.

Based on the successful complementation of the XP phenotype both *in vitro* and *in vivo,* adenoviral vectors could be proposed as an efficient tool for diagnosis and identification of XP patients' complementation groups. This hypothesis was recently tested and confirmed: with the use of adenoviruses carrying DNA repair genes, it has been possible to determine the complementation group of three Brazilian XP patients, now characterized as XP-C patients. To that end, adenoviral transduced cells from these patients have been submitted to UV treatment and then analyzed by simple assays, such as cell survival and UDS (Leite et al., 2009). This diagnosis has been performed using the patients' skin fibroblasts but the potential use of adenoviral vectors for this purpose becomes even more exciting, considering that the adenoviral transduction could be held in cells present in the patients' blood, thus becoming a faster and less invasive technique. Besides scientific and epidemiological goals, the identification of the gene defect may help to predict clinical prognosis for the XP patients and guide appropriate genetic counseling for their families. Direct gene sequencing can be performed to identify the mutated genes, but as there are eight potential candidate genes for XP, functional complementation assays are still used for the genetic diagnosis of these patients.

3.2 Investigating UV-induced cell responses employing photolyases

Photoreactivation is a very efficient DNA repair mechanism, which specifically removes the two main UV photoproducts. Photoreactivation is carried out by flavoproteins known as photolyases. These enzymes recognize and specifically bind to UV lesions, thus reverting them back to the undamaged monomers, using a blue-light photon as energy source (Brettel & Byrdin, 2010; Sancar, 2008). Interestingly, photolyases demonstrate a great efficiency for discriminating the target lesion, either CPDs or 6-4PPs, and so far no photolyase has been shown to be able to repair both lesions. Thus, enzymes that repair CPDs are referred to as CPD-photolyases, while 6-4PP-photolyases specifically repair 6-4PPs (Müller & Carell, 2009). Both classes of photolyases are evolutionarily related, but functionally distinct (Lucas-Lledó & Lynch, 2009). Curiously, genes encoding genuine photolyases have been lost somehow in the course of the evolution of placental mammals, including humans. Instead, these organisms retain cryptochromes, photolyase-homologous proteins that participate in the maintenance of circadian rhythm, but that do not keep any residual activity related to DNA repair (Partch & Sancar, 2005).

Previous studies have confirmed that the CPD-photolyase is active when delivered to human cells, reducing mutagenesis (You et al., 2001), preventing UV-induced apoptosis (Chiganças et al., 2000) and recovering RNA transcription driven by RNA polymerase II (Chiganças et al., 2002). These successful studies have motivated the adenoviruses-mediated expression of the CPD-photolyase from the rat kangaroo *Potorous tridactylus* and the plant 6-4PP-photolyase from *Arabidopsis thaliana* in human cells aiming to discriminate the precise role of UV-induced cellular responses in both NER-deficient and NER-proficient human cells. Employing immunofluorescence, immunoblot and local UV experiments, it has been possible to see that these enzymes are not only very specific for their lesions, but are also really fast to find them, colocalizing with regions of damaged DNA and other DNA repair enzymes in less than two minutes (Chiganças et al., 2004; Lima-Bessa et al., 2008).

Adenoviral-mediated photorepair of CPDs substantially prevented apoptosis in all UV-irradiated cell lines (both NER-deficient and NER-proficient cells), confirming the involvement of these lesions in cell death signaling, as previously reported. On the other hand, 6-4PP repair by the 6-4PP-photolyase decreased UV-induced apoptosis only in those cell lines deficient for both NER subpathways, causing minimal effect, if any, in NER-proficient cells, including those lacking polη. These results suggest that, when not efficiently repaired, 6-4PPs also have important biological consequences, triggering cell responses leading to the activation of apoptotic cascades. Interestingly, in CS-A cells (TC-NER deficient), a substantial attenuation of apoptotic levels could be again detected when CPDs were removed from the genome by the means of CPD-photolyase, while no detectable effect was observed as a consequence of photorepair of 6-4PPs, indicating that CPD lesions are the major UV-induced DNA damage leading to cell death, also in cells that are only proficient in GG-NER, the main subpathway of NER responsible for the removal of 6-4PPs in humans (Lima-Bessa et al., 2008).

These results suggest that CPDs and 6-4PPs may play different roles in UV-induced apoptosis depending on the repair capacity of human cells. In GG-NER proficient cells, the harmful effects of UV light seem to be predominantly due to the prolonged remaining CPDs in the genome caused by their slow removal by NER, with the minor participation of 6-4PPs (Lima-Bessa et al., 2008). Indeed, it has been reported that about 80–90% of 6-4PPs are removed from the human genome in the first 4 hours following UV exposure, whereas 40–50% of CPDs still remain to be repaired 24 hours later, probably due to the higher affinity of the XPC/hHR23B complex for 6-4PPs (Kusumoto et al., 2001). Thus, the lack of noticeable effects on UV-induced apoptosis in NER-proficient cells after 6-4PPs photorepair may be simply due to their fast repair by GG-NER. On the other hand, as for CPDs, the remaining of 6-4PPs in the genome seems to cause major disturbances in cell metabolism that lead to cell death. A summary of these results is shown in Figure 4.

To further confirm the idea that the roles of CPDs and 6-4PPs in UV-killing are related to the cellular repair capacity, authors have expressed these photolyases in TTD1V1 cells, a particular TTD cell line with a slower kinetics of 6-4PPs repair, eliminating about 50% and 70% of 6-4PPs at 6 and 24 hours post-UV treatment, respectively. Once again, repair of both lesions by the respective photolyase notably reduced apoptosis in these cells, even though the 6-4PP photorepair was less effective than seen for NER-deficient cell lines (Lima-Bessa et al., 2008). These photolyases were also used to identify a defect in the recruitment of downstream NER factors on certain XPD/TTD mutated cells, slowing down the removal of UV-induced lesions. As this recruitment was recovered by treatment with the histone deacetylase inhibitor trichostatin A, the data indicated that this defect is partially related to the accessibility of DNA damage in closed chromatin regions (Chiganças et al., 2008).

Another interesting finding came from assays investigating the time-dependent kinetics of the apoptosis commitment after UV treatment. Transduced XP-A cells were UV-treated and photoreactivated (to allow photorepair of the respective UV lesions) at increasing periods of time. Surprisingly, the data suggests that the initial trigger event to cell death after UV irradiation is relatively delayed, since photorepair of CPDs or 6-4PPs was able to reduce apoptosis even when photoreactivation was performed up to 8 hours after UV irradiation. After that, photoreactivation did not prevent UV-killing in these cells, indicating a commitment by events that irreversibly lead to cell death. These results are also in agreement with the indications that fast removed lesions (such as 6-PPs) do not activate apoptosis in NER-proficient human cells (Lima-Bessa et al., 2008). The main implication of all these findings is the fact that skin carcinogenesis in XP patients may also have 6-4PP lesions as important players, suggesting that tumors from these individuals are not only quantitatively different from those of normal people, but may also have different causative lesions. Transduction of XP knockout mice with adenoviral vectors carrying photolyase genes may help to address this question.

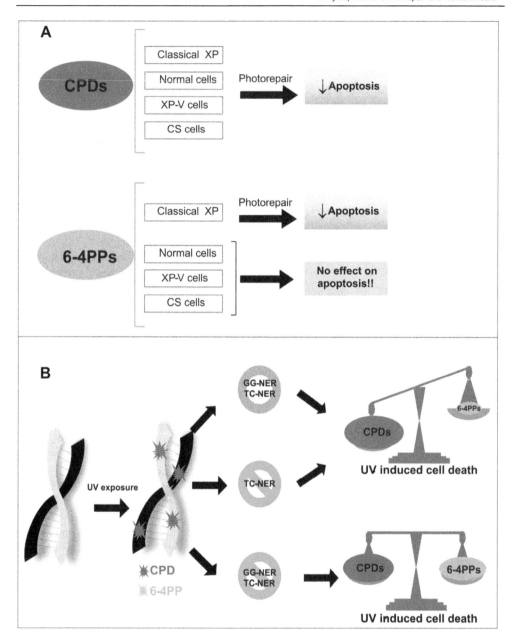

Fig. 4. Effects of photorepair of CPDs and 6-4PPs on UV-induced apoptosis. (A) Summary of the impact of the specific removal of CPDs and 6-4PPs by photorepair in human cell lines with different DNA repair capabilities. (B) Schematic representation of the main conclusions of the results shown in panel *A*. Those results clearly implicate that CPDs and 6-4PPs play different roles on UV-induced apoptosis depending on the cellular repair capacity.

4. Employing retroviral vectors for correcting XP phenotype

The first genetic analysis of XP patients was performed through somatic cell fusion followed by analysis of restoration of normal UDS. If somatic cell fusion complements XP genetic deficiency, it will then be positive for UDS activity. These experiments were able to identify the seven classical XP complementation groups and the variant group (Zeng et al., 1998). This implies that DNA repair deficiencies can, in fact, be corrected by the introduction of a normal copy of the affected gene, giving hope for the development of gene therapy protocols for XP patients. In fact, the introduction of a normal copy of the defective gene in XP cells can complement the DNA repair ability, as demonstrated by the delivery of conventional expression vectors, via calcium precipitation and microneedle injection (Mezzina et al., 1994).

In 1995, viral vectors were first used as gene delivery tools in DNA repair experiments (Carreau et al., 1995a). In this study, a LXPDSN retroviral vector carrying the wild-type XPD gene was capable of complementing primary fibroblasts of XPD patients with a long-term expression. A subsequent study showed that this complementation was gene-specific and that there was a long-term expression of the transgene (Quilliet et al, 1996). The use of retroviral vectors for DNA repair genes delivery was further validated in 1996 and 1997, when XP-A, XP-B, XP-C and TTD-D cells were also complemented with the aid of gene-specific retroviral vectors (Marionnet et al., 1996; Zeng et al., 1998).

The compilation of these results shows that the retroviral delivery of several DNA repair genes was able to specifically complement several deficiencies presented by XP, CS and TTD patients such as UDS, reduced catalase activity, UV-sensitivity, recovery of RNA synthesis, increased mutation frequency, stabilization of p53 (Dumaz et al., 1998) and deregulation of ICAM-1 (Ahrens et al., 1997).

Since XP patients already receive autologous graft transplants after massive skin tissue removal surgery (Atabay et al., 1991; Bell et al., 1983), most researches in the field of XP gene therapy focus on the three-dimensional skin reconstruction *in vitro*, using the patients' cells genetically corrected *ex vivo*. In this technique, the patients' fibroblasts and keratinocytes are cultured *in vitro* after a skin biopsy of a non-UV-irradiated area. Then, retroviral vectors are used to stably complement the genetic deficiency of these cells. Finally, the keratinocytes and the fibroblasts are used to three-dimensionally reconstruct the epidermis and dermis, respectively. This construct can then be used as a graft when the part of patient's damaged skin is removed in a necessary surgery. To that end, Arnaudeau-Bégard and co-workers managed to complement XP-C keratinocytes, recovering a wild-type phenotype and UV-resistance with the aid of a retroviral vector carrying a normal copy of the *XPC* gene (Arnaudeau-Bégard et al., 2003). Furthermore, Bergoglio and co-workers have also developed a selection method for genetically corrected keratinocytes that does not involve particles derived from microorganisms which could lead to immunological clearance of the transgene, using CD24 as an ectopic marker (Bergoglio et al., 2007).

In 2005, Bernerd and co-workers were able to reconstruct a three-dimensional skin model *in vitro* using fibroblasts and keratinocytes from a donor XP-C patient. With this model, they were able to see that the XP skin has peculiar characteristics: hypoplastic horny layers, decreased and delayed keratinocyte differentiation, epidermal invaginations, a generally altered proliferation control and fibroblasts with distinct morphology and orientation. Furthermore, the epidermal invaginations were proven to be related to alterations of both keratinocytes' and fibroblasts' functions and were characterized as epidermoid carcinoma-like structures (Bernerd et al., 2005). It is important to keep in mind that an XP skin biopsy might give us further and more precise knowledge of the XP skin physiology, but this is a delicate procedure which requires the patients' agreement.

Since the use of common retroviral vectors in gene therapy can be dangerous due to semi-random insertional mutagenesis, researchers have developed several self-inactivating-lentiviral vectors carrying DNA repair genes. These vectors were shown to efficiently transduce primary and transformed fibroblasts, complementing in a gene-specific manner XP-A, XP-C and XP-D cells. Furthermore, the recovery of normal levels of UV-resistance in the transduced cells was shown to be persistent for at least 3 months (Marchetto et al., 2006). The reconstruction of a genetically corrected, three-dimensional XP skin followed by the implantation of the graft on a patient (Figure 5) is still an ongoing chore that has to be taken very cautiously, always prioritizing the patient's well-being.

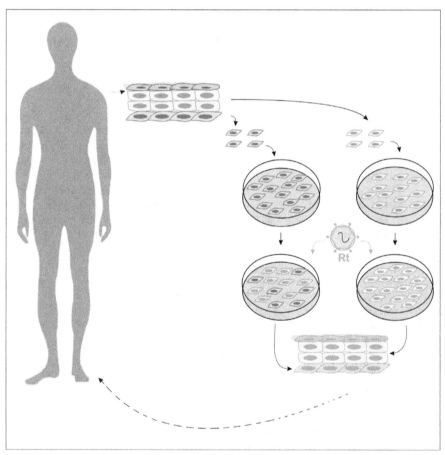

Fig. 5. Schematic representation of *ex vivo* gene therapy for XP patients using recombinant retrovirus (Rt). Skin-derived fibroblasts and keratinocytes from an XP patient are cultivated *in vitro*, and transduced with retroviral vector carrying the wild type *XP* cDNA. Transduced cells are then used to reconstruct the human skin *in vitro*, with a normal phenotype. Dashed line raises the possibility of engraftment of the reconstructed skin directly on XP patients.

It is also important to keep in mind that these grafts do not include melanocytes, responsible for the very common melanomas in these patients (Khavari, 1998), and that the skin will only be genetically complemented in the areas that receive the grafts, all the other areas of the body will still be extremely photosensitive since no paracrine effect is known for DNA repair proteins and that immunological clearance or gene silencing by cellular methylation can always prohibit a long-term transgene expression (Magnaldo & Sarasin, 2002). Importantly, several XP complementation groups also present other relevant symptoms, such as neurodegeneration, which will not be improved by the skin grafts. For those patients, another kind of gene therapy might be more efficient, such as the development of genetically corrected stem cells (ESs) (Magnaldo & Sarasin, 2002) or induced pluripotent cells (iPSCs, see below (Alison, 2009). Unfortunately, there is still no reference on that kind of research for xeroderma pigmentosum.

5. Host cell reactivation (HCR) as a tool for DNA repair research

The host cell reactivation (HCR) technique was first described in human cells by Protic-Sabljic and co-workers in 1985 (Protic-Sabljic et al., 1985). In this first work, the technique consisted of transducing cells with a plasmid containing a putative cDNA with a selective gene into XP cells to look for a reversion of the UV sensitivity due to gene complementation, allowing identification of the genes responsible for that phenotype.

Other studies have refined the technique which is now widely used as an indirect measure of cellular DNA repair capacity. Mostly, a plasmid containing a reporter gene such as luciferase (LUC) or chloramphenicol acetyltransferse (CAT) is treated with a genotoxic agent such as UV radiation and introduced in the cell where DNA repair capacity is to be evaluated. If the cell is able to remove the lesions from the plasmid, the reporter gene will be expressed. Different DNA repair rates can be addresses by differences on the amount of gene reporter expression at a certain time (Merkle et al., 2004). A schematic representation of HCR is shown in Figure 6.

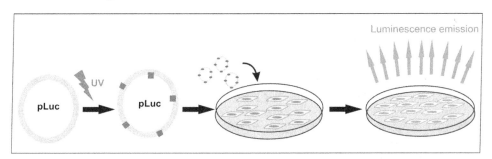

Fig. 6. Schematic representation of host cell reactivation (HCR) assay. A plasmid carrying a reporter gene (in this case, the luciferase gene) is UV-irradiated *in vitro* and then transfected into host cells. 48 hours later, the cellular DNA repair capacity is indirectly estimated by measurement of the reporter gene activity in the cellular extract.

In 1995, the HCR assay was further used to visualize the genetic complementation of mammalian expression vectors carrying the DNA repair genes *XPA*, *XPB*, *XPC*, *XPD* and *CSB*. In this study, plasmids containing LUC or CAT were UV irradiated and co-transfected with the plasmids containing each of the complementing genes of the DNA-repair deficient cells. Again, only the cells with the correct complementation were capable of removing the DNA damage in the reporter gene, allowing the expression of that protein. This technique facilitates the identification of the complementation group of a given patient, being particularly useful in cases of CS, TTD and some XP patients such as XP-E that present a normal UDS after UV treatment (Carreau et al., 1995b).

Recent data using the HCR assay has shown that the CS proteins are essential for the reversion of oxidated lesions (Pitsikas et al., 2005; Spivak & Hanawalt, 2006; Leach & Rainbow, 2011) and evidence obtained with HCR suggests that, unlike what was previously shown with UDS assays, DNA repair capacity in fibroblasts does not decrease with aging (Merkle et al., 2004). This reduction may however be cell type-specific and DNA repair pathway-specific since blood cells repair capacity decreases approximately 0.6% per year of age (Moriwaki et al., 1996). This technique is still widely used and its great advantage is that the DNA plasmids or the viral vectors are treated in a controlled manner, not being subject to the cell's global response to the same treatment. Further technique improvements will surely allow HCR to be used in different assays such as *in vivo*, yielding a better knowledge of the DNA repair pathways and their interactions with other pathways and physiological events.

6. Other treatments for xeroderma pigmentosum

6.1 General care

There is no treatment that has been proven so far to be 100% effective in all XP cases. The only palliative measure that patients can rely on is complete sun avoidance. This includes not only avoiding going out even on cloudy days and covering all exposed body areas such as skin and eyes, but also using special artificial lights that emit no UV wavelengths (Kraemer, 2008). Premalignant lesions, such as actinic keratoses, and malignant lesions must be quickly treated with topical 5-fluoracil or liquid nitrogen, imiquimod cream, electrodesiccation and curettage, surgical excision or chemosurgery, as needed. When extensive areas are damaged and have to be surgically removed, skin grafts from sun unexposed areas of the same patient should be used. When eyes are affected, methylcellulose eye drops or contact lenses can help prevent trauma and corneal transplantations might be needed in extreme cases (Kraemer, 2008).

When caring for XP patients, it is very important to keep in mind that the total sun avoidance also prevents the production of vitamin D in the skin, so dietary supplementation might be needed. Furthermore, the DNA repair deficiencies which prevent the repair of photolesions may also make individuals sensitive to other mutagens such as cigarette smoke, so patients should be protected against these agents (Kraemer, 2008).

Aside from removal of local lesions and total sun avoidance, two other palliative treatments might help improving the XP patient's quality of life: topical use of T4 endonuclease (Yarosh et al., 2001) and oral intake of retinoids (Campbell & DiGiovanna, 2006).

6.2 Topical use of T4 endonuclease

In 1975, Tanaka and co-workers demonstrated that the bacteriophage T4 endonuclease V is capable of making an incision 5' within a CPD lesion. The resulting DNA flap is recognized and removed by a 5'→3' exonuclease, leaving a gap that is filled by a DNA polymerase, using the undamaged single strand as a template. A DNA ligase then joins the repaired fragment to the parental DNA (Tanaka et al., 1975).

In the 80's, Yarosh's laboratory discovered that the T4 endonuclease V could be delivered into cells using 200 nm liposomes as a delivery vehicle. The anionic liposomes not only protect the cationic enzyme inside, but also promote the escape from a clatrin-coated endosome after cellular intake by destabilizing the vesicle's membrane with an acid pH. By cleaving DNA at the site of UV-induced lesions, the enzyme reverses the DNA repair defect of XP cells (Yarosh, 2002). Further work by the same group also showed that these T4N5 liposomes in a 1% hydrogel lotion when applied in cultured human fibroblasts, mouse dorsal back or cultured human breast skin is capable of delivering the enzyme into cells in less than one hour, being almost entirely restricted to the epidermis (Ceccoli et al., 1989; Kibitel et al., 1991).

An inverse correlation was later shown between the T4N5 dose and the level of CPDs that remained in the epidermis. This curve reached a plateau (at 0.5 µg/ml), probably due to saturation of the cell machinery for further repairing the damage after the initial incision by the T4 enzyme (Yarosh et al., 1994). These studies also showed that even in the higher dose of T4N5 liposomes, only ~50% of the CPD lesions were removed but that was capable of reducing the mutagenesis rate by 99% in transformed fibroblasts and 30% in primary fibroblast cell culture. These numbers are probably not only related to the number of remaining lesions, but also to the smaller size of the repair patch filled by BER compared to that needed in NER (Yarosh, 2002; Cafardi & Elmets, 2008).

Finally, after two phase I clinical trials (Yarosh et al., 1996 as cited in Cafardi & Elmets, 2008) and three phase II clinical trials (Wolf et al., 2000 and Yarosh et al., 1996 as cited in Cafardi & Elmets, 2008), in 2001 the T4N5 liposomes were tested in XP patients. The patients were instructed to apply 4-5 ml of the lotion containing 1 mg/ml of endonuclease everyday for a year. Except for lesion removal when necessary, and daily use of sunscreens of 15 SPF or higher, no concomitant treatments were allowed. The treatment was shown to be efficient, reducing the rate of actinic keratoses and basal-cell carcinomas to 68% and 30% respectively in the placebo and treatment groups, reducing tumor promotion and progression. The treatment was also capable of reducing some immunosuppressant molecules, such as interleukin-10 (IL-10) and tumor necrosis factor-α (TNF- α). Unfortunately, the treatment was only effective for patients under 18 years-old. This might be because XP patients older than that already had too much DNA damage in their cells that could not be reversed (Yarosh et al., 2001). Despite the promising results, there are currently no topical DNA repair enzymes approved by the FDA. Clinical trials are still being conducted to analyze the application of T4N5 liposomes in other deficiencies and immunosuppressed patients (Cafardi & Elmets, 2008).

6.3 Oral use of retinoids

Despite interventions such as sunlight avoidance and tumor removal, most of the XP patients continue to develop a large number of skin cancers. These high-risk patients may suffer from field cancerization that may happen when a wide field of the epithelium has been exposed to the same genotoxic agent and adjacent but not contiguous areas present genetic and morphological alterations that may lead to a carcinogenesis process. As the whole skin area has been exposed to sunlight, inducing independent tumors with different growth rates, this hypothesis may explain why the patients have a 30% increase in the chances of having a second basal cell carcinoma (BCC) and then a 50% increase of a third BCC (Campbell & DiGiovanna, 2006).

In XP patients, the oral use of retinoids might be beneficial, regardless of the strong side effects. In chemoprevention the goal is to identify early biological events in the epithelium which may lead to a carcinogenesis process and intervene with chemicals which will help stop or reverse the process (Campbell & DiGiovanna, 2006). Retinoids, also known as vitamin A, are the most studied chemopreventive agent for skin cancers, upper aerodigestive tract and breast and cervical cancers. The exact mechanisms through which the retinoids are capable of reducing cancer incidence are still unclear, but it has been shown that they are capable of altering keratinocytes' growth, increasing their differentiation status, affecting their cell surface and immune modulation. Retinoids mediate gene transcription by binding to two families of nuclear receptors, the retinoid acid receptors (RARs) and the retinoid X receptors (RXRs). Retinoids have only a mild effect on existing tumors, but can suppress the development of new lesions (Campbell & DiGiovanna, 2006). In 1988, it was shown in a three year study that isotretinoin in a dose up to 2 mg/day/Kg was able to reduce skin cancers in XP patients by 63%. Unfortunately, in the year following the discontinuation of the treatment there was an increase of 8.5% of cancer incidence in those patients with reference to the two years of treatment (Kraemer et al., 1988).

Furthermore, the constant use of retinoids can have severe side effects ranging from inflammation in existing tumors, dry skin and mucosa and hair loss to pancreatitis, osteoporosis, hyperostosis and myalgia among others. The retinoids' toxicity is dose related and cumulative, but most of the side effects can be prevented with constant check-ups and use of local special moisturizers (Campbell & DiGiovanna, 2006). Indeed, several retinoids can be used as chemopreventives. The two most common are isotretinoin and acitretin, the first having a shorter half-life and being the drug of choice for women due to retinoids' theratogenic potential, especially in fetuses (Campbell & DiGiovanna, 2006).

6.4 Potential effects of DNA repair adjuvants

The use of DNA repair adjuvants and antioxidants may also help reducing skin cancer incidence in XP patients. Some known DNA repair adjuvants are selenium, aquosum extract of *Urcaria tomentosa* and Interleukin-12 (IL-12) (Emanuel & Scheinfeld, 2007).

Selenium seems to interact with Ref-1, activating p53, inducing the DNA repair branch of the p53 pathway, in a BRCA1-dependent manner, dealing mainly with oxidative stress (Fisher et al., 2006). On the other hand, it has been already reported that high levels of selenium can be mutagenic, carcinogenic and possibly teratogenic (Shamberger, 1985), probably due to non-specific sulfur substitution on proteins and consequent TC-NER activity decrease (Abul-Hassan et al., 2004). Thus, special attention should be taken regarding the dose of dietary selenium supplementation.

The aquosum extract of *Urcaria tomentosa* (cat's claw) seems to increase the removal of CPDs and reduce oxidative damage, either by an increase in base excision repair (BER) or by an antioxidant property, reducing erythema and blistering after UV. Despite several studies *in vitro* and *in vivo*, the precise mechanisms are still unknown (Emanuel & Scheinfeld, 2007).

Another interesting finding is that, besides IL-12 being a strong immunomodulatory molecule, able to prevent UV-induced immunosuppression through IL-10 inhibition (de Gruijl, 2008), it is also capable of increasing DNA repair by inducing NER, as shown by the RNA level increase in some NER molecules (Schwarz et al., 2005).

6.5 Gene therapy targeted approaches: The use of meganucleases for correcting XP-C cells

There are several techniques to specifically target, substitute, or correct a gene, diminishing the chances of insertional recombination, such as the use of recombinases, transposons, zinc-finger nucleases, endonucleases and meganucleases (Silva et al., 2011). Meganucleases can function as RNA maturases, facilitating the maturation of their own intron or as specific endonucleases that can recognize and cleave the exon-exon junction sequence wherein their intron resides, creating a specific double strand break (DSB), giving rise to the moniker "homing endonuclease". The meganuclease function is probably related to the current status of its lifecycle (Silva et al., 2011).

Meganucleases can be used as gene targeting tools in several ways. Ideally, they can provide a true reversion of the mutation, but the efficacy of correction is invertionally correlated to the distance of the initial DNA DSB. Alternatively, it can insert a functional gene upstream of the mutated one or in a safe location where it will not induce insertional mutagenesis. Also, meganucleases can be used for introducing specific mutations for research purposes such as understanding the role of a gene or of a specific point mutation. Furthermore, meganucleases capable of targeting viral sequences are being researched as antiviral agents (Silva et al., 2011).

Recently, the design of a specific I-CreI meganuclease targeting for the *XPC* gene was able to specifically target two *XPC* sequences, showing *in vitro* for the first time that extensive redesign of homing endonuclease can modify a specific chromosome region without lost of specificity or efficiency (Arnould et al., 2007). These results are very promising for the development of future gene therapy strategies for XP patients.

6.6 Induced Pluripotent Cells (iPSCs) as gene therapy agents

In 2006, the induction of pluripotent cells (iPSCs) by the expression of Oct3/4, Sox2, c-Myc and Klf4 in fibroblasts gave hope for a new gene therapy using pluripotent cells that would not elicit an immunological response in the patient, since his own cells would be used to induce the iPSCs and that would not be confronted by ethical issues like the use of embryonic stem cells (Takahashi & Yamanaka, 2006). Since then, this technology has been improved and iPSCs have been induced in a variety of cell types from different species. Also, iPSCs have been differentiated to several different cell types, from fibroblasts to neurons (Sidhu, 2011).

Fanconi Anemina (FA) is a DNA repair related disease, where mutations in one of fourteen genes lead to extreme sensitivity to interstrand crosslinking agents. Patients show progressive bone marrow failure, congenital developmental abnormalities and early onset of cancers, mostly acute myelogenous leukemia and squamous cell carcinomas. Bone marrow transplantation is a palliative treatment for the secondary leukemia but no cure is currently available for FA patients (Kitao &.Takata, 2011). In 2009, Raya and co-workers were able to use lentiviral vectors to genetically correct fibroblast and keratinocytes from patients with various FA complementation group deficiencies and then induce their dedifferentiation into pluripotent stem cells. Interestingly, uncorrected FA cells did not generate iPSCs, indicating a role for DNA repair in nuclear reprogramming. Thus, the generated iPSCs had normal FA genes and have the potential of being used for gene therapy of the donor patients, with no risk of inducing immunological rejection (Raya et al., 2009). Hopefully soon FA patients and others will be able to benefit from this technology as a safe gene therapy approach.

7. Concluding remarks

Recombinant viral vectors were developed more than thirty years ago, and they have provided extremely useful tools to understand cell metabolism. This chapter focuses on their use to understand cells' responses to DNA damage, especially UV-irradiated DNA repair-deficient cells. These vectors provide means to interfere in these responses, affecting DNA metabolism and revealing important aspects of the DNA repair mechanisms. The discovery of RNA interference mechanisms in human cells offer still more opportunities to modify cells' responses by silencing specific DNA repair genes. Several libraries of viral vectors for the expression of small double-stranded RNA molecules (shRNA) targeting human genes are commercially available, and are already being used for understanding gene function. The use of such vectors to make cells deficient in more than one DNA repair pathway, using cells deficient in XP genes as hosts, for example, may help us to reveal the intricate network of interactions between the different metabolic pathways that contribute to genome maintenance after damage induction (Moraes, et al., 2011; in press). Moreover, the progress that has been made towards gene therapy for xeroderma pigmentosum, using these recombinant viral vectors is also discussed. Although the results indicate a series of limitations, and it is clear that there is still a long way to go, they make researchers go forward, giving a gleam of hope to these patients and their families.

8. Acknowledgements

KMLB has a post-doctoral fellowship from CAPES (Brasília, Brazil) and CQ has a PhD fellowship from FAPESP (São Paulo, Brazil). This research was supported by FAPESP (São Paulo, Brazil) and CNPq (Brasília, Brazil).

9. References

Abul-Hassan, K.S., Lehnert, B.E., Guant, L., & Walmsley, R. (2004). Abnormal DNA repair in selenium-treated human cells. *Mutation research*, V. 565, N. 1, pp. 45-51, ISSN 0027-5107

Alison, M.R. (2009). Stem cells in pathobiology and regenerative medicine. *The Journal of pathology*, V. 217, N. 2, pp. 141-143, ISSN 1096-9896

Ahrens, C., Grewe, M., Berneburg, M., Grether-Beck, S., Quilliet, X., Mezzina, M., Sarasin, A., Lehmann, A.R., Arlett, C.F., & Krutmann, J. (1997). Photocarcinogenesis and inhibition of intercellular adhesion molecule 1 expression in cells of DNA-repair-defective individuals. *Proceedings of the National Academy of Sciences of the United States of America (PNAS).*, V. 94, N. 13, pp. 6837-6841, ISSN 1091-6490

Armelini, M.G., Muotri, A.R., Marchetto, M.C., de Lima-Bessa, K.M., Sarasin, A., & Menck, C.F. (2005). Restoring DNA repair capacity of cells from three distinct diseases by XPD gene-recombinant adenovirus. *Cancer gene therapy*, V. 12, N. 4, pp. 389-396, ISSN 0929-1903

Armelini, M.G., Lima-Bessa, K.M., Marchetto, M.C., Muotri, A.R., Chiganças, V., Leite, R.A., Carvalho, H., & Menck, C.F. (2007). Exploring DNA damage responses in human cells with recombinant adenoviral vectors. *Human , & experimental toxicology*, V. 26, N. 11, pp. 899-906, ISSN 0960-3271

Arnaudeau-Bégard, C., Brellier, F., Chevallier-Lagente, O., Hoeijmakers, J., Bernerd, F., Sarasin, A., & Magnaldo, T. (2003). Genetic correction of DNA repair-deficient/cancer-prone xeroderma pigmentosum group C keratinocytes. *Human gene therapy*, V. 14, N. 10, pp. 983-996, ISSN 1043-0342

Arnould, S., Perez, C., Cabaniols, J.P., Smith, J., Gouble, A., Grizot, S., Epinat, J.C., Duclert, A., Duchateau, P., & Pâques, F. (2007). Engineered I-CreI derivatives cleaving sequences from the human XPC gene can induce highly efficient gene correction in mammalian cells. *Journal of molecular biology*, V. 371, N. 1, pp 49-65, ISSN 0022-2836

Atabay, K., Celebi, C., Cenetoglu, S., Baran, N.K., & Kiymaz, Z. (1991). Facial resurfacing in xeroderma pigmentosum with monoblock full-thickness skin graft. *Plastic and reconstructive surgery*, V. 87, N. 6, pp. 1121-1125, ISSN 0032-1052

Atkinson, H., & Chalmers, R. (2010). Delivering the goods: viral and non-viral gene therapy systems and the inherent limits on cargo DNA and internal sequences. *Genetica*, V. 138, N. 5, pp. 485-498, ISSN 0016-6707

Bell, E., Sher, S., Hull, B., Merrill, C., Rosen, S., Chamson, A., Asselineau, D., Dubertret, L., Coulomb, B., Lapiere, C., Nusgens, B., & Neveux, Y. (1983). The reconstitution of living skin. *Journal of investigative dermatology*, V. 81, N. 1 (suppl)., pp. 2s-10s, ISSN 0022-202X

Bergoglio, V., Larcher, F., Chevallier-Lagente, O., Bernheim, A., Danos, O., Sarasin, A., Rio, M.D., & Magnaldo, T. (2007). Safe selection of genetically manipulated human primary keratinocytes with very high growth potential usind CD24. *Molecular therapy*, V. 15, N. 12, pp. 2186-2193, ISSN 1525-0016

Bernerd, F., Asselineau, D., Frechet, M., Sarasin, A., & Magnaldo, T. (2005). Reconstruction of DNA repair-deficient xeroderma pigmentosum skin *in vitro*: a model to study hypersensitivity to UV light. *Photochemistry and photobiology*, V. 81, N. 1, pp. 19-24, ISSN 0031-8655

Brettel, K., & Byrdin, M. (2010). Reaction mechanisms of DNA photolyase. *Current opinion in structural biology*, V. 20, N. 6, pp. 693-701, ISSN 0959-440X

Cafardi, J.A., & Elmets, C.A. (2008). T4 endonuclease V: review and application to dermatology. *Expert opinion on biological therapy*, V. 8, N. 6, pp. 829-838, ISSN 1471-2598

Campbell, R.M., & DiGiovanna, J.J. (2006). Skin cancer chemoprevention with systemic retinoids: an adjunct in the management of selected high-risk patients. *Dermatologic therapy*, V. 19, N. 5, pp. 306-314, ISSN 13960296

Carreau, M., Quilliet, X., Eveno, E., Salvetti, A., Danos, O., Heard, J.M., Mezzina, M., & Sarasin, A. (1995a). Functional retroviral vector for gene therapy of xeroderma pigmentosum group D patients. *Human gene therapy*, V. 6, N. 10, pp. 1307-1315, ISSN 1043-0342

Carreau, M. Eveno, E., Quilliet, X., Chevalier-Lagente, O., Benoit, A., Tanganelli, B., Stefanini, M., Vermeulen, W., Hoeijmakers, J.H., Sarasin, A., & Mezzina, M. (1995b). Development of a new easy complementation assay for DNA repair deficiency human syndromes using cloned repair genes. *Carcinogenesis*, V. 16, N. 5, pp. 1003-1009, ISSN 0143-3334

Ceccoli, J., Rosales, N., Tsimis, J., & Yarosh, D.B. (1989). Encapsulation of the UV-DNA repair enzyme T4 endonuclease V in liposomes and delivery to human cells. *Journal of investigative dermatology*, V. 93, N. 2, pp. 190-194, ISSN 0022-202X

Chiganças, V., Miyaji, E.N., Muotri, A.R., de Fátima-Jacysyn, J., Amarante-Mendes, G.P., Yasui, A., & Menck, C.F. (2000). Photorepair prevents ultraviolet-induced apoptosis in human cells expressing the marsupial photolyase gene. *Cancer research*, V. 60, N. 9, pp. 2458-2463, ISSN 1538-7445

Chiganças, V., Batista, L.F., Brumatti, G., Amarante-Mendes, G.P., Yasui, A., & Menck, C.F. (2002). Photorepair of RNA polymerase arrest and apoptosis after ultraviolet irradiation in normal and XPB deficient rodent cells. *Cell death and differentiation*, V. 9, N. 10, pp. 1099-1107, ISSN 1350-9047

Chiganças, V., Sarasin, A., & Menck, C.F. (2004). CPD-photolyase adenovirus-mediated gene transfer in normal and DNA-repair-deficient human cells. *Journal of cell science*, V. 117, N. Pt 16, pp. 3579-3592, ISSN 0021-9533

Chiganças, V., Lima-Bessa, K.M., Stary, A., Menck, C.F., & Sarasin, A. (2008). Defective transcription/repair factor IIH recruitment to specific UV lesions in trichothiodystrophy syndrome. *Cancer research*, V. 68, N. 15, pp. 6074-6083, ISSN 1538-7445

Ciccia, A., & Elledge, S.J. (2010). The DNA damage response: making it safe to play with knives. *Molecular cell*, V. 40, N. 2, pp. 179-204, ISSN 1538-7445

Cleaver, J.E., Kaufmann, W.K., Kapp, L.N., & Park, S.D. (1983). Replicon size and excision repair as factors in the inhibition and recovery of DNA synthesis from ultraviolet damage. *Biochimica et biophysica Acta*, V. 739, N. 2, pp. 207-215, ISSN 0304-4165

Cleaver, J.E., Lam, E.T., & Revet, I. (2009). Disorders of nucleotide excision repair: the genetic and molecular basis of heterogeneity. *Nature reviews.Genetics*, V. 10, N. 11, pp. 756-768, ISSN 1471-0056

Costa, R.M., Chiganças, V., Galhardo, Rda.S., Carvalho, H., & Menck, C.F. (2003). The eukaryotic nucleotide excision repair pathway. *Biochimie*, V. 85, N. 11, pp. 1083-1099, ISSN 0300-9084

Daya, S., & Berns, K.I. (2008). Gene therapy using adeno-associated virus vectors. *Clinical microbiology reviews*, V. 21, N. 4, pp. 583-593, ISSN 0893-8512

de Boer, J., & Hoeijmakers, J.H. (2000). Nucleotide excision repair and human syndromes. *Carcinogenesis*, V. 21, N. 3, pp. 453-460, ISSN 0143-3334

de Gruijl, F. (2008). UV-induced immunosuppression in the balance. *Photochemistry and photobiology*, V. 84, N. 1, pp. 2-9, ISSN 0031-8655

Dong, B., Nakai, H., & Xiao, W. (2010). Characterization of genome integrity for oversized recombinant AAV vector. *Molecular therapy*, V. 18, N. 1, pp. 87-92, ISSN 1525-0016

Dumaz, N., Drougard, C., Quilliet, X., Mezzina, M., Sarasin, A., & Daya-Grosjean, L. (1998). Recovery of the normal p53 response after UV treatment in DNA repair-deficient fibrobalsts by retroviral-mediated correction with the XPD gene. *Carcinogenesis*, V. 19, N. 9, pp. 1701-1704, ISSN 0143-3334

Edelstein, M.L., Abedi, M.R., & Wixon, J. (2007). Gene therapy clinical trials worldwide to 2007- an update. *The journal of gene medicine*, V. 9, N. 10, pp. 833-842, ISSN 1521-2254

Emanuel, P., & Scheinfeld, N. (2007). A review of DNA repair and possible DNA-repair adjuvants and selected natural anti-oxidants. *Dermatology online journal*, V. 13, N. 3, pp. 10, ISSN 1087-2108

Fisher, J.L., Lancia, J.K., Mathur, A., & Smith, M.L. (2006). Selenium protection from DNA damage involves Ref1/p53/Brca1 protein complex. *Anticancer research*, V. 26, N. 2A, pp. 899-904, ISSN 0250-7005

Froelich, S., Tai, A., & Wang, P. (2010). Lentiviral vectors for immune cells targeting. *Immunopharmacology and immunotoxicology*, V. 32, N. 2, pp. 208-218, ISSN 0892-3973

Fousteri, M., & Mullenders, L.H. (2008). Transcription-coupled nucleotide excision repair in mammalian cells: molecular mechanisms and biological effects. *Cell research*, V. 18, N. 1, pp. 73-84, ISSN 1001-0602

Gerstenblith, M.R., Goldstein, A.M., & Tucker, M.A. (2010). Hereditary genodermatoses with cancer predisposition. *Hematology/oncology clinics of North America*, V. 24, N. 5, pp. 885–906, ISSN 0889-8588

Hall, K., Blair Zajdel, M.E., & Blair, G.E. (2010). Unity and diversity in the human adenoviruses: exploiting alternative entry pathways for gene therapy. *The Biochemical journal*, V. 431, N. 3, pp. 321-336, ISSN 0264-6021

Hanawalt, P.C. (2002). Subpathways of nucleotide excision repair and their regulation. *Oncogene*, V. 21, N. 58, pp. 8949-8956, ISSN 0950-9232

Hoeijmakers, J.H. (2009). Molecular origins of cancer: DNA damage, aging, and cancer. *The New England journal of medicine*, V. 361, N. 15, pp. 1475-1485, ISSN 0028-4793

Horibata, K., Iwamoto, Y., Kuraoka, I., Jaspers, N.G.J., Kurimasa, A., Oshimura, M., Ichihashi, M., & Tanaka, K. (2004). Complete absence of Cockayne syndrome group B gene product gives rise to UV-sensitive syndrome but not Cockayne syndrome. *PNAS*, V. 101, N. 43, pp. 15410–15415, ISSN 1091-6490

Howarth, J.L., Lee, Y.B., & Uney, J.B. (2010). Using viral vectors as gene transfer tools. *Cell biology and toxicology*, V. 26, N. 1, pp. 1-20, ISSN 0742-2091

Itin, P.H., Sarasin, A., & Pittelkow, M.R. (2001). Trichothiodystrophy: update on the sulfur-deficient brittle hair syndromes. *Journal of the American Academy of Dermatology*, V. 44, N. 6, pp. 891-920, ISSN 0190-9622

Iwakuma, T., Cui, Y., & Chang, L.J. (1999). Self-inactivating lentiviral vectors with U3 and U5 modifications. *Virology*, V. 261, N. 1, pp. 120-132, ISSN 0042-6822

Johnson, R.E., Kondratick, C.M., Prakash, S., & Prakash, L. (1999). hRAD30 mutations in the variant form of xeroderma pigmentosum. *Science*, V. 285, N. 5425, pp. 263–265, ISSN 0036-8075

Karalis, A., Tischkowitz, M., & Millington, G.W. (2011). Dermatological manifestations of inherited cancer syndromes in children. *The British journal of dermatology*, V. 164, N. 2, pp. 245–256, ISSN 0007-0963

Khavari, P.A. (1998). Gene therapy for genetic skin disease. *Journal of investigative dermatology*, V. 110, N. 4, pp. 462-467, ISSN 0022-202X

Kibitel, J.T., Yee, V., & Yarosh, D.B. (1991). Enhancement of ultraviolet-DNA repair in denV gene transfectants and T4 endonuclease V-liposome recipients. *Photochemistry and photobiology*, V. 54, N. 5, pp. 753-60, ISSN 0031-8655

Kitao, H., & Takata, M. (2011). Fanconi anemia: a disorder defective in the DNA damage response. *International journal of hematology*, V. 93, N. 4, pp. 417-424, ISSN 0925- 5710

Kraemer, K.H., DiGiovanna, J.J., Moshell, A.N., Tarone, R.E , & Peck, G.L. (1988). Prevention of skin cancer in xeroderma pigmentosum with the use of isotretinoin. *The New England journal of medicine*, V. 318, N. 25, pp. 1633-1637, ISSN 0028-4793

Kraemer, K.H., Patronas, N.J., Schiffmann, R., Brooks, B.P., Tamura, D., & DiGiovanna, J.J. (2007). Xeroderma pigmentosum, trichothiodystrophy and Cockayne syndrome: a complex genotype-phenotype relationship. *Neuroscience*, V. 145, N. 4, pp. 1388–1396, ISSN 0306-4522

Kraemer, K. H. (2008). Xeroderma pigmentosum. Gene reviews-NCBI Bookshelf, NBK1397, PMID: 20301571.

Kuluncsics, Z., Perdiz, D., Brulay, E., Muel B., & Sage, E. (1999). Wavelength dependence of ultraviolet-induced DNA damage distribution: involvement of direct or indirect mechanisms and possible artefacts. *Journal of Photochemistry and photobiology.B, Biology*, V. 49, N. 1, pp. 71–80, ISSN 1011-1344

Kusumoto, R., Masutani, C., Sugasawa, K., Iwai, S., Araki, M., Uchida, A., Mizukoshi, T., & Hanaoka, F. (2001). Diversity of the damage recognition step in the global genomic nucleotide excision repair in vitro. *Mutation research*, V. 485, N. 3, pp. 219–227, ISSN 0027-5107

Leach, D.M., & Rainbow, A.J. (2011). Early host cell reactivation of an oxidatively damaged adenovirus-encoded reporter gene requires the Cockayne syndrome proteins CSA and CSB. *Mutagenesis*, V. 26, N. 2, pp. 315-321, ISSN 1383-5718

Leite, R.A., Marchetto, M.C., Muotri, A.R., Vasconcelos, Dde.M., de Oliveira, Z.N., Machado, M.C., & Menck, C.F. (2009). Identification of XP complementation groups by recombinant adenovirus carrying DNA repair genes. *The journal of investigative dermatology*, V. 129, N. 2, pp. 502-506, ISSN 0022-202X

Lima-Bessa, K.M., Chigancas, V., Stary, A., Kannouche, P., Sarasin, A., Armelini, M.G., de Fatima Jacysyn, J., Amarante-Mendes, G.P., Cordeiro-Stone, M., Cleaver, J.E., & Menck, C.F. (2006). Adenovirus mediated transduction of the human DNA polymerase eta cDNA. *DNA repair*, V. 5, N. 8, pp. 925-934, ISSN 1568-7864

Lima-Bessa, K.M., Armelini, M.G., Chiganças, V., Jacysyn, J.F., Amarante-Mendes, G.P., Sarasin, A., & Menck, C.F. (2008). CPDs and 6-4PPs play different roles in UV-induced cell death in normal and NER-deficient human cells. *DNA repair*, V. 7, N. 2, pp. 303-312, ISSN 1568-7864

Lima-Bessa, K.M., Soltys, D.T., Marchetto, M.C., & Menck, C.F.M. (2009). Xeroderma pigmentosum: living in the dark but with hope in therapy. *Drugs of the Future*, V. 34, N. 8, pp. 665-672, ISSN 0377-8282

Liu, L., Lee, J., & Zhou, P. (2010). Navigating the nucleotide excision repair threshold. *Journal of cellular physiology*, V. 224, N. 3, pp. 585-589, ISSN 1097-4652

Lucas-Lledó, J.I., & Lynch, M. (2009). Evolution of mutation rates: phylogenomic analysis of the photolyase/cryptochrome family. *Molecular biology and evolution*, V. 26, N. 5, pp. 1143-1153, ISSN 0737-4038

Magnaldo, T., & Sarasin, A. (2002). Genetic reversion of skin disorders. *Mutation research*, V. 509, N. 1-2, pp. 211-220, ISSN 0027-5107

Marchetto, M.C., Muotri, A.R., Burns, D.K., Friedberg, E.C., & Menck, C.F. (2004). Gene transduction in skin cells: preventing cancer in xeroderma pigmentosum mice. *PNAS*, V. 101, N. 51, pp. 17759-17764, ISSN 1091-6490

Marchetto, M.C., Correa, R.G., Menck, C.F., & Muotri, A.R. (2006). Functional lentiviral vectors for xeroderma pigmentosum gene therapy. *Journal of biotechnology*, V. 126, N. 4, pp, 424-430, ISSN 0168-1656

Masutani, C., Kusumoto, R., Yamada, A., Dohmae, N., Yokoi, M., Yuasa, M., Araki, M., Iwai, S., Takio, K., & Hanaoka, F. (1999). The XPV (xeroderma pigmentosum variant). gene encodes human DNA polymerase eta. *Nature*, V. 399, N. 6737, pp. 700-704, ISSN 0028-0836

Menck, C.F., Armelini, M.G., & Lima-Bessa, K.M. (2007). On the search for skin gene therapy strategies of xeroderma pigmentosum disease. *Current gene therapy*, V. 7, N. 3, pp. 163-174, ISSN 1566-5232

Marionnet, C., Quilliet, X., Benoit, A., Armier, J., Sarasin, A., & Stary, A. (1996). Recovery of normal DNA repair and mutagenesis in trichothiodistrophy cells after transduction of the XPD human gene. *Cancer research*, V. 56, N. 23, pp. 5450-5456, ISSN 1538-7445

Mátrai, J., Chuah, M.K., & VandenDriessche, T. (2010). Recent advances in lentiviral vector development and applications. *Molecular therapy*, V. 18, N. 3, pp. 477-490, ISSN 1525-0016

Merkle, T.J., O'Brien, K., Brooks, P.J., Tarone, R.E., & Robbins, J.H. (2004). DNA repair in human fibroblasts, as reflected by host-cell reactivation of a transfected UV-irradiated luciferase gene, is not related to donor age. *Mutation research*, V. 554, N. 1-2, pp. 9-17, ISSN 0027-5107

Mezzina, M., Eveno, E., Chevallier-Lagente, O., Benoit, A., Carreau, M., Vermeulen, W., Hoeijmakers, J.H., Stefanini,M, Lehmann,A.R., Weber, C.A., & Sarasin, A. (1994). Correction by the ERCC2 gene of UV-sensitivity and repair deficiency phenotype in a subset of trichothiodistrophy cells. *Carcinogenesis*, V. 15, N. 8, pp. 1493-1498, ISSN 0143-3334

Michelfelder, S., & Trepel, M. (2009). Adeno-associated viral vectors and their redirection to cell-type specific receptors. *Advances in genetics*, V. 67, pp. 29-60, ISSN 0065 -2660

Moraes, M.C.S., Cabral-Neto, J.B., & Menck, C.F. (2011). DNA repair mechanisms protect our genome from carcinogenesis. *Frontiers in bioscience*, in press, ISSN 0143-3334

Moriwaki, S., Ray, S., Tarone, R.E., Kraemer, K.H., & Grossman, L. (1996). The effect of donor age on the processing of UV-damaged DNA by cultured human cells: reduced DNA repair capacity and increased DNA mutability. *Mutation research*, V. 364, N. 2, pp. 117-123, ISSN 0027-5107

Müller, M., & Carell, T. (2009). Structural biology of DNA photolyases and cryptochromes. *Current opinion in structural biology*, V. 19, N. 3, pp. 277-285, ISSN 0959-440X

Muotri, A.R., Marchetto, M.C., Zerbini, L.F., Libermann, T.A., Ventura, A.M., Sarasin, A., & Menck, C.F. (2002). Complementation of the DNA repair deficiency in human xeroderma pigmentosum group A and C cells by recombinant adenovirus-mediated gene transfer. *Human gene therapy*, V. 13, N. 15, pp. 1833-1844, ISSN 1043-0342

Narayanan, D.L., Saladi, R.N., & Fox, J.L. (2010). Ultraviolet radiation and skin cancer. *International journal of dermatology*, V. 49, N. 9, pp. 978–986, ISSN 00119059

Partch, C.L., & Sancar, A. (2005). Cryptochromes and circadian photoreception in animals. *Methods in enzymology*, V. 393, pp. 726-745, ISSN 0076-6879

Pitsikas, P., Francis, M.A., & Rainbow, A.J. (2005). Enhanced host cell reactivation of a UV-damaged reporter gene in pre-UV-treated cells is delayed in Cockayne syndrome cells. *Journal of photochemestry and photobiology. B, Biology*, V. 81, N. 2, pp. 89-97, ISSN 1011-1344

Protic-Sabljic, M., Whyte, D., Fagan, J., Howard, B.H., & Gorman, C. M., Padmanabhan, R., & Kraemer, K.H. (1985). Quantification of expression of linked cloned genes in a simian virus 40-transformed xeroderma pigmentosum cell line. *Molecular and cellular biology*, V. 5, N. 7, pp. 1685-1693, ISSN 0270- 7306

Quilliet, X., Chevallier-Lagente, O., Eveno, E., Stojkovic, T., Destée, A., Sarasin, A., & Mezzina, M. (1996). Long-term complementation of DNA repair deficient human primary fibroblasts by retroviral transduction of the XPD gene. *Mutation research*, V. 364, N. 3, pp. 161-169, ISSN 0027-5107

Rastogi, R.P., Richa, Kumar, A., Tyagi, M.B., & Sinha, R.P. (2010). Molecular mechanisms of ultraviolet radiation-induced DNA damage and repair. *Journal of nucleic acids*, ISSN 2090-0201

Raya, A., Rodríguez-Pizà, I., Guenechea, G., Vassena, R., Navarro, S., Barrero, M.J., Consiglio, A., Castellà, M., Río, P., Sleep, E., González, F., Tiscornia, G., Garreta, E., Aasen, T., Veiga, A., Verma, I.M., Surrallés, J., Bueren, J., & Izpisúa Belmonte, J.C. (2009). Disease-corrected haematopoietic progenitors from Fanconi anaemia induced pluripotent stem cells. *Nature*, V. 460, N. 7251, pp. 53-59, ISSN 0028-0836

Rosenberg, S.A., Aebersold, P., Cornetta, K. Kasid, A., Morgan, R.A., Moen, R., Karson, E.M., Lotze, M.T. Yang, J.C., Topalian, S.L., Merino, M.J., Culver, K., Miller, D., Blaese, M., & Anderson, W.F. (1990). Gene transfer into humans – immunotherapy of patients with advanced melanoma, using tumor-infiltrating lymphocytes modified by retroviral gene transduction. *The New England journal of medicine*, V. 323, N. 9, pp. 570-578, ISSN 0028-4793

Sancar, A. (2008). Structure and function of photolyase and in vivo enzymology: 50th anniversary. *The Journal of biological chemistry*, V. 283, N. 47, pp. 32153-32157, ISSN 0021-9258

Schmidt, M., Voutetakis, A., Afione, S., Zheng, C., Mandikian, D., & Chiorini, J.A. (2008). Adeno-associated virus type 12 (AAV12).: a novel AAV serotype with sialic acid- and heparin sulfate proteoglycan-independent transduction activity. *Journal of virology*, V. 82, N. 3, pp. 1399-1406, ISSN 0022-538X

Schuch, A.P., da Silva Galhardo, R., de Lima-Bessa, K.M., Schuch, N.J., & Menck C.F. (2009). Development of a DNA-dosimeter system for monitoring the effects of solar-ultraviolet radiation. *Photochemical , & photobiological sciences*, V. 8, N. 1, pp. 111-120, ISSN 1474-905X

Schwarz, A., Maeda, A., Kernebeck, K., van Steeg, H., Beissert, S., & Schwarz, T. (2005). Prevention of UV radiation-induced immunosuppression by IL-12 is dependent on DNA repair. *The Journal of experimental medicine*, V. 201, N. 2, pp. 173-179, ISSN 0022-1007

Seregin, S.S., & Amalfitano, A. (2009). Overcoming pre-existing adenovirus immunity by genetic engineering of adenovirus-based vectors. *Expert opinion on biological therapy*, V. 9, N. 12, pp. 1521-1531, ISSN 1471-2598

Shamberger, R.J. (1985). The genotoxicity of selenium. *Mutation research*, V. 154, N. 1, pp. 29-48, ISSN 0027-5107

Sidhu, K.S. (2011). New approaches for the generation of induced pluripotent stem cells. *Expert opinion on biological therapy*, V. 11, N. 5, pp. 569-579, ISSN 1471-2598

Silva, G., Poirot, L., Galetto, R., Smith, J., Montoya, G., Duchateau, P., & Pâques, F. (2011). Meganucleases and other tools for targeted genome engineering: perspectives and challenges for gene therapy. *Current gene therapy*, V. 11, N. 1, pp. 11-27, ISSN 1566-5232

Sinha, R.P., & Häder, D.P. (2002). UV-induced DNA damage and repair: a review. *Photochemical , & photobiological sciences*, V. 1, N. 4, pp. 225–236, ISSN 1474-905X

Spivak, G. (2005). UV-sensitive syndrome. *Mutation research*, V. 577, N. 1-2, pp. 162-169, ISSN 0027-5107

Spivak G., & Hanawalt, P.C. (2006). Host cell reactivation of plasmids containing oxidative DNA lesions is defective in Cockayne syndrome but normal in UV-sensitive syndrome fibroblasts. *DNA repair*, V. 5, N. 1, pp. 13-22, ISSN 1568-7864

Stefanini, M., Botta, E., Lanzafame, M., & Orioli, D. (2010). Trichothiodystrophy: from basic mechanisms to clinical implications. *DNA repair*, V. 9, N. 1, pp. 2-10, ISSN 1568-7864

Suzumura, H., & Arisaka, O. (2010). Cerebro-oculo-facio-skeletal syndrome. *Advances in experimental medicine and biology*, V. 685, pp. 210-214, ISSN 0065-2598

Takahashi, K., & Yamanaka, S. (2006). Induction of pluripotent stem cells from mouse embryonic and adult fibroblast cultures by defined factors. *Cell*, V. 126, N. 4, pp. 663-676, ISSN 0092-8674

Tanaka, K., Sekiguchi, M., & Okada, Y. (1975). Restoration of ultraviolet-induced unscheduled DNA synthesis of xeroderma pigmentosum cells by the concomitant treatment with bacteriophage T4 endonuclease V and HJV (Sendai virus). *PNAS*, V. 72, N. 10, pp. 4071-4075, ISSN 1091-6490

Voigt, K., Izsvák, Z., & Ivics, Z. (2008). Targeted gene insertion for molecular medicine. *Journal of molecular medicine*, V. 86, N. 11, pp. 1205-1219, ISSN 0946-2716

Wang, J., Faust, S.M., & Rabinowitz, J.E. (2011). The next step in gene delivery: molecular engineering of adeno-associated virus serotypes. *Journal of molecular and cellular cardiology*, V. 50, N. 5, pp. 793-802, ISSN 0022-2828

Weidenheim, K.M., Dickson, D.W., & Rapin, I. (2009). Neuropathology of Cockayne syndrome: evidence for impaired development, premature aging, and neurodegeneration. *Mechanisms of ageing and development*, V. 130, N. 9, pp. 619-636, ISSN 0047-6374

Wolf, P. Maier, H., Mullegger, R.R., Chadwick, C.A., Hofmann-Wellenhof, R., Soyer, H.P., Hofer, A., Smolle, J., Horn, M., Cerroni, L., Yarosh, D., Klein, J., Bucana, C., Dunner K. Jr., Potten, C S., Hönigsmann, H., Kerl, H., & Kripke, M.L. (2000). Topical treatment with liposomes containing T4 endonuclease V protects human skin *in vivo* from ultraviolet-induced upregulation of interleukin-10 and tumor necrosis factor-α. *Journal of investigative dermatology*, V. 114, N. 1, pp. 149-156, ISSN 0022-202X

Yarosh, D, Bucana, C., Cox, P., Alas, L., Kibitel, J., & Kripke, M. (1994). Localization of liposomes containing a DNA repair enzyme in murine skin. *Journal of investigate dermatology*, V. 103, N. 4, pp. 461-468, ISSN 0022-202X

Yarosh, D., Klein, J., Kibitel, J., Alas, L., O'Connor, A., Cummings, B., Grob, D., Gerstein, D., Gilchrest, B.A., Ichihashi, M., Ogoshi, M., Ueda, M., Fernandez, V., Chadwick, C., Potten, C.S., Proby, C.M., Young, A.R., & Hawk, J.L. (1996). Enzyme therapy of xeroderma pigmentosum: safety and efficacy testing of T4N5 liposome lotion containing a prokaryotic DNA repair enzyme. *Photodermatology, photoimmunology , & photomedicine*, V. 12, N. 3, pp. 122-130, ISSN 0905-4383

Yarosh, D., Klein, J., O'Connor, A.O., Hawk, J., Rafal, E., & Wolf, P. (2001). Effect of topically applied T4 endonuclease V in liposomes on skin cancer in xeroderma pigmentosum: a randomized study. *Lancet*, V. 357, N. 9260, pp. 926-929, ISSN 0140-6736

Yarosh, D.B. (2002). Enhanced DNA repair of cyclobutane pyrimidine dimers changes the biological response to UV-B radiation. *Mutation research*, V. 509, N. 1-2, pp. 221-226, ISSN 0027-5107

You, Y.H., Lee, D.H., Yoon, J.H., Nakajima, S., Yasui, A., & Pfeifer GP. (2001). Cyclobutane pyrimidine dimers are responsible for the vast majority of mutations induced by UVB irradiation in mammalian cells. *The Journal of biological chemistry*, V. 276, N. 48, pp. 44688-44694, ISSN 0021-9258

Zeng, L., Sarasin, A., & Mezzina, M. (1998). Retrovirus-mediated DNA repair gene transfer into xeroderma pigmentosum cells: perspectives for a gene therapy. *Cell biology and toxicology*, V. 14, N. 2, pp. 105-110, ISSN 0742-2091

Permissions

The contributors of this book come from diverse backgrounds, making this book a truly international effort. This book will bring forth new frontiers with its revolutionizing research information and detailed analysis of the nascent developments around the world.

We would like to thank Dr. Sonya Vengrova, for lending her expertise to make the book truly unique. She has played a crucial role in the development of this book. Without her invaluable contribution this book wouldn't have been possible. She has made vital efforts to compile up to date information on the varied aspects of this subject to make this book a valuable addition to the collection of many professionals and students.

This book was conceptualized with the vision of imparting up-to-date information and advanced data in this field. To ensure the same, a matchless editorial board was set up. Every individual on the board went through rigorous rounds of assessment to prove their worth. After which they invested a large part of their time researching and compiling the most relevant data for our readers. Conferences and sessions were held from time to time between the editorial board and the contributing authors to present the data in the most comprehensible form. The editorial team has worked tirelessly to provide valuable and valid information to help people across the globe.

Every chapter published in this book has been scrutinized by our experts. Their significance has been extensively debated. The topics covered herein carry significant findings which will fuel the growth of the discipline. They may even be implemented as practical applications or may be referred to as a beginning point for another development. Chapters in this book were first published by InTech; hereby published with permission under the Creative Commons Attribution License or equivalent.

The editorial board has been involved in producing this book since its inception. They have spent rigorous hours researching and exploring the diverse topics which have resulted in the successful publishing of this book. They have passed on their knowledge of decades through this book. To expedite this challenging task, the publisher supported the team at every step. A small team of assistant editors was also appointed to further simplify the editing procedure and attain best results for the readers.

Our editorial team has been hand-picked from every corner of the world. Their multi-ethnicity adds dynamic inputs to the discussions which result in innovative outcomes. These outcomes are then further discussed with the researchers and contributors who give their valuable feedback and opinion regarding the same. The feedback is then collaborated with the researches and they are edited in a comprehensive manner to aid the understanding of the subject.

Apart from the editorial board, the designing team has also invested a significant amount of their time in understanding the subject and creating the most relevant covers. They scrutinized every image to scout for the most suitable representation of the subject and create an appropriate cover for the book.

The publishing team has been involved in this book since its early stages. They were actively engaged in every process, be it collecting the data, connecting with the contributors or procuring relevant information. The team has been an ardent support to the editorial, designing and production team. Their endless efforts to recruit the best for this project, has resulted in the accomplishment of this book. They are a veteran in the field of academics and their pool of knowledge is as vast as their experience in printing. Their expertise and guidance has proved useful at every step. Their uncompromising quality standards have made this book an exceptional effort. Their encouragement from time to time has been an inspiration for everyone.

The publisher and the editorial board hope that this book will prove to be a valuable piece of knowledge for researchers, students, practitioners and scholars across the globe.

List of Contributors

Vaidehi Krishnan, Baohua Liu and Zhongjun Zhou
Department of Biochemistry, The University of Hong Kong, Hong Kong

Augusto Nogueira, Raquel Catarino and Rui Medeiros
Molecular Oncology & Virology - Portuguese Institute of Oncology, Portugal

Rui Medeiros
CEBIMED, Faculty of Health Sciences of Fernando Pessoa University, Portugal
ICBAS, Abel Salazar Institute for the Biomedical Sciences, Portugal

Augusto Nogueira and Rui Medeiros
Portuguese League Against Cancer (LPCC-NRNorte), Portugal

Marie-jo Halaby and Razqallah Hakem
The Ontario Cancer Institute, Canada

Li Li
Department of Oncology, Johns Hopkins University School of Medicine, USA

Carine Robert and Feyruz V. Rassool
Department of Radiation Oncology and Greenebaum Cancer Center, University of Maryland School of Medicine, Baltimore, MD, USA

Joost P.M. Melis, Mirjam Luijten and Harry van Steeg
National Institute of Public Health and the Environment Laboratory for Health Protection Research, The Netherlands

Joost P.M. Melis, Leon H.F. Mullenders and Harry van Steeg
Leiden University Medical Center, Department of Toxicogenetics, The Netherlands

Carolina Quayle and Carlos Frederico Martins Menck
Dept. of Microbiology, Institute of Biomedical Sciences, University of Sao Paulo, Brazil

Keronninn Moreno Lima-Bessa
Dept. of Cellular Biology and Genetics, Institute of Biosciences Federal University of Rio Grande do Norte, Brazil

Printed in the USA
CPSIA information can be obtained
at www.ICGtesting.com
JSHW011349221024
72173JS00003B/247

9 781632 410009